Women and
Culture Series

The Women and Culture Series is dedicated to books that illuminate the lives, roles, achievements, and status of women, past or present.

Fran Leeper Buss
Dignity: Lower Income Women Tell of Their Lives and Struggles
La Partera: Story of a Midwife

Valerie Kossew Pichanick
Harriet Martineau: The Woman and Her Work, 1802–76

Sandra Baxter and Marjorie Lansing
Women and Politics: The Visible Majority

Estelle B. Freedman
Their Sisters' Keepers: Women's Prison Reform in America, 1830–1930

Susan C. Bourque and Kay Barbara Warren
Women of the Andes: Patriarchy and Social Change in Two Peruvian Towns

Marion S. Goldman
Gold Diggers and Silver Miners: Prostitution and Social Life on the Comstock Lode

Page duBois
Centaurs and Amazons: Women and the Pre-History of the Great Chain of Being

Mary Kinnear
Daughters of Time: Women in the Western Tradition

Lynda K. Bundtzen
Plath's Incarnations: Woman and the Creative Process

Violet B. Haas and Carolyn C. Perrucci, editors
Women in Scientific and Engineering Professions

Sally Price
Co-wives and Calabashes

Patricia R. Hill
The World Their Household: The American Woman's Foreign Mission Movement and Cultural Transformation 1870–1920

Diane Wood Middlebrook and Marilyn Yalom, editors
Coming to Light: American Women Poets in the Twentieth Century

Leslie W. Rabine
Reading the Romantic Heroine: Text, History, Ideology

Joanne S. Frye
Living Stories, Telling Lives: Women and the Novel in Contemporary Experience

E. Frances White
Sierra Leone's Settler Women Traders: Women on the Afro-European Frontier

Catherine Parsons Smith and Cynthia S. Richardson
Mary Carr Moore, American Composer

Barbara Drygulski Wright, editor
Women, Work, and Technology: Transformations

Women, Work, and Technology

Women, Work, and Technology
Transformations

Edited by
Barbara Drygulski Wright and
Myra Marx Ferree
Gail O. Mellow
Linda H. Lewis
Maria-Luz Daza Samper
Robert Asher
Kathleen Claspell

68.384

The University of Michigan Press
Ann Arbor

Library of Congress Cataloging-in-Publication Data

Women, work, and technology.

(Women and culture series)
Primarily papers presented at a conference held
at the University of Connecticut in Oct. 1984,
sponsored by the Project on Women and Technology.
Includes bibliographies and index.
1. Women—Exployment—Effect of technological
innovations on—Congresses.   I. Wright, Barbara
Drygulski, 1945–   .   II. University of Connecticut.
Project on Women and Technology.   III. Series.
HD6052.W566   1987   331.4   87-16236
ISBN-0-472-09373-8 (alk. paper)
ISBN 0-472-06373-1 (pbk.: alk. paper)

Acknowledgments

The genesis of this book is not one but several stories. For that reason, thanking everyone who contributed is a happy occasion both for recalling some early history and for looking to the future. The core of this collection is a set of papers which were originally presented at the conference "Women, Work and Technology," held at the University of Connecticut in October, 1984. The conference, in turn, was the first large-scale public activity of the Project on Women and Technology. The project grew out of the desire of women in Storrs for a larger, more visible feminist scholarly community, out of their ambitions for the Women's Studies Program and the Women's Center at University of Connecticut, and out of their conviction that a feminist analysis of technology could make an important contribution to the state and the region.

So to acknowledge all the effort that this book represents, it is necessary to work backward a bit, first to the group of women, led by Diana Woolis of the Women's Center and Joan Hall of the Women's Studies Program, who began meeting during the 1982–83 academic year to discuss the feasibility of a long-term research and outreach project. It was that group, looking at the resources and professional interests on campus as well as the concentration of high-tech businesses in Connecticut and the Northeast, that made the crucial decision to focus on women and technology.

In the fall of 1983 the Women's Studies Program moved ahead with the project. About three thousand needs-assessment questionnaires were mailed, enthusiastic responses poured in, and at the urging of Katherine Jones-Loheyde, then assistant dean in the School of Education, we began to plan a national conference on women, work, and technology. The Division of Extended and Continuing Education assigned Deb Huntsman and Kathleen Brainard to help us with the technical planning for the conference; their enthusiasm for the project and their technical expertise, together with the financial support of the division, contributed immeasurably to the success of the conference. The conference also received support from John DiBiaggio, then president of the University of Connecticut, from the Connecticut Project on Equal Education Rights, and from the Network for the Advancement of Women in Technical and Analytical Fields.

The planning committee that worked so hard to solicit papers, screen them, plan sessions, and organize the conference ultimately became the editorial collective of this book, though we lost Claudia Wolk and Laverne Gordon to other projects. Colleagues tended to roll their eyes and shake their heads when told that seven of us were going to edit the book together, but that skepticism—to give a polite name to it—has proven quite unwarranted. On the contrary, disagreements were never irresolvable, and the book profited enormously from the disciplinary perspective, the special skills, and the contacts that each member of the group contributed. Maria-Luz Daza Samper kept us mindful always of the implications for labor, Bob Asher safeguarded historical accuracy, and Linda Lewis kept us on track with her careful attention to group process; Kathy Claspell measured theory against her practical experience as an office worker and graduate assistant, Gail Mellow developed a knack for putting her editorial finger on the crux of the argument, and Myra Ferree maneuvered us out of many a cul-de-sac with her unfailing sense of what should be there in the argument but was not—yet.

By the end of the process, we had all learned a great deal from each other—and of course from our contributors, who deserve a special word of thanks for bearing up with so much grace under the pressure of various deadlines and delays. Elaine Hall provided valuable and timely assistance in the checking of references. For the blemishes that remain I assume full responsibility.

As the labor on this book comes to an end, however, the efforts of the Project on Women and Technology continue, supported not only by the University of Connecticut but by grants from Richardson-Vicks, GTE, and others. A second conference, focusing on women, health, and technology, was held in the fall of 1986, and a second volume based on that conference is forthcoming. A third conference, dealing with women, technology, and education, is planned for the fall of 1988, while work goes forward on several other fronts. The project is conceived as both a scholarly and an action-oriented endeavor. Thus we hope to promote academic research through the creation of a data archive and eventually a research institute on women and technology; at the same time, however, consulting teams, course development, and fact sheets for use by schools, unions, businesses, and other groups are also in the planning. The goal of all these efforts is to move both women and technology into a more humane and equitable twenty-first century.

Barbara Drygulski Wright

Contents

Introduction

Barbara Drygulski Wright

In the last twenty-five years, science and technology have increasingly become the object of critical examination. Yet gender issues have been largely overlooked in mainstream scholarship on the history, philosophy, and social consequences of science and technology. These fields have themselves often excluded women and devalued the female, but their gender biases have generally been taken as "natural" and thus have not seemed to require any explanation. Similarly, the impact of technology was until recently neglected in much of the literature on women and work. Happily, this situation is beginning to change. Contemporary historians and philosophers of science and technology are increasingly viewing their subjects in a social and economic context that includes women and feminist perspectives; sociological and economic research on women and work, meanwhile, is broadening its traditional concern with sex segregation, wage discrimination, and limited employment opportunity to include the effects of workplace technologies. The present volume, a collection of scholarly essays that concentrate precisely on the interactions between women, work, and technology, offers a contribution to that growing body of literature.

The subject of this book is technological development and its relationship to women workers. We recognize that throughout the world, women labor in many settings for many different kinds of rewards, and a truly comprehensive definition of women's work must include reproduction and agricultural and household labor, as well as paid employment outside the home. In this collection, however, we have chosen to focus primarily on workplace technology and paid labor in the United States and Western Europe. The volume is strongly interdisciplinary and thus provides a variety of models and perspectives for studying the historical, economic, and ideological contexts of technological change. Some of the articles in this collection use quantitative methods to examine gender and race stratification in jobs being transformed by new technologies, while others help to rescue a tradition of women inventors or theorists from oblivion. Still others are concerned with values and with qualitative changes wrought by technology in women's lives. Some articles present original research, while others are review essays. In three sections that focus on the history of women's association with workplace technologies, on the transformation of the work process through new technologies, and on issues of access, equity, and action, this volume attempts to illustrate the sometimes contradictory meanings of technological change and the opportunities as well as the problems that technology can create for women workers.

What these articles share is the fresh, close look they take at very specific groups of women and what these women have done—as inventors of technology or as users, as theorists or as strategists. The collection demonstrates how the impact of technology differs not only according to women workers' race and class but also according to many other factors, such as type of industry, level of skills, size and organization of the workplace, power relations, and women's ability to capitalize on technological advances. In emphasizing the diversity of experience among various groups of women, the articles in this book help to explode the myths of universality and biological or technological determinism.

In the following pages, I will situate this book in the context of earlier feminist literature that has looked at women, work, and technology; clarify the theoretical assumptions of the volume; and attempt to extrapolate feminist critiques of science to the related but somewhat different problem of technology.

Some Predecessors

Though this collection may focus more sharply than others on women, work, and technology, it is not without its family tree. Previous scholarship has contributed significantly to our understanding of women's participation in the creation of new technologies and the relationship of women and work as the workplace is transformed by technology. The following literature review is not intended to be exhaustive, but simply to provide an overview and a useful orientation for readers unfamiliar with the field.

Technology and Women's Work, by Elizabeth Faulkner Baker, is an early milestone. It remains an important book today, as Judith McGaw observes, because despite its weaknesses it provides "the best and often the only historical treatment of technological change and women's work in many enterprises" (McGaw 1982, 806). Published in 1964, Baker's book traced a parallel history of technology in the workplace and steadily increasing levels of female employment. While Baker's chief concern was automation, with its tendency to deskill work, depress wages, and lead to layoffs, she also noted the potential impact of the computer on office work and wrote, almost clairvoyantly, "observers seem to agree that the displacement of workers will go farthest and fastest in the office, and that . . . women clerical workers may be the largest affected group" (Baker 1964, 220). In the infancy of the "paperless office," Baker diagnosed stress, poor working conditions, and displacement as serious problems; she recommended as antidotes wider opportunities for women in nontraditional fields, an "Equal-Pay Law" (411), and unionization of female white-collar workers.

Her book does reflect some of the assumptions of the period. For example, Baker seemed to accept the prospect that for most women, employment and workplace ambitions would remain secondary to home responsibilities, and she assured her readers that women could achieve prominence in their fields "without sacrificing their femininity" (vii). She tended to view numerical gains somewhat simplistically as signs of progress, and she credited new technology with enabling women to move into new occupations. Nevertheless, Baker was respectful of women's abilities and realistic about the external barriers women faced. She saw them negotiating "a zigzag road in man's domain, beset with obstacles—social, economic, physical and psychological. For women have been contending not only with the difficulties of the new work itself but also with the problems of establishing their rights to have it" (vii).

The book offers a gratifying contrast to the attitude toward women in science and engineering professions otherwise expressed during the early 1960s, when the view prevailed that women were inferior to men, if not in raw ability, then in motivation and commitment. It was that, and not discrimination, that supposedly accounted for the smaller numbers of women scientists and engineers and their lesser prominence. Bruno Bettelheim, in his keynote address at a symposium sponsored by the MIT Association of Women Students in October, 1964, asserted, "we must start with the realization that, as much as women want to be good scientists or engineers, they want first and foremost to be womanly companions of men and to be mothers" (Mattfeld and Van Aken 1965, 15). Some women on the program, including Alice Rossi and Vivianne Nachmias, vehemently disagreed with Bettelheim; and Jessie Bernard argued that marriage was generally overrated as a design for living. Others, however—including closing speaker Erik Erikson—warmly concurred.

Historical scholarship on women and American technology was reviewed by Judith A. McGaw in 1982. She noted that in the six years since 1976, when Ruth Schwartz Cowan first argued that the female experience of technological change was significantly different from the male experience, there had been an extraordinary flowering of research on women in the history of technology, as well as in two related subdisciplines, the history of science and the history of medicine. McGaw's review concentrated on technology's relationship to "the segregated and exploitative world of women's employment" and "technology's role in women's place, the home"; but she also referred to the literature on reproduction and on women as scientists and developers of technology (1982, 799–800).

Surveying the history of technology and women's work, McGaw observed that "most early scholarship depicted technology as an agent of change, drawing women into paid employment and transforming tasks so that men's jobs were reassigned to women. By contrast, recent studies present the story of technology and women's work as a tale of continuity, despite superficial change" (804). Those underlying continuities are: wage discrimination ("women were almost always paid less than men even for the same work"); sex segregation ("women rarely performed the same tasks as men"); and the perception, on the part of both women and men, that women were merely transitory members of the labor force (Cowan, cited in McGaw 1982, 804).

The research presented in this volume builds on the scholarly foundation outlined by McGaw, and by necessity it deals with the continuities first defined by Cowan. Beyond this, however, it also takes a critical and differentiated stand toward those continuities, examines change inspired by the interaction of technology and social values *within* those continuities, and looks at the social as well as technological forces that have been marshaled not only to enforce but also to break those continuities. Thus one contribution demonstrates how the female work force in the airline industry became far less transitory as a result of both technological and social changes; the end effect was greater autonomy for largely female flight attendants' unions. Another contribution examines the choice of technology in relation to the construction of *male* gender in the printing industry; what emerges is not a static view of workers being fitted to preexisting sex-role stereotypes, but a dynamic and ongoing construction and reconstruction of female *and* male gender, as well as shifting assignments for male and female workers.

In other fields besides history, numerous publications have appeared in recent years that deal with women's economic roles, trends in labor force participation, investment in human capital, occupational segregation, and similar topics, but they touch on technology only sporadically. This is clearly reflected in Shirley Harkess's review of the sociological and economic research on women's employment from 1977 to 1983 (1984, 3). Harkess surveys a voluminous literature dealing with white-collar workers (professionals, managers and administrators, sales workers, and clericals), blue-collar craft workers and operatives, and service workers (in law enforcement, food service, household work, and other areas). In her review, technology does not emerge as a consistent theme of current research, but it is mentioned occasionally in the context of office work, factory automation, and job loss. On her crowded agenda for future research, Harkess specifically calls for an investigation of the ways in which technology can "have a discriminatory effect" (515). Similarly, technology per se is not a central theme in the papers presented at the conference "Ingredients for Women's Employment Policy" held at the State University of New York at Albany in spring of 1985 (Bose and Spitze 1987), but the collection does include a study of the factors affecting young women's nontraditional occupation choices.

Some recent collections on women and work, e.g., Stromberg and Harkess, *Women Working* (1978), Reskin, *Sex Segregation in the Workplace* (1984) and Wallace, *Women in the Workplace* (1982), are primarily concerned with such issues as women's labor force participation, affirmative action, relations between work and family, career advancement, nontraditional blue-collar work for women, and ways to improve women's opportunities; within this framework, technology figures only tangentially. Other books, however, have focused more explicitly on technology in a variety of work settings and have offered important insights, both into the effects of workplace technologies and into the kinds of questions that scholars may profitably investigate. For example, in Sacks and Remy's *My Troubles Are Going to Have Trouble with Me* (1984), an entire section is devoted to "Technology and the Changing Shapes of Women's Work." The section includes two articles on office work as well as an account of the way technology was used in a meat packing plant to thwart affirmative action.

A similar collection, *Work, Women and the Labour Market* (1982), edited by Jackie West and published in Britain, contains an article by West that focuses on women's office work. West's astute assessment of a British government report on the impact of new technology should alert readers to the bias in similar reports from other sources, public and private, in the United States and elsewhere. She writes that the Department of Employment's 1979 report

> clearly represents managerial objectives, hidden within a broader argument that "new" technology will not have devastating effects. It plays down the labour-saving effects of micro-electronics which along with control are the most obvious advantages to management. Instead it stresses that increased productivity is the key to competitiveness and growth. . . . In addition, the use and development of the new technology is seen to require specialist skills, currently in short supply. It thus entails, by implication, an increase in, not dispossession of, the knowledge and experience of workers. (62)

Also passed over in silence in this report is the differential impact of the new technologies on women. West contrasts this conventional wisdom about the value of technological innovation with evidence of its actual effect on women workers from the civil service and finance sectors, and she concludes that women's work is particularly vulnerable. While the main purpose of West's collection is to present an overview of women's employment in contemporary Britain, to illuminate the differences and similarities in women's and men's experience in the labor market, and to examine the way class and gender relations are interwoven in the production process, technology emerges as a consistent, if not dominant, theme.

Still another perspective is provided by Ann Game and Rosemary Pringle in *Gender at Work* (1984), which first appeared in Australia. The authors contend that gender is fundamental to the way that work is organized and work is central in the social construction of gender. The purpose of the book is to show how the concepts of masculine and feminine are produced in relation to each other through work, with technological change providing a useful backdrop for studying this process. Game and Pringle view gender, like other power relations, as something constantly renegotiated and recreated, and they find this process particularly visible at points where work is being reorganized and new technology introduced. Their six occupational studies, which cover manufacturing, banking, retailing, computing, nursing, and housework, trace in intriguing detail the shifting lines between what is considered appropriate "men's" or "women's" work. Some of these occupations are clearly more affected by new technologies than others; from all of them, however, the authors conclude that the sexual division of labor is a structural feature of modern capitalism. They argue moreover that the fusion of technology with patriarchy has invariably worked to reaffirm sexual divisions of labor rather than to reduce them and thus has consistently disadvantaged women. While Game and Pringle reject the more conventional, optimistic reading of technological determinism, they seem to embrace an equally deterministic negative reading of technological impact.

At the same time, several books have appeared that deal with the connections between women and science. Rossiter's *Women Scientists in America* (1982), together with several contributions in Trescott's *Dynamos and Virgins Revisited* (1979) and Stanley's article in Rothschild's *Machina ex Dea* (1983), makes an important contribution to the compensatory history of women in science and technology. Other works, such as Lowe and Hubbard's *Woman's Nature* (1983), Bleier's *Science and Gender* (1984), Keller's *Reflections on Gender and Science* (1985) and

Fausto-Sterling's *Myths of Gender* (1985) subject scientific method and the assumption of "scientific objectivity" to rigorous feminist critiques. Merchant's *The Death of Nature* (1980) traces the mechanistic and masculinist characteristics of modern Western science to the emergence of a new epistemology and methodology in the early seventeenth century. In Harding's *The Science Question in Feminism* (1986), these works and many others form the basis of a "second-order" inquiry into the limitations not only of traditional science, but also of the feminist literature *about* science (Martin 1986). In a more practical vein, Haas and Perrucci's *Women in Scientific and Engineering Professions* (1984) examines the careers of women in these fields and concludes, first, that it is discrimination and not lack of ability that has held women back from recognition and achievement equal to men's; and second, that serious problems remain in this period of transition and improving opportunities for women. The book closes with an examination of the masculinist and capitalist biases that inform science and technology today and argues that women should not adopt these biases but rather seek to change science and technology.

Together these books powerfully refute biological determinism as an explanation for the rarity of women in scientific, technical, or other male-dominated fields today, and at the same time they reveal an abundance of social, political, economic, and ideological determinants. With the exception of Trescott, it is not the purpose of these books to address the relationship between women, work, and technology; nevertheless, they do suggest reasons why technology in the workplace may be so very problematic for women—reasons addressed later in this introduction and in the articles that follow.

There are three books that come closest to the present volume in structure and purpose. Martha Moore Trescott's pioneering collection, *Dynamos and Virgins Revisited* (1979), is historical in orientation and grew out of presentations by women members of the Society for the History of Technology. The book was organized to elaborate on the four major topics set forth by Cowan in her opening article, "From Virginia Dare to Virginia Slims": "women as bearers and rearers of children," "women as workers," "women as homemakers," and "women as anti-technocrats." Surveying evidence of persistent discrimination in the paid workplace as well as increasing hours of housework for women at home, Trescott concluded, "it is clear that whether in the home or outside, technological change has not enabled women to rise above proletarian status" (12). Trescott noted further that education and socialization tended to make women "anti-technocrats," even as technology became more pervasive in both public and private spheres, and that, particularly in traditionally female areas such as housework and child care, changes in societal attitudes lagged far behind the development of technologies that, theoretically at least, could facilitate change. In view of these glaring contradictions, Trescott prophetically suggested that study of the history of women and technology might help to answer one of the "big questions" in the history of technology: does technology dictate to society, or do social values determine the course of technological change and "progress"?

Whereas the Trescott book spans the eighteenth to the early twentieth centuries and is largely concerned with traditional manufacturing and homemaking technologies, Jan Zimmerman's *The Technological Woman* (1983) surveys the impact of new technologies on contemporary women's lives and is very much concerned with women's relationship to high technology in the future. The contributions, which concentrate on the prosaic reality of automobiles and plumbing, word processors and electricity, reveal the extent to which old values—based on race, sex, class, and age, for example—are replicated in the design and application of new technologies. Work is also part of women's everyday reality, and like the Trescott book, this one construes women's work in the broadest possible terms. Thus there are sections devoted to household labor and reproduction as well as to paid labor. The book draws three main conclusions: first, that technology is not gender-free; second, that women have a long and important, albeit largely invisible, history of achievement in technological innovation; and third, that technological determinism is a myth. Thus the Zimmerman book lends important support to Trescott's theses; our own collection strengthens the case further.

Joan Rothschild's *Machina ex Dea* (1983), finally, opens with a meticulous documentation of the exclusion of women from the history of technology and redresses that omission by providing feminist perspectives on the social context, the content, and the methodology of technology. The first section on women, technology, and production accomplishes several things: it reestablishes women as active contributors in the development and implementation of technological innovation; it examines the problem of access for women to nontraditional technical professions; it demonstrates a connection between technological innovation and work degradation; and it questions the extent to which household technologies have liberated women from the household—or from the traditional role of housewife. The book then examines the values that underlie modern science and technology and closes with alternative feminist visions of a future with—or without—technology. In the afterword, Rothschild recommends further research in the three areas of historical analysis, women and work, and epistemology and values. The present collection, which provides a magnified view of the same set of problems raised in the first part of her book, may be regarded as a continuation of Rothschild's work.

Some Definitions

The assumptions this collection begins from and the conclusions it ultimately reaches may be suggested or corroborated by the feminist literature just cited; but they are by no means commonly accepted in the academy or by policymakers, in the media, or in society at large. On the contrary, precisely the views that are treated here as myths—technological determinism, biological determinism, and the belief that technology is neutral or essentially beneficial—enjoy wide popular acceptance, although they are rejected by feminists as well as by critics of technology whose analysis is not gender-based.

What is technological determinism, first of all, and why do the contributors to this volume reject it? Technological determinism is the view that technological discoveries and applications occur according to their own inner necessity, from laws that govern the physical and biological world, and that they, in turn, unilaterally affect social reality. From the perspective of technological determinism, human beings have few alternatives in their response to technology besides enthusiastic or resigned acceptance. In contrast to this view, many critics of technology, such as Ellul, Dubos, Toffler, Pacey, and Winner, have emphasized the extent to which social, political, and economic forces first promote some kinds of technological research while inhibiting others and then shape new technologies into a particular pattern of development, use, and accessibility that reinforces the cultural and ideological values of that society. Feminists have reached a similar diagnosis; they are particularly concerned, moreover, with the ways in which new technologies serve to reinforce dominance based not only on class or race but on sex, age, and sexual preference (Zimmerman 1983, 116; Game and Pringle 1984, 17).

Biological determinism is the view that biology predetermines the differences between human beings; the corollary of this view is that since certain differences are programmed in the genes, there is essentially nothing society can do to eradicate inequality. Biological determinism has been used in the past to explain inequality between classes or races, and most recently it has enjoyed renewed popularity as an explanation for differences between male and female levels of achievement, particularly in mathematics, science, and technology. Although it is clear that at present men dominate most professions, particularly scientific and technical ones, at least in North America and Western Europe, the reasons for this are open to debate. Feminist scholars, for example, Lowe, Hubbard, Bleier, and Fausto-Sterling, argue that biological and social factors influencing male and female development are so inextricably intertwined that it is virtually impossible to say to what extent current patterns of male and female behavior are determined by one set of factors or the other. They assume that given equal education and equal opportunity, as well as a less blatantly masculinist notion of science, women will enter and succeed at science in the same numbers as men. In the feminist view, there is a great deal individuals and societies can do to reach this goal. With a few notable exceptions—for example, Illich, Pacey, and Gravender—male critics of technology have generally been unconcerned about the absence of women from science and technology.

This brings the discussion around to feminist assertions of masculine bias in science and technology. The Western ideology of science contends that science is supremely objective and value-free, while technology is beneficial or at least neutral. This liberal view has not gone undisputed by critics of technology, whether male or female, but it is currently the dominant view in the United States and is reflected, for example, in a speech by Henry Steele Commager, who assured his audience at a forum entitled "Values and Higher Education" that "science and technology are neither benign nor malign, but neutral" (1985, 9). Commager argues that it is only when science enters service to a cause such as "irrational nationalism" that it becomes dangerous.

The philosopher Elizabeth Minnich challenges that conventional view by pointing out what she has called "three anomalies." First, of all disciplines, science has the greatest raw power over our lives; second, science enjoys support from government and private enterprise that runs to hundreds of millions of dollars per year and far exceeds anything other disciplines receive; and third, those who engage in science are overwhelmingly white middle-class males (Minnich 1984). She suggests, in effect, that science is already in service to social, political, and economic causes that are all the more dangerous because they go largely unrecognized. Other critics of technology approach the problem from different angles. Rene Dubos, for example, recommends implementation of technology based not on what is technically possible, but on what is socially desirable; Alvin Toffler, similarly, calls for technology to be evaluated in terms of personal fulfillment and aesthetic achievement. Arnold Pacey argues for a shift from the unspoken but nearly absolute priority of "technical virtuosity" to the inclusion of "user values."

Knotted and tangled with political, economic, and social considerations is the issue of gender bias. As Marian Lowe writes, "science is seen as male, as an essentially masculine activity, not only because historically almost all scientists have been men, but also because the attributes of science itself are defined as the attributes of males" (Zimmerman 1983, 8). Thus science is seen as objective rather than subjective, active rather than passive, logical rather than intuitive, rational rather than emotional, powerful rather than powerless. Since the beginning of modern science and most clearly since the mid-nineteenth century, the attributes ascribed to scientists have been the stereotypical attributes of males, the scientific production of knowledge reflecting a stereotypically male way of relating to the world (Rothschild 1981; Trescott 1979).

If the genderedness of science has been overlooked by male scientists as well as the general public because of the tendency to view the male as the norm, it has not been so easily overlooked by feminists or those interested in women in science. Elizabeth Fee has outlined a variety of responses to this problem (1983, 14). One is to claim that women can be both female and male, as J. H. Mozans did in his historical survey, *Woman in Science* (1913). The difficulty with this response is that it accepts the masculine bias as indispensable to scientific methodology and places the burden of adjustment, a double burden of gender, squarely on the woman who wants to become a scientist. A second response is to deny there are any significant differences between women and men, and to argue that apparent differences are the result of discrimination or socialization. Thus women may be helped by counseling, support groups, compensatory math and science instruction, or special technical training for nontraditional work. This may be viewed as a liberal "minimizer" interpretation, one that again leaves the ideology of science untouched and implicitly puts the burden of proof on individual women.

A third strategy, the one Fee herself embraces, is to accept the dichotomy between male and female—but with an important difference. Fee goes on to revalue female qualities and styles of relating as fundamental to human experience; if they are left out of science, then science is "partial" in two senses: it includes only a *part,* the masculine part, of human experience; thus it is also *biased* toward male concerns. To correct this bias, she argues for a new vision of science that will incorporate female values. Joan Rothschild (1981) argues similarly for the inclusion of female values in technology. Evelyn Fox Keller takes yet another approach: changing science, she contends, will depend "less on the introduction of a specifically female culture into science than on the rethinking of sexual polarities and the abandonment of a sexual division of intellectual labor altogether" (Keller 1983, 143). In other words, she believes there are at present real differences in the ways males and females think and relate, and that science has suffered from the exclusion of female traits. These differences are not inherent in male and female human beings, however, any more than a masculine bias is indispensible to science. A breaking down of sexual polarities would facilitate the emergence of "feminine" subthemes in science, just as it would allow all individuals greater freedom to develop currently male- or female-identified intellectual and personality traits. Science would move from masculinist to fully human if the paradigm of scientific thinking could be expanded to formally include intuition and empathy rather than being limited to an objectivist illusion of distance from the object of scientific inquiry. Models of self-modifying process, which reflect currently feminine modes of relating to the external world, would replace unidirectional models of causality and dominance (Gravender 1986, 24).

This is the context of feminist debate within which our collection of articles on women, work, and technology is embedded and to which the volume hopes to contribute. But a largely unexamined issue in all this work is the relationship between science and technology. It is to this relationship we now turn.

"Fraternal" Twins?

In discussions of "science and technology," technology always seems to get short shrift. The feminist critique of science has been brave, brilliant, and enormously significant, but it has also been guilty of conflating science and technology. "Science and technology" has become a kind of stock phrase, an obligatory pairing, and when the phrase must be abbreviated, it is technology that is omitted or forgotten. Clearly there are problems with this common usage. While science and technology are related, they are not identical, and what applies to science does not necessarily follow for technology. Yet the effect of this linguistic—and perhaps theoretical—habit is to obscure the very real distinctions between science and technology.

The implications of the phrase "science and technology" are three-fold. First, it suggests that whatever is true of science applies equally to technology, and thus it discourages an investigation of the relationship between the two and the ways in which they differ. Second, it seems to reflect an intellectual bias toward the study of science as more abstract yet more basic, more important and thus more interesting; in other words, it seems to reflect the very hierarchical relationship within the sciences and between science and technology that feminist theorists have criticized.

Finally, the formula "science and technology" implies that science somehow came first and that technology is merely a practical spin-off. Yet this is clearly inaccurate. Not only did a vast array of technologies exist before the emergence of modern, Western-style science; such mechanical technologies actually functioned as the precondition for the emergence of modern science. Carolyn Merchant's *The Death of Nature* (1980) is subtitled *Women, Ecology and the Scientific Revolution*. Interestingly, there is only the briefest reference to technology per se in the index, yet the underlying thesis of the book is that in the sixteenth and seventeenth centuries a "mechanistic" or technological approach to nature became established and not only stimulated "scientific" investigation of natural phenomena but also led to the exploitation of nature and the pollution of the natural environment, to unrestrained commercial expansion, and to increased socioeconomic subordination of women. In other words, although the book is ostensibly about science, technology plays an absolutely central role in it. It is technology that supplies the original model for the view of the natural world modern science embraces, and it is through technology that the link from science to the economy is established, ensuring that science is financially secured (Merchant 1980, 193; Mumford 1934, 25). In addition, the really revolutionary aspect of the knowledge upon which the new science is based is that it comes not from classical or occult sources, but from practical experience and the observation of everyday life.

Of course there are real similarities between science and technology; in Lewis Mumford's words, "science and technics form two independent yet related worlds: sometimes converging, sometimes drawing apart" (52). Thus it would be counterproductive in distinguishing between them to construct a whole new set of dichotomies. A more fruitful approach is to imagine the two as partially overlapping fields. When technology is examined in its own right and then compared to science, we find that in some ways the two share the same characteristics, in some cases an analogy may be drawn from one to the other, and in some cases they are quite different.

One of the most fundamental distinctions that can be drawn between science and technology is that science is the production of new knowledge, whereas technology is the attempt to achieve specific ends or perfect specific processes. Modern science follows a model of *abstract* rationalism: that is, discrete pieces of information are abstracted from the natural world independent of context and then manipulated mathematically to formulate laws and rules for the behavior of natural phenomena (Merchant 1980, 227–33). Technology, however, is an expression of *instrumental* rationalism: its purpose is not so much to discover new knowledge as to find new applications for knowledge that already exists.

If science serves knowledge, technology serves utility; if science above all wants its discovery to be "right," technology wants its discovery to work. What they share, at least in the mainstream view, is conscious manipulation of the natural world and a simplistic view of causality as linear, additive, and unidirectional, together with a method that is biased toward reductionism rather than holism, toward domination rather than interaction (Gravender 1986, 22, 24–25; Pacey 1983, 34).

Both science and technology also enjoy an extraordinary level of ideological support, quite apart from the tangible financial support they receive from governments or businesses. The dominant belief in contemporary Western societies is that both science and technology are driven by their own inner imperative, and citizens of modern, developed countries are educated to accept the notion that the playing out of this imperative is not merely good but the most noble and illustrious part of their cultural heritage. The imagery used to convey this message is as vivid as any adventure tale. In the West, the tireless scientific pursuit of knowledge "for its own sake," regardless of the costs or consequences, has a heroic and virile flavor about it, evoking the glory of martyrs for the cause of science like Galileo or Harvey in their struggles against the Catholic church or social convention. Little taught and seldom remembered is the other side of this story, the execution in the fifteenth, sixteenth, and seventeenth centuries of millions of female healers and midwives as witches.

Similarly, Goethe's Faust is driven to extend the limits of the technologically possible: he rejects classical "book learning" at the beginning of the drama, and in the closing pages, at the time of his death, he is engaged in a massive land reclamation project. This "Faustian striving," as it has become mythologized in Western consciousness, appears not merely as the quintessentially human activity but as a form of participation in divinity that virtually guarantees redemption regardless of the sins and abuses committed. Enhanced by the liberating moment that was undeniably present in the emergence of modern science, scientific knowledge has been raised to the status of a philosophical ideal; likewise, technological "know-how" has been mythologized all out of proportion to the good it is actually able to accomplish.

Of course, the representation of science and technology as unqualified good constitutes ideology rather than fact. It is an extremely powerful ideology in its own right and also justifies the economic, political, and gender interests that are served by contemporary technology. These interests are further served by a second assumption: the identity of interests between people and government or people and business. In the United States, this is expressed in slogans like "What's good for business is good for America," in the notion of "trickle-down" economics, or in the ideal of a government "of the people, for the people, by the people." Ideologically, science and technology are "right" until proven otherwise—and often even after.

But what does it mean to be "right" in terms of science and technology? Modern Western science claims that it is objective and value-free, and that this is the only way to arrive at correct results. "Objectivity" may be understood on several levels. Epistemologically, it means predictability and replicability independent of the individual scientist. On a personal level, "objectivity" is understood as a split between scientific rationalism and any emotion or social commitment, along with the conviction that scientific detachment is superior to feeling (Fee 1983, 18). It is "cancellation of self" (Keller 1983, 132) and dedication to ideas. On a political or social level, finally, "objectivity" entails a rigid separation between the production of knowledge and the uses to which that knowledge may be put (Fee 1983, 17). The scientific enterprise is represented as the pursuit of knowledge for its own sake, without thought for political repercussions or economic rewards. The problem with this "objectivist illusion," as Evelyn Fox Keller calls it (1983, 134), is that it blinds scientists to the very real influence that subjective, economic, and political factors have on the questions they are able to formulate and the answers they are able to accept.

Technology, too, claims a kind of objectivity, but because technology is based on an instrumental rationalism, rather than the abstract rationalism of science, its notion of "objectivity" is constructed differently. For technology, epistemology is not central; instead, the "objectivity" of technology is operational and economic. It requires not distance and abstraction but the solution of real problems in a concrete environment. As an individual, the engineer is expected to display not intellectual detachment so much as "hard-headed realism"; being "hard," "tough," and "objective" in the technological fields means filtering out considerations beyond feasibility, profitability, and "building it right" (see Layton 1971, 53–78). In a curious analogy to scientific "objectivity," technological "objectivity" requires not only "cancellation of self" but a more explicit cancellation of other people; it requires not dedication to ideas so much as dedication to objects and objectives. Like the scientist, the engineer is supposed to maintain distance between the work at hand and its social or economic impact. Maintaining that distance is more challenging and contradiction-ridden for technology, however, since it operates not in the sheltered environment of a laboratory but on building sites and shop floors, in mines and offices. Technology is more clearly tied to the economic interests of firms or governments and more directly confronted with the social consequences of application. Though protected to some extent by the mystique of the expert, as is science, technology is also more exposed to criticism from lay sources and even to the pirating of its inventions for alternative ends.

In science, when new knowledge is generated, it is subjected to a control process: critical evaluation and empirical testing by the rest of the scientific community. But what is the control process for technological innovations? The first question is quite simply whether the device or process *works* as it was supposed to, and the second, whether it produces the intended economic benefit. The ultimate "proof" of modern technology is its economic profitability, tested according to the supposedly objective and disinterested logic of the economic marketplace. Much as modern science seeks simple, unified laws for natural phenomena that can be formulated as mathematical principles, so modern technologies are ultimately proven "effective" or "correct" by the mathematics of the profit-and-loss statement. However, just as scientific "objectivity" masks certain biases embedded in the scientific method, so too the calculation of economic profitability does not occur without a certain amount of manipulation. "Correctness" and "success" are measured in terms of benefit to the firm or sponsoring government, not in terms of nature or society. Thus specific, potentially very real costs—for example, workers' compensation for injury or illness, the impoverishment of women and children, depletion of natural resources, or environmental cleanup—never get factored in at all (see Bush 1983, 164–65).

In Western culture, science and the scientist are strongly identified with images of masculinity, and this is equally true of technology; but the particular stereotype of masculinity differs for science and technology. Consequently, the particular set of polarities that each constructs in relation to femininity also differs. Both the scientific and the technological mind are viewed as active, rational, and logical, whereas the feminine has traditionally been viewed as passive, emotional, and intuitive. Both science and technology pride themselves on being hard, cold, and impersonal, whereas the feminine is presumably soft, warm, and insistently personal. Both science and technology are alienated from nature, but for slightly different reasons: science wishes to penetrate nature's secrets, while technology's task is to manage and exploit nature. Women, by contrast, are frequently identified with nature; they, like nature, must be penetrated and managed. Both science and technology seek power and dominance; the exercise of power, however, is viewed as incompatible with femininity.

But if science wears a white lab coat, technology wears a hard

hat and has slightly dirty fingernails. If science, in the popular imagination, seems to stand outside of and above everyday life, technology
prides itself on standing squarely and aggressively in the middle of
things. While science is an ascetic and idealistic seeker after truth,
technology is a rough-and ready can-do type, a realist who makes
things happen. While science merely seeks intellectual dominance
over nature, technology seeks tangible material and economic dominance; moreover, because technology is "in touch with reality" in a
way that science cannot be, technology enjoys more authority to organize, exert power, and impose its will on society. Science may be a
little absentminded and eggheaded, but technology cannot afford that
luxury.

As different as these two roles are, they both have an unmistakably
masculine aura about them, and traditional conceptions of femininity do
not fit easily with either. If women are "too practical" for science, they
are "too idealistic" for technology. Women are often presumed to be
intellectually unsuited for science and mathematics, and at the same
time both intellectually *and* physically unsuited for technology, which
may require work in dirty, dangerous surroundings or distant locations.
In relation to the masculine stereotype of technology, it is women's
supposed moral superiority, their sensitivity and ability to empathize
with others, that disqualifies them vis-à-vis the presumably coarser but
stronger, hardier, more self-interested and therefore more "realistic"
male. In relation to the masculine stereotype of science, however,
women are too earthy, too bound to their own hearth and family; they
lack the greatness of spirit or intellect to transcend the particularity of
their own situation and support more general or abstract goals.

What this pattern represents is not merely a series of bipolar antithe-
ses between male and female, but a veritable *encircling* of the "appropriate" female domain and a restriction on female mobility beyond it—
literally and metaphorically—in *all* directions, as women are denied
access both to the technological *vita activa* and to a secularized, scientific
vita contemplativa. To view this phenomenon as a series of Cartesian
dualisms, as has commonly been done (see, e.g., Harding 1986, 142;
Rothschild 1983, x–xi; Lowe and Hubbard 1983, 11–12), is to view it too
simplistically. For women to enter and change scientific or technical
fields may thus require that they do battle not on a single front, against a
single construction of masculine and feminine, but on several fronts
simultaneously. In other words, the ideological problem women face in
gaining full access to science and technology is perhaps more complex
than we have heretofore acknowledged.

Transforming Technology

The difficulty in challenging the masculine bias of science and technology is that one thereby challenges the economic and political status quo, as well as centuries of tradition. Fortunately, feminist voices are not the only ones crying in the wilderness. Since the late 1960s and early 1970s, as we have seen, another critique of technology has emerged that is not gender-based but has focused on many of the same characteristics of technology as the more recent and more radical feminist critique. Jerry Gravender speaks for many of us when he wonders "what it is about the method of technology that results in technologists—and the rest of us—always being surprised by negative consequences" (1986, 20). He and other critics of technology focus on three problem areas: the "ideal of objectivity," "reductionistic" methodology, and the will to dominate and control. Feminist critiques of technology fault the same three tendencies, link them to Western gender ideology, and offer a provocative alternative.

What would a less masculinist, more fully human technology be like? Barbara McClintock's life and work have implications not only for science, as Keller has pointed out, but for technology as well. In McClintock's work, Keller finds examples of themes that are not alien to science, but "subthemes"—not dominant, but with a long tradition. According to Keller, McClintock's chief criticism of conventional science is that it lacks "respect for the system" and awareness of its own "tacit assumptions." McClintock believes that too often researchers want to impose an answer. McClintock herself has developed an extraordinary degree of respect and empathy for the organisms she works with and pays them a kind of attention Keller describes as "almost nurturant." She views the subjects of her research not as isolated phenomena but as elements constantly in delicate interaction with their environment. By paying attention to the individual and by developing a "feeling for the organism," by "forgetting" herself, "letting the material tell you what to do," and following an interactive rather than a "master control" model, McClintock has been able to make discoveries that are as unconventional and as original as her scientific style (Keller 1983, 139–43).

In other words, McClintock challenges the conventional notion of scientific objectivity. She does not isolate her subjects from their context, nor does she distance herself from that context; on the contrary, she has been able to see most vividly and fully when she became "part of the system" and the chromosomes became her "friends." McClintock has approached her subjects not with arrogance but with respect and affection. At present, the traditional methodology of science is to isolate the object of inquiry from its physical context; technology, in close analogy to science, seeks to solve problems by breaking them down into small units and examining them in isolation from a larger and more complex context. Yet in doing so technology isolates itself not only from the physical but from the social context, in which a particular device will have not only a functional but also a social impact. While science, at least theoretically, can operate in relative isolation from society, this isolation is even more illusory in the case of technology.

Clearly, technology needs to develop more respect for the natural and physical environment in which it operates. More respectful and affectionate attention to the whole physical "system" might lead to smaller, less intrusive and disruptive, more appropriate technologies. It might result in a technology that complements and enhances nature rather than exploiting or damaging it. "Forgetting" instrumental and economic interests and "letting the material tell you what to do" at the beginning of a technological endeavor could make an enormous difference in the amount of damage control and cleanup we are forced to deal with afterward. Instead of a one-directional imposition of will and then a desperate reaction to resulting disaster, there could be a delicate interaction between technology and its physical context. This, however, would require of technology more humility and less faith in after-the-fact technological fixes.

But beyond that, even more than science, technology must acknowledge the social environment of which it is a part and learn to respect the interests not only of business or government but those of the "nonexperts," both workers and consumers, who are affected by technology. Instead of imposing a given solution, technology must learn to proceed with empathy and affection—not only toward the natural and physical environment but *also* toward the people and institutions that comprise the social context. By developing the capacity for genuine interaction, by forgetting its "professional" or "expert" status and giving up the distance between itself and the material, by letting the social environment tell it what to do, quite literally by *listening* to people instead of dismissing them, technology could be changed from the roots up.

This collection of articles reflects both the current "main theme" in technology and a variety of "subthemes." For the most part, it details the effects of the polarization and exclusion that characterize workplace technology today; but it also celebrates those women who have contributed to technology or have turned it to their benefit against all odds. It acknowledges the relief from drudgery that technologies have sometimes provided women, without ignoring the associated costs. In the final section, readers may begin to catch a glimpse of a world in which women not only have some control over the implementation of technology but also influence educational and economic structures and participate in the very definition of technology. The authors are not so rash as to believe we are now in the midst of a transition to the inclusion of female-associated, generally neglected values in our practice of science and technology; but they suggest the potential for such a transformation—if we understand what we are about and take appropriate action.

The collection is intended to convey specific information about the interactions between women, work, and technology. Beyond that, however, it is our hope that it may accomplish several other purposes, as well: to stimulate further research on women and technology; to encourage women and men who do not fit the current stereotypes of science and technology in the belief that there may be room for them after all; and to suggest the outlines, however faint, of the more fully human technology and the more humane workplace that may yet come to be.

REFERENCES

Baker, Elizabeth Faulkner. 1964. *Technology and woman's work*. New York: Columbia University Press.
Bleier, Ruth. 1984. *Science and gender: A critique of biology and its theories on women*. New York: Pergamon Press.
Bose, Christine, and Glenna Spitze, eds. 1987. *Ingredients for women's economic policy*. Albany: State University of New York Press.
Bush, Corlann Gee. 1983. Women and the assessment of technology: To think, to be, to unthink, to free. In *Machina ex dea*, 151–70. *See* Rothschild 1983.
Commager, Henry Steele. 1985. Science, nationalism and the academy. *Academe* 71, no. 6:9–13.
Commoner, Barry. 1971. *The closing circle: Nature, man and technology*. New York: Knopf.
Cowan, Ruth Schwartz. 1983. *More work for mother: The ironies of household technology from the open hearth to the microwave*. New York: Basic Books.
Dubos, Rene. 1970. *Reason awake: Science for man*. New York: Columbia University Press.
Ellul, Jacques. 1965. *The technological society*. New York: Knopf.
———. 1980. *The technological system*. New York: Continuum Books.
Falk, Richard. 1971. *This endangered planet: Prospects and proposals for human survival*. New York: Random House.
Fausto-Sterling, Anne. 1985. *Myths of gender: Biological theories about women and men*. New York: Basic Books.
Fee, Elizabeth. 1983. Women's nature and scientific objectivity. In *Woman's nature*, 9–28. *See* Lowe and Hubbard 1983.

Game, Ann, and Rosemary Pringle. 1984. *Gender at work*. London: Pluto Press.

Gravender, Jerry. 1986. Technology assessment and women. Lecture delivered at the University of Connecticut Health Center, Apr. 3.

Haas, Violet B., and Carolyn C. Perrucci, eds. 1984. *Women in scientific and engineering professions*. Ann Arbor: University of Michigan Press.

Harding, Sandra. 1986. *The science question in feminism*. Ithaca: Cornell University Press.

Harkess, Shirley. 1984. Women's occupational experiences in the 1970's: Sociology and economics. *Signs* 10, no. 3:495–516.

Jensen, Joan M., and Sue Davidson, eds. 1984. *A needle, a bobbin, a strike: Women needleworkers in America*. Philadelphia: Temple University Press.

Keller, Evelyn Fox. 1983. Women, science, and popular mythology. In *Machina ex dea*, 130–46. *See* Rothschild 1983.

————. 1985. *Reflections on gender and science*. New Haven: Yale University Press.

Layton, Edwin T., Jr. 1971. *The revolt of the engineers: Social responsibility and the American engineering profession*. Cleveland: Press of Case Western Reserve University.

Lowe, Marian, and Ruth Hubbard, eds. 1983. *Woman's nature: Rationalizations of inequality*. New York: Pergamon Press.

McGaw, Judith A. 1982. Women and the history of American technology. *Signs* 9, no. 2:798–828.

Martin, Jane Roland. 1986. Questioning the question. *Woman's Review of Books* 4, no. 3 (Dec.): 17–18.

Mattfeld, Jacquelyn A., and Carol G. Van Aken. 1965. *Women and the scientific professions*. Cambridge, Mass.: MIT Press.

Merchant, Carolyn. 1980. *The death of nature: Women, ecology, and the scientific revolution*. San Francisco: Harper and Row.

Minnich, Elizabeth. 1984. On truth and equity: A modest proposal for educational excellence. Lecture delivered in Storrs, Conn., Mar. 19.

Mozans, J. H. [1913] 1974. *Woman in science*. Reprint, with introduction by Mildred Dressenhaus. Cambridge, Mass.: MIT Press.

Mumford, Lewis. 1934. *Technics and civilization*. New York: Harcourt, Brace and Co.

Pacey, Arnold. 1975. *The maze of ingenuity: Ideas and idealism in the development of technology*. New York: Holmes and Meier.

————. 1983. *The culture of technology*. Cambridge, Mass.: MIT Press.

Reskin, Barbara F., ed. 1984. *Sex segregation in the workplace: Trends, explanations, remedies*. Washington, D.C.: National Academic Press.

Rossiter, Margaret W. 1982. *Women scientists in America: Struggles and strategies to 1940*. Baltimore: Johns Hopkins University Press.

Roszak, Theodore. 1969. *The making of the counter-culture*. New York: Doubleday and Co.

————. 1974. The monster and the titan: Science, knowledge, and gnosis. *Daedalus* 103, no. 3 (Summer): 17–32.

Rothschild, Joan. 1981. A feminist perspective on technology and the future. *Women's Studies International Quarterly* 4, no. 1:65–74.

————, ed. 1983. *Machina ex dea: Feminist perspectives on technology*. New York: Pergamon Press.

Sacks, Karen Brodkin, and Dorothy Remy, eds. 1984. *My troubles are going to have trouble with me: Everyday trials and triumphs of women workers*. New Brunswick, N.J.: Rutgers University Press.

Stanley, Autumn. Women hold up two-thirds of the sky: Notes for a revised history of technology. In *Machina ex dea*, 3–22. *See* Rothschild 1983.

Stromberg, Ann H., and Shirley Harkess, eds. 1978. *Women working: Theories and facts in perspective*. Palo Alto: Mayfield Publishing Co.

Toffler, Alvin. 1970. *Future shock*. New York: Random House.

————. 1980. *The third wave*. New York: William Morrow and Co.

Trescott, Martha Moore, ed. 1979. *Dynamos and virgins revisited: Women and technological change in history*. Metuchen, N.J.: Scarecrow Press.

Wallace, Phyllis, ed. 1982. *Women in the workplace*. Dover, Mass.: Auburn House.

West, Jackie, ed. 1982. *Work, women and the labour market*. Boston: Routledge and Kegan Paul.

White, Lynn. 1971. *Dynamo and virgin reconsidered: Essays in the dynamism of western culture*. Cambridge, Mass.: MIT Press.

Winner, Langdon. 1977. *Autonomous technology: Technology-out-of-control as a theme in political thought*. Cambridge, Mass.: MIT Press.

————. 1986. *The whale and the reactor: The search for limits in an age of high technology*. Chicago: University of Chicago Press.

Ziman, John. 1978. *Reliable knowledge: An exploration of the grounds for belief in science*. Cambridge: Cambridge University Press.

————. 1984. *An introduction to science studies: The philosophy and social aspects of science and technology*. Cambridge: Cambridge University Press.

Zimmerman, Jan, ed. 1983. *The technological woman: Interfacing with tomorrow*. New York: Praeger Publishers.

Part 1
Historical Perspectives

Introduction

Robert Asher

The essays in the historical section of this volume focus on the way the work of women was altered by new production technologies in the nineteenth and early twentieth centuries. As the authors demonstrate, women successfully adapted to new work technologies and shifting job requirements. Women also invented many important manufacturing technologies. Unionized and unorganized women struggled against unsafe and unhealthy working conditions created by industrial technologies and opposed the legal and institutional exclusion of women from the machine-operating and managerial jobs that were created by economic growth and technological change.

In this section, the authors examine the dynamic interaction between technological change and social change, the dialectic of gender struggles and class struggles, and the consequent transformations in the gender-based division of labor. Historically, the impact of technological change on women's (and men's) work has often been negative. But women have actively tried to take advantage of the real opportunities for advancement created by technological "progress." The new technologies of the Industrial Revolution were diffused in a social setting marked by a polarized, gender-based division of labor in which women were given jobs and roles that brought them lower financial rewards and a lower social status than those men gained from their economic activities. Business owners adopted new machinery and organizational schemes that advanced the division of labor, creating large numbers of new, highly specialized jobs that were performed by low-paid workers. Women wage earners were hired for these jobs in disproportionate numbers. The fortunate minority of male workers who latched onto the smaller number of high-paying machine-operating, machine-repairing, and managerial jobs that were also created by mechanization and economic growth tried to exclude women from these occupational strata. Male workers trying to justify this exclusion manipulated gender stereotypes of work and workers, as did employers seeking to hire women workers at lower wages than male workers.

Most early human societies had gender-based divisions of labor. While women could and did perform every type of work that men did, women generally concentrated on food gathering while men focused on hunting. In these societies, the status of women's and men's work was approximately equal because the economic activities of women were essential to day-to-day survival. But with the emergence of more productive technologies, economic and social stratification intensified; men began to control the majority of the economic activities that produced surplus goods that were exchanged in the marketplace. Men increasingly aggrandized economic and political power at the expense of women (Appelbaum 1984; Collier and Rosaldo 1981; Leibowitz 1978; Sacks 1979).

After 1500, as technological change accelerated in Western Europe and its New World colonies, the gender-based division of labor continued to evolve. By the eve of the Industrial Revolution in the United States and Western Europe, married men had obtained sole legal authority over all productive property owned by their wives. Within agricultural families, women generally had control over the activities of the house and the yard. Although women did work in the fields, they exercised much less control than men over decisions concerning the growing and marketing of crops (Jones 1987). In the large numbers of households that produced handicrafts, men and women often performed the same type of skilled labor, e.g., spinning, weaving, stocking knitting, and sewing (Thirsk 1978). But there is some evidence that by the early nineteenth century, household shoe production in the United States was characterized by a polarized, gender-based division of labor in which women did most of the "binding" (sewing together the leather pieces that formed the upper part of a shoe) while men monopolized leather cutting and the task of attaching the upper part of the shoe to the innersole, tasks that received the highest wages and were assigned to men when shoe production was moved into factories (Mulligan 1986).

Carol Haddad's opening essay of the historical section shows that the development of mechanized commodity production severely disrupted the household production system that had allowed women to exercise considerable control over their economic activities. The lower production costs of machine-made commodities forced many women out of the household system and into factory jobs, which offered them a way of continuing to bring in income for themselves or the support of their families. Women factory workers in the United States operated machinery that made shoes, thread, cloth, boxes, pins, and other commodities. Haddad challenges the notion that this work was liberating, pointing out that it was tedious and exhausting and did not free women from the traditional expectation that their primary adult roles would be those of wife and mother. Such expectations were also part of the argument employers used to justify paying working women lower wages than men for the same work (e.g., operating shoe-lasting machines) and for hiring large numbers of women to work in the lowest paying jobs available in most industrial and service occupations. Since employers assumed that the typical working woman was not the *primary* family wage earner, they reasoned she did not need as much income as male workers, who were assumed to be the chief breadwinners for their families (Beechey 1978; Kessler-Harris 1982). Ironically, although innumerable women in the United States and Europe worked as machine operatives, in the twentieth century in several Third World countries women have been excluded from partly mechanized commercial, agricultural, and mineral extraction jobs on the grounds that they were not competent to operate machinery.

Turning to the development of modern, automated production technologies in the years after World War II, Haddad points out that many of the occupations in which women comprise a substantial proportion of the labor force—especially retail and clerical work—can be expected to be severely affected by technological unemployment, in which more efficient technologies displace workers. Such technologies frequently standardize and downskill work while reducing appreciably the control that workers exercise over their jobs. Women manufacturing workers, especially in the Third World, are also exposed to many toxic chemicals that cause occupational diseases. Electronic monitoring has enabled employers to force workers (most frequently women), whether they are employed in blue- or white-collar jobs, to increase their work pace substantially. Meanwhile, most of the new professional and managerial jobs that are being created by technological change are held by men.

Women workers in the United States, Europe, and the Third World have often turned to labor unions to agitate for shorter hours, higher pay, a slower work pace, safer and healthier working conditions, and an end to employment discrimination. Strong governmental opposition to unions impeded these efforts in the past, as it still does in Third World nations where independent unions are illegal and workers are often forced to join government-sponsored unions. From the mid-nineteenth century to the present, unions of skilled male workers have often refused to admit women or, if they did, placed them in separate locals that were assigned an inferior status. Although large numbers of women factory laborers in the United States were ignored by the mainstream labor movement in the early years of the twentieth century, the women nevertheless staged militant strikes. Often socialist and anarchist labor organizers, both female and male, were the only unionists who would aid women factory workers (Kessler-Harris 1982).

Ava Baron offers a finely detailed case study of the way concepts of gender were manipulated in the newspaper publishing industry during the struggle between men and women for access to skilled typesetting jobs in both the hand- and machine-composition eras. Baron points out that during the era of hand composition, male typesetters viewed their jobs as masculine because the jobs required skill and brought high wages, enabling them to be the main supporters of their families. When employers began training women (in the 1850s and 1860s) to do straight composition, male printers believed (correctly) that employers were trying to undermine the wages of the men by increasing the supply of workers with typesetting skills. While unionized male printers tried to justify their attempts to exclude women on the grounds that the print-shop environment would undermine the femininity of women, employers maintained that printing work was feminine because it was light, clean, and intellectual. Upon failing to exclude women, the male printers admitted them to their union and insisted that the women be paid the same wages as men, viewing their action as fulfilling a male obligation to protect women.

When the Linotype machine was introduced in the early 1890s, employers sought to hire women operators, whom employers hoped to pay less than men. Employers claimed that the Linotype was similar to the typewriter, a machine that supposedly did not require skilled operators. Employers claimed that Linotype operating was pleasant and respectable work and that women operators would be neater and more industrious than men. The male printers favored the Linotype over other available typesetting machines because its intrinsic characteristics enabled them to develop a rationale to justify excluding women from typesetting jobs. They shifted their argument from the assertion that typesetting work embodied gender to the notion that only workers embodied gender and that male workers could do work that women could not do. The male printers argued that the Linotype machine required an operator who could rapidly make the decisions necessary to justify the right-hand margin of the columns being set, had a great deal of stamina, would be able to endure the heat and fumes generated by the Linotype's molten lead, and could lift heavy weights. They claimed that only men had these physical and mental abilities. Most publishers appear to have cut a deal with the unionized male printers, tolerating the exclusion of women in return for a pledge by the men to accept mechanization without opposition and to refrain from attempting to restrict output on Linotype machines. The employers thus cleverly turned the printers' assertion of superior male stamina against them. The unionized male printers barred women from apprenticeship programs and lobbied successfully in some states (along with other unions that sought to exclude women from various labor markets) to pass legislation banning night work for women. Women typesetters resisted and managed to obtain repeal of some of these laws, but they still were not able to obtain many Linotype jobs after 1905.

Carole Srole's analysis of the gender division of labor in office work begins in the pretypewriter era. As the size of offices in business firms and government grew in the 1860s and thereafter, the male clerk's multi-faceted job was subdivided, and the occupation of copyist was created. Women were excluded from the middle-rank clerical and bookkeeping jobs that men still monopolized but were hired for the lower-paying clerical jobs. These, unlike the entry-level jobs available to men, did not give the worker experiences that would facilitate promotion to marketing and managerial positions. The development of a new technology, the typewriter, did not alter the role assigned to women in the office hierarchy. From the outset, employers viewed the typewriter as a tool to be used primarily by female copyists. Women who had learned typing were frequently assigned to jobs that involved typing only and were at the bottom of the office pay scale.

Women still wanted to train as typists, however, to obtain entry into office work, because they saw the work as more pleasant and higher in status than factory work, and because they believed (optimistically) that a typist job could be a stepping-stone to better-paying clerical jobs like bookkeeper and accountant. When shorthand was developed, Eliza Boardman Burnz and others like her took the lead in training women as stenographers. Employers began to hire stenographers as letter-writing specialists. This represented an intensification of the division of labor, since stenographers performed a task that formerly had been only *part* of the duties of the well-paid male clerk. Employers now hired fewer clerks and more stenographers, who were paid better wages than typists but received less than male clerks had under the previous division of labor.

In the years when office work was a male bastion, employers had justified excluding women by implying that they were unsuited for office work. As the demand for office workers increased markedly after the Civil War, it became necessary to hire women, and managers who had previously accepted the exclusion of women from the office began to argue that clerical work was feminine and *was* appropriate for women. Women stenographers (and later typists) were touted as superior to men because the women were more nimble, more painstaking, more obedient, and brought a feminine caring and cheerfulness to the office. Male

managers also believed that their status was enhanced by having a stenographer to whom they could "dictate" and that the presence of "inferior" women workers highlighted the power of the "superior" man.

Patricia Klein's study of lead poisoning addresses another facet of
exclusion. She examines women's exclusion from occupations in which
exposure to toxic chemicals supposedly is more harmful to female workers than to males due to the chemicals' effects on women's reproductive functions. As Klein shows, the exclusion of women from particular
trades often preceded the development of scientific rationales. But as
medical science progressed and physicians began to study the impact of
industrial toxins on workers, evidence that these substances had adverse effects on reproduction was used to justify continued discrimination against women workers as well as protective labor laws that
banned the employment of pregnant women or women who might
become pregnant. Rather than removing the lead hazards in printing,
pottery making, and battery manufacturing, government and private
industry have preferred to remove women workers from the work environment. But policymakers have often ignored medical evidence suggesting that males exposed to lead could also transmit birth defects to
their offspring.

Klein's description of Alice Hamilton, the pioneer American industrial physician, in her efforts to deal with the health problem of women
workers' exposure to lead, reveals the complexity of the tactical decisions facing professionals who were not hostile, in principle, to the
employment of women. Hamilton never hesitated to criticize government policymakers who ignored the adverse effects of lead exposure on
the male reproductive system. And she spoke out boldly in advocating
safety measures, not exclusion, to reduce the deleterious effects both
sexes experienced upon exposure to lead in the workplace. Nevertheless, discouraged by the difficulty of securing legislation that would markedly reduce the exposure of all workers to lead, by 1919 Hamilton was
willing to accept female exclusion as the *only* way to prevent women
workers, at least, from being exposed to high levels of lead.

Industrial society has generally underestimated the economic and
social contributions made by women, and especially by wage-earning
women. This tendency reflects, in part, a failure to appreciate the skills
that were (and are) necessary to produce efficiently in so-called semiskilled and unskilled blue-collar and white-collar jobs for which employers have hired many women. This classification, formulated by the U.S.
Census Bureau, suggests that only "skilled" jobs (which have been
largely the preserve of men) require ingenuity and refined manual skills.
But as Kenneth Kusterer (1978) has shown, "semiskilled" and "un-

skilled" jobs, which have constituted the bulk of the jobs created as technological change constantly eliminates existing jobs and fashions new ones, entail considerable problem-solving ability and physical skill, especially if maximum productive efficiency is to be achieved. Downgrading the capabilities of women who labor in such jobs distorts our understanding of how an industrial society prospers and advances.

Autumn Stanley's essay documents another aspect of the tendency to ignore and undervalue the significant economic activities of women. Stanley discusses the underrepresentation, in historical accounts of invention, of the achievements of women inventors, and especially women who developed new machinery for heavy industrial processes. Large numbers of nineteenth-century women were granted patents on their inventions of new consumer products and manufacturing machinery. In the late 1880s, Charlotte Smith, a women's rights activist, launched a determined and successful effort to get the U.S. Patent Office to acknowledge the activity of women by compiling a catalog of women's inventions. Stanley has found, however, that the Patent Office's 1890 catalog of inventions by women omitted many items, especially the *machines* that women developed. Even more telling, the Patent Office avoided the use of *any* category for manufacturing in its 1890 catalog of women's inventions. Stanley concludes that this pattern of oversight reflects the assumption by Patent Office personnel that "women invent, if at all, mainly in the so-called domestic areas."

Industrialization based on an accelerating rate of technological innovation arose in the West within societies that were already patriarchal. It is thus hardly surprising that women were generally relegated to the low-wage interface between human producers and technology (Hartmann 1979). The women's movement has frequently mounted legal and political challenges against wage discrimination and gender-based exclusion. In the last two decades, feminist efforts to raise the consciousness of women and secure legislation aimed at reducing sex discrimination have begun to open up many traditionally male-dominated *professions* to women. But working-class women have made only modest inroads into high-paying jobs in the blue- and white-collar industries, especially those jobs that rely less on hand skills than on knowledge of electronics, mathematics, and metalworking. During the last decade, businesses have been adopting technologies that have reduced levels of work skill more often than they have enhanced them. As the proportion of "skilled," high-paying jobs shrinks, the legacy of pervasive exclusion of women from such jobs will continue to create barriers for women as they compete with men for work that is creative, pays well, and offers the worker a degree of freedom.

REFERENCES

Applebaum, Herbert. 1984. *Work in non-market and traditional societies.* Albany: State University of New York Press.

Beechey, Veronica. 1978. Women and production: A critical analysis of some sociological theories of women's work. In *Feminism and materialism,* ed. Annette Kuhn and Ann Marie Wolpe. Boston: Routledge and Kegan Paul.

Collier, Jane F., and Michelle Z. Rosaldo. 1981. Politics and gender in simple societies. In *Sexual meanings,* ed. S. Ornter and H. Whitehead. Cambridge: Cambridge University Press.

Hartmann, Heidi. 1979. Capitalism, patriarchy, and job segregation by sex. In *Capitalist patriarchy and the case for socialist feminism,* ed. Z. Eisenstein. New York: Monthly Review Press.

Jones, Lu Ann. 1987. "Everything we had." In *Cotton mill people: An oral history of the textile South, 1880–1940,* ed. Christopher B. Daly, Jacquelyn Dowd Hall, Lu Ann Jones, James L. Leloudis III, Robert Korstad, and Mary Murphy. Chapel Hill: University of North Carolina Press.

Kessler-Harris, Alice. 1982. *Out to work: A history of wage-earning women in the United States.* New York: Oxford University Press.

Kusterer, Kenneth C. 1978. *Know-how on the job: The important working knowledge of "unskilled" workers.* Boulder: Westview Press.

Leibowitz, Lila. 1978. *Females, males, families: A biosocial approach.* North Scituate, Mass.: Duxbury Press.

Mulligan, William H., Jr. 1986. From artisan to proletarian: The family and the vocational education of the shoemaker in the handicraft era. In *Life and labor: dimensions of American working-class history,* ed. C. Stephenson and R. Asher. Albany: State University of New York Press.

Sacks, Karen. 1979. *Sisters and wives: The past and future of sexual equality.* Westport, Conn.: Greenwood Press.

Thirsk, Joan. 1978. *Economic policy and projects.* Oxford: Clarendon Press.

Technology, Industrialization, and the Economic Status of Women

Carol J. Haddad

Technological change is often hailed as a signpost of human progress and a vehicle for human liberation. When introduced in a context of industrialization, technology is credited with raising the economic status of societies that have embraced it, on a global basis. Its proponents contend that it has brought greater wealth and opportunity to all by promising the entry of more people into the paid work force and by raising the skill levels and workplace autonomy of those already working. Consequently, women are seen as reaping tremendous benefits from the introduction of new technology.

There is, however, another side to this coin. Critics of technological change argue that although technology is capable of bestowing the benefits described above, its historic and current applications suggest that such outcomes are far from inevitable. Critics further contend that the implementation of technological change has often served to reinforce and intensify existing differentials in economic status. Hence, women are seen as losing ground in this scenario. A central question emerges from these conflicting analyses: what *is* the effect of technological change upon the economic status of women?

Before answers to this question can be fully explored, however, some clarifications are necessary. First, what is meant by "technology"? Second, what is meant by "economic status of women"? Technology is a term that represents many things to many people. It encompasses human innovations as ancient, modern, and diverse as the stone tools of the First Ice Age, ploughs, factory assembly lines and robots, space satellites, nuclear warheads, genetic engineering, and microwave ovens. Ellul (1964) defines technology in its broadest sense to mean not merely machines or procedures but "the *totality of methods rationally arrived at and having absolute efficiency* (for a given stage of development) in *every* field of human activity" (xxv).

However, because this paper will focus on technology pertaining to the work process in the context of modern industrialization and development, I have chosen to define technology more narrowly. Throughout this paper, the terms "technology" and "technological change" will mean the following: devices and systems applied to work processes for the stated purpose of improving efficiency by increasing output while reducing human labor input. This definition includes tools and implements, mechanization, automation, integrated production systems, and microelectronic-based technology.

Defining what is meant by the "economic status of women" is a more difficult task. Rosaldo (1973) and Sanday (1973) view women's "status" as a function of their participation in public spheres of activity and their control over strategic resources. Other scholars, notably Whyte (1976), have argued that "cross-culturally, there appears to be no such thing as *the* status of women." Those who subscribe to this philosophy view status as a composite of economic, political, cultural, religious, and legal factors, varying through time and across regions. Consequently, operational definitions of women's economic status are difficult to construct because there is little agreement among scholars as to which indicators of status are paramount (Buvinic 1976). Even "economic status," seemingly a narrower concept, can be measured in a variety of ways. Indicators include (but are not limited to) the following: property ownership (including land, capital, durable and luxury goods, stocks, etc.), control over property and resources, employment in the paid labor force, salary level, skill level,[1] opportunity for promotion, control over the work process, and job classification.

In examining the impact of technology on the economic status of women, I have limited my analysis to three of these indicators: income and control over resources, skill level, and control over the work process. I focus on these because they seem most basic and salient, and because it is particularly these factors that are most affected by the introduction of new technologies. I also examine the impact of technology on gender-based divisions of labor.[2] Women's participation in the paid labor force, while important, is an insufficient measure of economic status in my opinion and will be regarded only in the context of the previously mentioned indicators. Most importantly, this article explores the question of women's economic status and its relation to technology both historically *and* cross-culturally. Such examination is critical to a determination of whether there is universality in technology's impact on women, or whether its impact is culture bound. In the final section, I suggest strategies to enhance women's economic power and control.

The United States

Women in a Preindustrial Economy

The economy of the preindustrial United States was heavily dependent upon family farming and home production. Women functioned as skilled workers: they spun and dyed yarn, which they then wove into cloth; grew, preserved, and prepared food; shoed horses; sewed uppers onto leather soles; and served as healers and midwives. Some white women operated sawmills and gristmills, printing presses, slaughter-houses, stores, and inns (Wertheimer 1977). Native women were gener-ally responsible for cultivation and production of goods, while men hunted and defended territory. Black women cooked, cleaned, sewed, raised children, and worked in the fields for their white enslavers (Hull, Scott, and Smith 1982).

Economic status for women of this period is difficult to measure, for a number of reasons. One is that economic status and sexual divisions of labor varied according to race and marital status. While historians con-tinue to debate the existence and extent of gender-based divisions of labor in preindustrial society, the labor of white, married women in this period centered around household subsistence production, while that of their husbands was directed toward the marketplace. White women with-out husbands were more likely to enter the "masculine" sphere by be-coming entrepreneurs (e.g., tavern-keepers), or to support themselves by becoming domestic workers (Matthaei 1982). Black slave women worked in the fields alongside men; women's duties on plantations in-cluded plowing, hoeing, shoveling, and tree felling (Matthaei 1982; Da-vis 1981).

Another difficulty in determining women's economic status in this period is that it was, to some extent, determined by legal, political, social, and religious factors. For example, inheritance and property laws generally kept property out of the hands of women. Still, although women of this period may not have been the owners of property, white women, at least, enjoyed control over resources (the means of produc-tion) and over the work process. Black slave women obviously had little or no control in these respects. Whether they labored in the private (subsistence) sphere or in the public sphere, white women had control over how to weave fabric, grow and preserve food, and operate their inns and taverns. Furthermore, both black and white women were val-ued for their work skills. Sexual divisions of labor, which were less prevalent among black slaves than whites during this period,[3] had far more to do with familial authority structures and degree of participation in the public sphere than with the nature of the work itself.

The First Industrial Revolution

Mechanization promoted a radical transformation of the production pro-cess. Early in the nineteenth century, mills and factories began to replace homes and small shops as centers of production, and wage labor began to replace family and slave labor. Despite its potential for improving working conditions and living standards, the machine was not well received by all who witnessed its introduction. A speaker at the 1878 meeting of the American Social Science Association lamented:

> It has broken up and destroyed our whole system of household and family manufactures as done by our mothers, when all took part in the labor and shared in the product, to the comfort of all; and has compelled the daughters of our country and town to factory operations for 10 to 12 hours a day in the manufacture of cloth they may not wear. . . .
>
> It has . . . compelled all working men and women to a system of communal work, where . . . they are forced to labor . . . with no voice, no right, no interest in the product of their hands and brains, but subject to the uncontrollable interest and caprice of those who too often know no other motive than that of avarice. . . .
>
> It has thrown out of employment substantially one-half of the working classes. . . . [4]

Women's control over resources and production declined as it became easier to buy cheaply the goods that they had labored long and hard to produce for their households. Consequently, many women turned to factory work to support themselves or contribute to the family income. By 1840, although less than 10 percent of the population held manufacturing jobs, women comprised 50 percent of this sector's work force, and they outnumbered men in shoe factories and textile mills (Kessler-Harris 1982).

Because of the influx of women into factory production during this period, it is commonly believed that the Industrial Revolution liberated women from their traditional roles in the home by providing them with permanent, paid employment and thus greater social and economic status. But as at least one historian has observed, this premise is built upon faulty assumptions. First, not only had unmarried women worked prior to industrialization, e.g., in cottage industries or as domestics; they were *expected* to perform such work until they married. Second, mill and factory employment of young women did not alter societal expectations about their traditional roles as wives and mothers. Women's factory and mill work was viewed as "secondary," and sex bias prevailed in wage rates, classification schemes, training, and promotion as well as in hiring and retention practices favoring sixteen- to twenty-five-year-old unmarried women (Scott 1982).

Technology of the early industrial era profoundly affected the utilization of workers' skills and altered gender-based divisions of labor. Mechanization and routinization permitted the breakdown of skilled work into relatively unskilled functions that were minute pieces of the entire production process. In industries that replaced household production formerly performed and controlled by women, technological change permitted men's employment in large numbers.

The manufacture of textiles serves as perhaps the best example. In the cotton industry, females were thought to outnumber males by 110 percent in 1832. By the end of the nineteenth century, women sixteen years of age and older comprised only 42 percent of the work force in that industry (Baker 1964). The 1905 U.S. Census reported that

> the number of places in which women can profitably be employed in a cotton mill in preference to men or on an equality with them, steadily decreases as the speed of machinery increases and as the requirement that one hand shall tend a greater number of machines is extended. Accordingly we find that without any concert of action—perhaps unconsciously to the general body of manufacturers—there is a slow but steady displacement of women by men. (Baker 1964, 17)

Although the assumption that women were less capable than men of handling production speedup deserves to be challenged, this quotation is revealing of attitudes that contributed to women's work segregation and displacement. Technology facilitated the displacement of women in other areas of the textile industry as well, notably in the woolen and knit goods industries following the introduction of power looms. In short, according to one historian, technology in textile manufacturing had, by the turn of the century, "pushed men in at the top, women down, and children out" (Baker 1964, 23).

Conversely, in industries that had once been the province of skilled white males, technology gave women new opportunity. This "opportunity" was a mixed blessing, however, for although women (and children) found work in these industries, the wages they earned and the skill classifications they were assigned were generally the lowest in the factory hierarchy. The shoe industry is an interesting case in point.

Throughout the eighteenth century, shoemaking had been a skilled domestic trade controlled by men. Wives and daughters of the master craftsmen participated in the production process as "binders" but unlike their sons and brothers had no access to the apprenticeship system. By the 1830s, as production moved from the cottage to central craft shops, binding and decorating operations continued to be performed in the home by women and children, but for piece-rate pay. The development of the factory system in this industry, which began before mechanization and was spurred by the introduction of the McKay and Singer stitching machines, took women's employment out of the home but did little to alter gender-based divisions of labor, despite the fact that by 1900 forty-eight different occupations existed in the stitching room alone (Dewey 1900, 1198–1201).

> Men still did the cutting, earning about $3 a day in Lynn, and they continued to do the work of sewing uppers to the soles, using the McKay machines instead of the old laborious hand sewing or pegging. For operating the new machine they received from $25 to $40 a week. Women and girls were still almost exclusively engaged in fitting and sewing uppers, earning at this time from $7 to $14 a week. (Abbott 1909, 173–74)

Yet evidence of gender-based wage differentials also exists where women performed the *same* work as men. For example, lasting, which was done in preparation for the sewing together of soles and uppers on the McKay machine, was performed by both men and women; however, the women earned from twelve to twenty dollars per week for this work, while the men earned from thirty-six to forty dollars (Abbott 1909, 173–74; see also U.S. Bureau of the Census 1900, vol. 7, pt. 1, xcvii, cxix). Hence the theory that women earned less than men because they performed easier, lighter work is an inadequate explanation of the gender-based wage differential that existed in the shoe industry at the turn of the century. This point is reinforced in the writing of Horace B. Davis (1940), who noted that

> where both men and women are employed at essentially the same occupation the women earn only half to two-thirds as much as the men. . . . There is thus a strong indication that the differential is due to sex alone, and not the fact that women do "lighter, less straining types of work." (111)

One traditional argument made by proponents of technology is that, historically, it has prompted a large influx of women into the paid labor force. Indeed, statistics from this period would seem to substantiate this claim. Again, using the shoe industry as an example, data from table 1 reveal that the number of women aged sixteen years and older working in this industry increased by 97 percent between 1880 and 1905, years characterized by increased mechanization and standardization of the industry.

It is important to note, however, that an equally large, if not larger, proportion of women worked in this industry prior to the time it underwent mechanization and standardization. These were the women stitch-

TABLE 1.   Number of Persons Employed in the Shoe Industry, 1880–1905

Year	Men	Women	Children under 16	Percentage of Women Employed	Total Number of Employees
1880	82,547	25,122	3,483	23	111,152
1890	91,406	39,849	2,435	30	133,690
1900	90,415	46,894	4,521	33	141,830
1905	95,257	49,535	5,132	33	149,924

Source. Abbott 1910, 178.

ers and binders who labored in their own homes and consequently were not counted in government or industry statistics. Abbott (1910) challenged the notion that women made tremendous employment gains during the mechanization of the shoe industry; she argued instead that although women might now work in factories instead of cottages, and sew on machines instead of by hand, they were still doing essentially the same work of sewing uppers. Moreover, work that had been done *exclusively* by women prior to establishment of the factory system now was shared with men (179–80).

In other lines of work, feminization did occur. One of them was office work. As the demand for paperwork increased due to the growth of urban populations and commerce, routine clerical work (typing, filing, and stenography) was separated from administrative work. This change, which was facilitated by the widespread introduction of the typewriter and the telephone, transformed office work from a predominantly male occupation offering the prospect of advancement into the executive hierarchy to a female-dominated service industry. By 1910, 83 percent of all stenographers and typists were women (Scott 1982).

The examples presented thus far suggest that early industrial technology had a detrimental impact on women's control over resources and production and did little to improve women's income. Not only did this technology fail to eradicate preexisting gender-based divisions of labor; it even created new divisions in certain industries. Discussion of technology's impact on the economic status of women in this early industrial period is not complete, however, without mention of its impact on two additional phenomena—skill level and control over the work process.

The breaking down of complex tasks into fragmented, standardized production processes requiring relatively little or no skill was certainly an outcome, if not the intent, of the introduction of new technology into various industries.[5] Although most of the writing on this subject focuses on the breakdown of crafts*men's* skills and their replacement by the work of unskilled women and children, women also experienced a reduction in both their skill level and their control over the work process as production was moved from the home to the mechanized factory. "Where their labor at home had been highly skilled and self-regulated," writes Kessler-Harris, "employment outside it required leaving their skills behind and obeying another's clock" (1982, 29). The textile industry, discussed above, is one example of this phenomenon. Another is the cigar industry. Although cigar making in the United States is commonly thought to have been a male craft occupation in its earliest days, it was originally a home industry controlled by women. In the early eighteenth century, farmers' wives and daughters in Connecticut, Pennsylvania, and other tobacco-growing states rolled cigars in their homes and peddled or bartered them at country stores.

Then, during the first half of the nineteenth century, immigrant men from Cuba and later from Germany who were highly skilled in cigar making virtually took over the industry, producing high-quality cigars that could compete with those imported from Spain and Germany. By the 1880s, Bohemian immigrant women, manufacturing cigars in their New York tenement homes, were being used by employers to break the monopoly held by skilled males. This process was completed a decade later with the introduction of machinery that allowed employers to use low-paid female operatives to replace skilled male cigar makers (Baxandall, Gordon, and Reverby 1976). This is one of the few industries in which technology enabled women to dominate employment after having been displaced. However, technology did *not* lead to the rehiring of the *same* group of women, and it did not enable the second group to control the work process or achieve the level of skill the first group of women enjoyed.

The Second Industrial Revolution

The mechanization of the early industrial era gave birth to subsequent generations of technology, such as automation and the integrated, self-regulating production systems of the 1940s and 1950s. These latter systems can be regarded as extensions of the first wave of industrialization, for they are variations on the theme of mechanization. In contrast, microelectronic technology, originally developed for space and military use and subsequently applied to the workplace, has radically transformed the work process. Its sophistication, rapid development, and broad range of application have prompted some observers to regard its arrival as a second "industrial revolution."

As was true in the first Industrial Revolution, today's new technology is being introduced in a context of occupational sex segregation, which in some cases predated the implementation of new technology and in other instances has followed it. Women are most heavily concentrated precisely in those industries that have been or are expected to be most dramatically affected by new technology. For example, women comprise 96.3 percent of typists, 93.5 percent of bank tellers, 92.9 percent of telephone operators, 80.5 percent of clerical workers, and 71.2 percent of retail workers (U.S. Department of Labor 1982).

The telephone industry has been experiencing the introduction of microelectronic technology slowly but steadily over the past twenty-five years. Gone are the old cord switchboards that operators once used to connect calls.[6] The old system was replaced in the mid-1960s with the new Traffic Service Position System (TSPS). TSPS involves pushing buttons on a computerized console to connect operator-assisted calls or to calculate charges. The new system has its advantages. It is physically easier to manipulate, it automatically performs the calculations that operators formerly had to make, and it has greatly improved productivity: an operator averaged 20 calls per hour under the old system; with TSPS the average has jumped to 100 calls per hour (Howard 1980). These benefits are not without some costs, however.

Under the cord switchboard system operators had some control over the pace of their work; TSPS routes calls to operators in unending succession. A flashing light on the "call-waiting" box alerts supervisors to calls not answered within ten seconds. Operators are also timed by computer to determine how long they spend on individual calls (Howard 1980; Asher 1983). According to Ronnie Straw, research director for the Communications Workers of America (CWA), TSPS "allows for the elimination of local phone offices, paces the flow of calls to the individual operator, catalogues the operator's average work time for each call, predicts the future flow of calls, schedules the operator's breaks, and in general welds the operator to the equipment" (Straw 1981).

Union sentiment on this subject was perhaps best expressed on T-shirts sported by CWA members at a working women's leadership school.[7] The shirts featured a drawing of the Statue of Liberty wearing headphones, wrapped in telephone cord, and stating, "Give me your tired, your poor, your hungry . . . but make it fast—I only have 22 seconds." Operators are monitored (without their knowledge) not only for speed but also for courtesy and accuracy (Howard 1980). It is little wonder that stress has reached epidemic proportions in this industry, and that "more and more telephone workers have turned to drugs to put the lid on stress" (Howard 1981).

The retail industry has experienced various forms of technological change within the past few years. One of the most pervasive changes has been the introduction of electronic scanners, which have replaced traditional cash registers at checkout lanes. These computerized machines are capable of "reading" Universal Product Code symbols, which appear as a series of black and white bars on retail products. It has been estimated that the entire industry will convert to scanner use by the end of the 1980s (Burns 1982). Scanners are capable of more than adding up the prices of goods that are moved across their electronic "eyes." They eliminate the need for item pricing (unless state law requires it), automatically inventory stock, and enable stores to operate more "efficiently"—that is, with fewer employees.

Moreover, scanners are capable of recording cashiers' speed, accuracy, and number and length of pauses. This provides store managers and employers with tremendous control over the work process. Employees of a Michigan department store chain have already begun to experience the ill effects of such a system. Each week, charts are posted in the stores showing production and error rates of each cashier, identified by name. Store managers typically write comments next to employees' names, such as "Very good!" or "Come and see me immediately." This practice is a source of humiliation and job stress for cashiers, and posted data can be used to encourage "speedup" and to foster rivalry among employees.

The arrival of microelectronic technology into offices has facilitated the most recent phases of work "rationalization" in the clerical industry. Vincent Giuliano (1982) describes the organization of offices as having "evolved" through three stages: "preindustrial," "industrial," and "information age." In the preindustrial model, which dates back to the turn of the century, secretaries perform a variety of tasks with a fair degree of autonomy. Human relationships are valued, and little emphasis is placed on systematic work organization or modern technology. Most small offices continue to operate in this fashion. The industrial model is akin to a "pink-collar" assembly line: tasks are fragmented and standardized. Human relationships take second place to office "efficiency." This model is commonly found in high-output settings such as insurance claims offices. The information age model is meant to combine the human orientation of the preindustrial office with the efficiency of the industrial office through the use of microelectronic information technology. Despite his accuracy in describing the first two models, Giuliano, an executive with Arthur D. Little, Inc., takes a rather idealistic view of work organization in the information age: "the machine is paced to the needs and abilities of the person who works with it. . . . The job is no longer tied to the flow of paper across a designated desk; it is tied to the worker himself" (85).

While office technology is perfectly capable of providing the kind of autonomy that Giuliano describes, present applications suggest that for the great majority of clerical workers, work is becoming more standardized and less skilled as a result of new technology. Secretaries, whose jobs once encompassed far more than typing, are increasingly being transformed into "word processing operators" (Machung 1983). Gregory (1982) has described the ways in which deskilling can follow the implementation of new technology, using the example of a midwestern corporate headquarters:

> Secretarial jobs were broken down into component parts when word-processing equipment was brought into the department. As a result, one woman does electronic filing all day, another handles correspondence all day, and so on. The company requires that each woman complete a "tour of duty" of several months in each subtask in order to be considered for promotion. In other words, each woman must be promoted four times to get back where she started. (85)

In addition to its impact on worker skill, new office technology has also had a noticeable impact on worker autonomy. Feldberg and Glenn (1983) studied the impact of technology and work reorganization on the jobs of customer service clerks in a utility company. They discovered that after the introduction of computer terminals, the work of the customer service clerks broadened to encompass a series of fragmented tasks formerly performed by several clerks. On the surface, it would appear that technology in this case facilitated a transformation of the work process from an "industrial" model to Giuliano's utopian "information age" model, because of the broadening of the scope of work performed by customer service clerks. However, this positive feature is offset by increased supervision and electronic monitoring. Specific procedures and time frames accompany each portion of the job, and the volume of work and error rate of each clerk are tabulated by computer.

Electronic monitoring of this type often results in the establishment of arbitrary production standards, which may be used as a basis for disciplining or even terminating employees who fail to keep up with production quotas set by management. Wernecke (1983) cites the example of the firing of two Blue Cross/Blue Shield workers for their failure to meet an experimental quota for processing insurance claims on a visual display unit. Fortunately for the workers, they were represented by a union and were able to take the case before an arbitrator, who reinstated them.

Proponents of office technology might argue that the previous examples are atypical, and that new technology most often results in the elevation of white-collar workers from low-level clericals to technicians, supervisors, and managers. Indeed, debate about the numbers of upper-level jobs that are created by technology (Levin and Rumberger 1983) and observations about the shrinking of middle management (Kuttner 1983; "A new era for management" 1983) notwithstanding, new technology can and does create professional and technical white-collar jobs. However, as Feldberg and Glenn (1983) have noted, these new jobs have become the province of men, while low-level clerical jobs have become increasingly feminized. Moreover, technological change has been found to decrease women's chances for upward mobility, since it eliminates many of the more highly skilled clerical and middle-level jobs. The data presented by Feldberg and Glenn (1983) suggest that technological change has served to increase preexisting sex stratification among white-collar workers.

In summary, current applications of new technology to industries and occupations in which women are heavily concentrated have served to reduce worker skill and control over the work process and have intensified preexisting sexual divisions of labor, despite their potential for improving the economic status of women. Thus, the trends that emerged in the first Industrial Revolution have persisted through the second.

Developing Countries[8]

Precolonial Societies and Colonialization

The introduction of new technology into various societies has often occurred within the larger context of "development," and more specifically development under colonial or imperial rule. Western history texts are filled with accounts of "civilized" people taking up "the white man's burden" in the hope of bringing Christianity and "progress" to "untamed heathens" in various parts of the world. As one modern Western scholar has observed,

> in the arrogance of modern achievement we tend to regard . . . [various] forms of technical asistance to underdeveloped and developing countries as a charitable endowment, an act of generosity by the highly advanced countries to the "backward" countries, forgetting that many of those countries had advanced civilization and what we would now call "technology" when the ancestors of the Industrial Revolution were running around painted in woad. (Ritchie-Calder 1972, 65)

Undoubtedly, the white men bent on spreading Western civilization and technology to peoples around the rest of the globe were unaware that the ancient Hindus were producers and exporters of steel, that the Nabateans of Palestine could produce bountiful crops in desert wilderness, and that the ancient Chinese had mastered silk production (Ritchie-Calder 1972). Ignorance of the rich histories and cultures of "primitive" nations was generally matched by an ignorance of their economic and social structures and the existing relationships between women and men. Consequently, economic development and Western technologies were often introduced in ways that indiscriminately replaced traditional structures and values with white Western ones.

As Boserup (1970) discovered, the economic status of women often suffered as a result. In precolonial African societies characterized by shifting cultivation, women performed most of the tasks connected with food production.[9] Because farming was done on a subsistence, not a cash-crop, basis, and because there was no land ownership, this system provided women with almost complete control over resources and production. But as population density increased and plough cultivation was introduced, women often experienced a dramatic shift in their status. Men became the sole operators of the plough, even where hoeing had formerly been women's work. Plough cultivation also resulted in higher crop yields and cash-crop production, leading to a further division of labor and erosion of women's economic status:

> In Uganda women began the cultivation of cotton, yet in 1923 the European director of agriculture in the territory had stated that "cotton growing could not be left to the women and old people," and one decade later most of the men were growing cotton and coffee, and importing hired labor from the other tribes to do most of the work. In those parts of Uganda where cultivation continued to be done mainly by women, the Europeans neglected to instruct the female cultivators when they introduced new agricultural methods, teaching only the men in an agricultural setting of traditional female farming, with particularly unfortunate results in regions with large male emigration. (Boserup 1970, 54–55)

Boserup's conclusions are shared by Seidman (1981). She notes that in precolonial African societies, women commanded "significant decision-making powers about what to produce and how to produce it" (112). Nor was women's control over the work process limited to farming; women and men "worked together, using long-established technologies, to produce iron tools, salt, soap, textiles" (112). Yet not only were African women denied knowledge of new farming techniques following imposition of colonial rule; as landholdings were individualized to encourage higher crop output, women were generally denied title to the land and bank credit, even where they performed the bulk of the farm labor.

The preceding examples have focused on women in precolonial African societies; studies of other precolonial areas also confirm a pattern of lowered female economic status following the introduction of new technology (Dauber and Cain 1981; D'Onofrio-Flores and Pfafflin 1982; Nash and Fernandez-Kelly 1983). Chaney and Schmink (1976), in their study of Latin American women, have offered an explanation for this phenomenon: "It is widely recognized that the 'technological imperative' carries with it a set of sex-role prescriptions. . . . Women are considered incapable of handling or understanding complex machinery, and thus often are deprived of access to useful tools" (175). Parallels can be drawn between the economic status of women in precolonial developing countries and that of women in the preindustrial United States: both groups of women maintained considerable control over the production of subsistence goods and the resources that enabled such production. However, erosion of Third World women's economic status occurred not only as a result of industrialization and new technology, but also as a result of colonial rule and the client status of their respective countries.

Dependent Industrialization

The industrialization of developing countries has largely occurred in a context of dependence upon industrialized countries for finance capital and technology transfer. Indeed, the dominant countries have fostered such dependence. In the early stages of western capital expansion, this relationship provided dominant countries with raw materials and markets for their manufactured goods. More recently, Western-based multinational corporations have exported production of consumer goods to developing countries; finished goods are usually then shipped to the industrialized countries for consumption.

Although it is commonly believed that technology transfer benefits developing countries, another school of thought on this subject contends that technology has reinforced the structures of Western dominance and has served to widen the gap between rich and poor nations. This view was expressed by Morehouse (1979), who described science and technology as "primary instruments of power and social control" used by the "major industrialized countries" to maintain their "dominance" (387). Similarly, D'Onofrio-Flores (1982) explains that alternative native technologies are rejected or marginalized, while Western-style technologies become a component in the inequalities between social classes, between regions, and between the developed and underdeveloped countries (14). This leads to "dependent" development of Third World nations.

In this context, technology's impact on the economic status of women obviously varies according to such factors as the economic structure and stage of industrialization of the country or region, as well as the class, education, and training of the women in question. Nonetheless, some trends have been identified by Davidson Nicol, speaking as Under Secretary General of the United Nations, who noted that in general, "technology aggravates the existing disparities in earnings and in sociopolitical efficacy between men and women." "Modernization" leads to "a female concentration in domestic-related roles, non-market productive roles, and labour-intensive activities." Men, on the other hand, universally appear to take over "women's work" when production shifts from subsistence to a market economy; similarly, when an operation becomes mechanized, it also "becomes a male preserve. For women, this translates into the loss of control over the means of production and over economic resources as well as reduced possibilities for the provision of food and care for their families. Often it means harder work for longer hours with less appropriation of the economic returns to their own labor" (D'Onofrio-Flores and Pfafflin 1982, x). These points are best illustrated by examining the economic status of women in regions that have switched from subsistence to market production and are entering the early stages of industrialization.

We have already seen how women's economic status in African societies suffered as technology and cash-crop production were introduced. Similarly, women who had controlled the production and sale of pottery, handicrafts, textiles, and other home-produced goods experienced a loss of income as mechanized factories took over the production of these items. For example, "the introduction of large-scale breweries in Africa . . . undercut women's income from home-brewed traditional beer" (Tadesse 1982, 93). In Ghana, pottery making was primarily the work of women until the introduction of the potter's wheel, when men took over the industry. Because women lacked the money to buy a wheel, as well as training in the new technique, they were unable to take advantage of the mechanized process (NGO Task Force on Roles of Women 1981, 232).

Factory production of consumer goods meant far more than the loss of income for women engaged in home production. During the early period of industrialization, employers generally preferred to hire men over women, in order to avoid the cost of "special benefits" for female employees such as maternity leave, child care, and/or measures to protect health (Boserup 1970). Moreover, when women were employed in factories they usually were the first to lose their jobs to automation. The decline of female employment in the tobacco, textile, chemical, rubber, paper, and food industries between 1946 and 1965 coincided with increased male employment in chemical, paper, rubber, and metal industries during this same period (Chinchilla 1977).

The trend toward displacement of women following mechanization has been evident outside the factories as well. In Bolivia, women's employment in tin mining had increased steadily from 1880 to 1940, at which point "new methods displaced female workers, who were replaced by male workers in the sink-and-float-plants" (Tadesse 1982, 96–97). Similarly, rural women in Java, Indonesia, who had been employed to hand pound rice were displaced when mechanized rice-hulling processes were introduced. As a result, the women "lost a highly remunerative source of income. They are now forced to work longer hours at other jobs, if such can even be found" (Cain 1981, 134).

The undermining of women's sources of income and their control over production as a result of mechanization and industrialization is further illustrated by events in Curaçao. Prior to industrialization, black women enjoyed high economic and social status. They "performed many of the agricultural tasks, engaged in crafts such as weaving straw hats for export, and sold the agricultural products, fish, homemade foodstuffs, and handicrafts" (Abraham-Van Der Mark 1983, 375). The establishment of a Shell oil refinery on the island caused dramatic changes in the local economy, and consequently in the status of women. Industrialization brought an end to agriculture and crafts, in which women had previously played a leading role. Traditionally female small trade was taken over by foreign males, and consumer goods that had been produced and sold by women were replaced by machine-made products. Whereas women's access to subsistence activities became more and more limited, men enjoyed full employment. This in turn led to an increase in the gap between men's and women's earnings. "For those without formal training or education—that is, the large majority—possibilities to earn money were limited to domestic work, selling sweets and cakes, and the trade in legal and illegal lottery tickets" (Abraham-Van Der Mark 1983, 377).

It should be clear from the foregoing discussion that as industrialization and mechanization penetrated developing countries, women generally suffered a decline in their economic status. Moreover, interesting parallels can be drawn between the economic status of women in the developing world and that of women in the United States during the early stages of industrialization. In both cases women exerted considerably more control over the means of production and the work process before the introduction of new technology resulted in a diminution of subsistence home production.

Multinationals and World Market Production

Whereas industrialization in its early stages resulted in the displacement of women from their traditional employment activities, the trend toward world market production that began in the mid-1960s has resulted in increased factory employment for women. World market production or "offshore sourcing" by multinational corporations refers to production of manufactured goods in developing countries for consumption in industrialized countries.[10] As Lim (1981) has noted, "offshore sourcing is concentrated in labor-intensive industries, or in high technology industries with some labor-intensive processes, all of which have traditionally employed women in the home countries of the multinationals, and do the same overseas" (182). The phenomenon of world market production can be viewed as a form of technological change when "technology" is defined in its broadest sense to include changes in production processes.

In order to examine the economic status of women working in global factories, it is first necessary to understand the nature of world market production. Contrary to popular belief, the production that is exported from Western-based multinational corporations to developing countries is generally not highly technical or highly skilled in nature. According to Fernandez-Kelly, "advanced industrial nations such as the United States retain control over research and development, technological expertise, decisions affecting production, and the distribution of financial outflow" (1983, 19). Moreover, production processes that are relocated to the Third World "are standardized, repetitive, call for very little modern knowledge, and are highly labour intensive. In many cases . . . the production processes are assembly-type operations which have proved difficult and/or costly to mechanise further" (Elson and Pearson 1984, 19).

World market factories are most attracted to countries that combine the highest production output with the lowest possible labor costs. It is not surprising, therefore, that "wages in world market factories are often ten times lower than in comparable factories in developed countries, while working hours per year are up to 50% higher" (Elson and Pearson 1984, 21). Additionally, governments in host countries offer attractive incentives to the multinationals to encourage investment in their countries. These include the establishment of "free trade" or "export processing zones" and the passage and enforcement of laws prohibiting union organizing, strikes, and other labor activities. In many cases, these repressive measures are enforced through political dictatorships and martial law (Lim 1981, 183).

Women, especially young single women with less than twelve years of formal schooling, comprise 85 to 90 percent of the work force in export processing zones (Fernandez-Kelly 1983). This preference is explained in an investment brochure distributed in the United States by the Malaysian government:

> The manual dexterity of the oriental female is famous the world over. Her hands are small and she works fast with extreme care. Who, therefore, could be better qualified by nature and inheritance to contribute to the efficiency of a bench-assembly production line than the oriental girl? No need for a Zero Defects program here! By nature, they "quality control" themselves. (Lim 1981, 184)

Critics nevertheless find manual dexterity an insufficient explanation for employers' preference for women in the global factories. Fernandez-Kelly notes that in both the past and the present men have worked in occupations that required a high level of manual skill, for example as brain surgeons or pianists. She argues that women are hired to perform tedious and low-paying assembly work for political and economic reasons, not psychological or anatomical ones (Fernandez-Kelly 1983, 21). Women are preferred in global factories quite simply because they are the cheapest available labor. It has been estimated that women's wages in world market factories are 20 to 50 percent lower than the earnings of men in comparable jobs (Elson and Pearson 1984). In Malaysia and Singapore, women's factory wages start at two dollars per day, with women earning approximately one-third less than men (Lim 1981).

Apart from low wages, women of the global factory experience instability of employment and lack of vertical (and sometimes horizontal) job mobility. In addition, the labor-intensive work that they perform is fragmented, repetitive, and highly regulated. The electronics industry, one of the largest employers of women in world market production, provides an illustration: according to Lim, "the work is intense and meticulous, involving looking through a highly magnifying microscope for 8 hours a day, in a rigidly regulated environment. Output goals are constantly raised, and productivity incentive schemes [are] designed by the companies" (Lim 1981, 187).

Proponents of world market production assert that employment in global factories liberates women from restrictive, patriarchal social structures and provides them with economic and social independence. However, Lim suggests that such employment does little to improve women's economic status, since "low-paid, dead-end, unstable jobs provide only small and temporary income gains" and the employment of women in multinational subsidiaries "is based on their inferior labor market status," which gives these women a "comparative advantage" of sorts over higher skilled, better paid workers (189).

In summary, there are remarkable similarities in the ways that technological change and industrialization have detrimentally affected women's economic status in "developing" and industrialized countries. The job conditions that women experienced in the Lowell cotton mills and Lynn shoe factories 150 years ago are being replicated today in factories throughout the developing world. Only the technology has advanced, not the status of the women who operate it.

Strategies for the Future

The problems described thus far are not the result of technology itself, for technology can indeed be utilized in ways that improve the quality of life and work for all people. Still, experience has taught us that this will not happen automatically; people who are being adversely affected by the development, implementation, and transfer of technology will have to *make* it happen.

The first step is to define what is appropriate technology. Women of developing nations have already begun to do this. At the 1980 Copenhagen conference sponsored by the United Nations Decade on Women, a number of recommendations to governments and UN organizations emerged, among them:

> to provide women with the necessary skills and appropriate technologies to enable them to participate better in the process of subsistence food production;
> to supply rural women with the appropriate technology and training to enable them to improve their traditional small-scale village industries;
> to create and strengthen the infrastructure needed to lighten the workload of rural women through the application of appropriate technology, whilst insuring that such measures do not result in the occupational displacement of women. (Carr 1982, 2)

In order for these strategies to be implemented, it is clear that women must be involved as full and equal partners in the development process.

Women of industrialized nations are also grappling with the issue of appropriate technological development and application. A central theme in the evolving dialogue on this subject is that technology *must* be implemented in ways that do not perpetuate sex-based role definitions or historic patterns of discrimination and control. In our society, as Jan Zimmerman points out, women's control over their lives is primarily determined by their economic power (1979, 20). Thus technology, to quote Corlann Gee Bush, "is an equity issue. [It] has everything to do with who benefits and who suffers, whose opportunities increase and whose decrease, who creates and who accommodates." If women are to "revalence" technology, Bush argues, they must "develop ways to assess the equity implications . . . and develop strategies for changing social relationships as well as mechanical techniques" (1983, 163).

If women are to have any control at all over technology, they must struggle for equal access to education and they must work to eliminate sex biases in education, training, and retraining ("Do schools teach computer anxiety?" 1982; Duley-Morrow 1983; Giese 1980). Another important source of protection in the face of new technology is unions, but clearly this would have to be a global phenomenon to be most effective. An obvious problem is that many of the industries that are being most adversely affected by technology are not organized; indeed, in the developing world, union organizing is frequently illegal and subject to brutal repression. It is also becoming clear that new technology itself can be utilized in ways that discourage unionization, for example through homeworking, or by creating part-time and temporary jobs and new job classifications that are exempt from bargaining units. Nevertheless, unions in the United States and in Europe have made some progress in protecting workers against the adverse effects of technology (Meyer 1983).[11] However, their effectiveness could be heightened by better utilization of existing networks to promote international trade union solidarity, not just among industrialized nations but between developed and developing ones.

Women must be ever vigilant in ensuring that technology is employed in ways that enrich the quality of life, on a global basis. Such an outcome requires greater awareness of the universality of women's economic and social oppression,[12] information sharing about technology's impact on women in various countries, and a commitment to global solidarity. A step in this direction was taken in June, 1983, with the holding of the "International Women and New Technology Conference" in Geneva, Switzerland. The conference attracted women from Hong Kong, the Philippines, India, Malaysia, Japan, Canada, the United States, the United Kingdom, West Germany, Denmark, France, the Netherlands, Italy, Norway, Sweden, the Dominican Republic, Switzerland, and Belgium. Participants shared information about technology's impact on women in their own countries, developed strategies for action and research, and laid the groundwork for the creation of an international network on women and new technology.

Of course, global networking per se is no guarantee of global solidarity. World economic recession fuels the divisive ideology of competition. Great discrepancies of wealth within and between nations, as well as strong cultural differences, serve to widen the chasm. Hope for the improvement of women's status rests in a recognition of the commonalities underlying the differences. Only when women forge connections with one another that are as integrated as the circuits they assemble will they be able to exert control over the technology that now controls them.

NOTES

The author gratefully acknowledges the critical comments of Dr. Barbara Wright, University of Connecticut, and Dr. Margot Duley, Denison University, on earlier drafts of this article.

1. The term "skill" has myriad meanings in academic literature, and even governmental measures of occupational status are based on subjective assumptions about the relative value of certain kinds of work. For a discussion of this latter point, see Caplow 1954. Throughout this paper, my use of "skill" is most closely approximated by a definition constructed by Veronica Beechey: "in general terms, skilled labour can be objectively defined as labour which combines conception and execution, and involves the possession of particular techniques" (Beechey 1982, 63).

2. The existence of gender-based or sexual divisions of labor has been well established in historical, economic, sociological, and feminist literature and is accepted as a given by this author. Among the many resources on this subject are: Barrett 1980; Phillips and Taylor 1980; Elson and Pearson 1984.

3. Black slave women and children worked in southern textile, hemp, and tobacco factories in large numbers. They also worked in "heavy" industries such as sugar refining, rice milling, transportation, and lumbering. Black slave women also served on the work crews in the construction of southern canals and railroads (Davis 1981, 10; Matthaei 1982, 88).

4. Quoted in the Bay City, Michigan, *Evening Press,* July 21, 1885.

5. Resources on this issue are far too numerous to list. In particular, see Montgomery 1979; Zimbalist 1979.

6. Apparently the old cord switchboard system is still used in rural parts of the United States.

7. The author observed these shirts at the 1983 Midwest School for Women Workers sponsored by the University and College Labor Education Association.

8. Characterizations of countries as "developed" and "developing" utilized in

this article refer strictly to the wealth of nations as measured by gross national product, annual average per capita income, and degree of industrialization. While some may use these terms to denote degrees of "progress" or "civilization," this author does not.

9. Men's contribution to this system of farming was generally in the form of tree felling.

10. Sometimes the goods are only assembled in the developing countries and are returned to the parent corporation for finishing. In other cases (notably in the automobile industry), component parts are produced abroad, and final assembly is done in the factories of the parent corporation.

11. These efforts are described quite extensively in my article "Technological Change and Reindustrialization: Implications for Organized Labor" (Haddad 1984); see also Kennedy, Craypo, and Lehman 1982.

12. For specific examples of this, and suggestions on how to integrate the study of the cross-cultural status of women into various academic disciplines, see Duley and Edwards 1986.

REFERENCES

Abbott, E. [1910] 1969. *Women in industry*. New York: D. Appleton.
Abraham-Van Der Mark, E. E. 1983. The impact of industrialization on women: A Caribbean case. In *Women, men and the international division of labor,* ed. J. Nash and M. P. Fernandez-Kelly. Albany: State University of New York Press.
A new era for management. 1983. *Business Week,* Dec. 5, 50–97.
Asher, R. 1983. *Connecticut workers and technological change.* Storrs: Center for Oral History, University of Connecticut.
Baker, E. F. 1964. *Technology and woman's work.* New York: Columbia University Press.
Barrett, M. 1980. *Women's oppression today.* London: New Left Books.
Baxandall, R., L. Gordon, and S. Reverby. 1976. *America's working women: A documentary history, 1600 to the present.* New York: Vintage Books.
Beechey, V. 1982. The sexual division of labour and the labour process: A critical assessment of Braverman. In *The degradation of work? Skill, deskilling and the labour process,* ed. S. Wood, 54–78. London: Hutchinson.
Boserup, E. 1970. *Women's role in economic development.* New York: St. Martin's Press.
Burns, W. 1982. Changing corporate structure and technology in retail food. In *Labor and technology. See* Kennedy, Craypo, and Lehman 1982.
Bush, C. G. 1983. Women and the assessment of technology: To think, to be, to unthink, to free. In *Machina ex dea: Feminist perspectives on technology,* ed. J. Rothschild. New York: Pergamon Press.
Buvinic, M. 1976. *Women and world development: An annotated bibliography.* Washington, D.C.: Overseas Development Council.

Cain, M. L. 1981. Java, Indonesia: The introduction of rice processing technology. In *Women and technological change in developing countries. See* Dauber and Cain 1981.

Caplow, T. 1954. *The sociology of work.* Minneapolis: University of Minnesota Press.

Carr, M. 1982. Has anything changed for women? *Appropriate Technology* 9, no. 3:1–4.

Chaney, E. M., and M. Schmink. 1976. Women and modernization: Access to tools. In *Sex and class in Latin America,* ed. J. Nash and H. Safa. New York: Praeger Publishers.

Chinchilla, N. S. 1977. Industrialization, monopoly capitalism, and women's work in Guatemala. *Signs* 3, no. 1:38–56.

Dauber, R., and M. L. Cain, eds. 1981. *Women and technological change in developing countries.* Boulder: Westview Press.

Davis, A. Y. 1981. *Women, race and class.* New York: Random House.

Davis, H. B. 1940. *Shoes: The workers and the industry.* New York: International Publishers.

Dennison, M. 1983. Computer gap separates girls from boys. *Detroit Free Press,* Aug. 3, 1-B.

Dewey, D. R. 1900. Special report on employees and wages. In *Twelfth census of the United States. See* U.S. Bureau of the Census 1900.

D'Onofrio-Flores, P. M. 1982. Technology, economic development, and the division of labour by sex. In *Scientific-technological change and the role of women in development. See* D'Onofrio-Flores and Pfafflin 1982.

D'Onofrio-Flores, P. M., and S. M. Pfafflin, eds. 1982. *Scientific-technological change and the role of women in development.* Boulder: Westview Press.

Do schools teach computer anxiety? 1982. *Ms.,* Dec., 15.

Duley, M., and M. I. Edwards, eds. 1986. *The cross-cultural study of women.* New York: Feminist Press.

Duley-Morrow, M. 1983. Educational war zones. *Michigan Voice,* July, 5.

Ellul, J. 1964. *The technological society.* New York: Vintage.

Elson, D., and R. Pearson. 1984. The subordination of women and the internationalisation of factory production. In *Of marriage and the market: Women's subordination internationally and its lessons,* ed. R. Pearson, A. Whitehead, and K. Young. London: Routledge and Kegan Paul.

Feldberg, R. L., and E. N. Glenn. 1983. Technology and work degradation: Effects of office automation on women clerical workers. In *Machina ex dea,* ed. J. Rothschild. New York: Pergamon Press.

Fernandez-Kelly, M. P. 1983. Gender and industry on Mexico's new frontier. In *The technological woman: Interfacing with tomorrow,* ed. J. Zimmerman. New York: Praeger Publishers.

Giese, E. H. 1980. *You see the cat walking . . . .* Milford, Mich.: Michigan Project on Equal Rights.

Giuliano, V. E. 1982. The mechanization of office work. *Scientific American* 247, no. 3 (Sept.): 149–64.

Gregory, J. 1982. Technological change in the office workplace and implications for oganizing. In *Labor and technology. See* Kennedy, Craypo, and Lehman 1982.

Haddad, C. 1984. Technological change and reindustrialization: Implications for organized labor. In *Labor and reindustrialization: Unions, workers and corporate change,* ed. D. Kennedy. College Park, Pa.: Department of Labor Studies, Pennsylvania State University.

Howard, R. 1980. Brave new workplace. *Working Papers,* Nov.–Dec., 21–31.

———. 1981. Drugged, bugged and coming unplugged. *Mother Jones* 6, no. 7 (Aug.): 39–59.

Hull, G. T., P. B. Scott, and B. Smith. 1982. *All the women are white, all the blacks are men, but some of us are brave.* Old Westbury, N.Y.: Feminist Press.

ILO (International Labour Office). 1978. *General report and training requirements in the textile industry in light of changes in the occupational structure.* Tenth Session. Geneva.

Kennedy, D., C. Craypo, and M. Lehman, eds. 1982. *Labor and technology: Union response to changing environments.* College Park, Pa.: Department of Labor Studies, Pennsylvania State University.

Kessler-Harris, A. 1982. *Out to work: A history of wage-earning women in the United States.* Oxford: Oxford University Press.

Kuttner, B. 1983. The declining middle. *Atlantic Monthly,* July, 60–72.

Levin, H. J., and R. W. Rumberger. 1983. *The educational implications of high technology.* Project Report no. 83-A4. Stanford: Institute for Research on Educational Finance Governance, Stanford University.

Lim, L. Y. C. 1981. Women's work in multinational electronics factories. In *Women and technological change in developing countries. See* Dauber and Cain 1981.

Machung, A. 1983. Turning secretaries into word processors: Some fiction and a fact or two. In *Office automation: Jekyll or Hyde?* ed. D. Marschall and J. Gregory. Cleveland: Working Women Education Fund.

Matthaei, J. A. 1982. *An economic history of women in America.* New York: Schocken Books.

Meyer, R. 1983. Collective bargaining strategies on new technology: The experience of West German trade unions. In *Office automation: Jekyll or Hyde?* ed. D. Marschall and J. Gregory. Cleveland: Working Women Education Fund.

Montgomery, D. 1979. *Workers' control in America.* Cambridge: Cambridge University Press.

Morehouse, W. 1979. Science, technology, autonomy and dependence: A framework for international debate. *Alternatives* 4, no. 3 (Jan.): 387–412.

NGO Task Force on Roles of Women. 1981. Roles of women: UNCSTD background discussion paper. Cited in *Women and technological change in developing countries. See* Dauber and Cain 1981.

Nash, J., and M. P. Fernandez-Kelly, eds. 1983. *Women, men and the international division of labor.* Albany: State University of New York Press.

Nicol, D. 1982. Introduction to *Scientific-technological change and the role of women in development. See* D'Onofrio-Flores and Pfafflin 1982.

Phillips, A., and B. Taylor. 1980. Sex and skill: Notes towards a feminist economics. *Feminist Review* 6 (Oct.): 79–88.

Ritchie-Calder, L. 1972. Technology in focus: The emerging nations. In *Technology and culture: An anthology,* ed. M. Kranzberg and W. H. Davenport. New York: Schocken Books.

Rosaldo, M. Z. 1973. Woman, culture, and society: A theoretical overview In *Woman, culture, and society,* ed. M. Z. Rosaldo and L. Lamphere. Stanford: Stanford University Press.

Sanday, P. R. 1973. Female status in the public domain. In *Woman, culture, and society,* ed. M. Z. Rosaldo and L. Lamphere. Stanford: Stanford University Press.

Scott, J. W. 1982. The mechanization of women's work. *Scientific American* 247, no. 3 (Sept.): 166–87.

Seidman, A. 1981. Women and the development of "underdevelopment": The African experience. In *Women and technological change in developing countries. See* Dauber and Cain 1981.

Straw, R. J. 1981. *Statement on the human impact of technological change.* Washington, D.C.: Communications Workers of America.

Tadesse, Z. 1982. Women and technology in peripheral countries: An overview. In *Scientific-technological change and the role of women in development. See* D'Onofrio-Flores and Pfafflin 1982.

Tinker, I. 1981. New technologies for food-related activities: An equity strategy. In *Women and technological change in developing countries. See* Dauber and Cain 1981.

U.S. Bureau of the Census. 1900. Twelfth census of the United States. Vol. 7, *Manufactures.* Washington, D.C.: GPO.

U.S. Department of Labor. 1982. *Labor Force Statistics* 1 (Sept.): 664–81.

Wernecke, D. 1983. *Microelectronics and office jobs: The impact of the chip on women's employment.* Geneva: International Labour Office.

Wertheimer, B. M. 1977. *We were there: The story of working women in America.* New York: Pantheon.

Whyte, M. K. 1976. The status of women: Partial summary of a cross-cultural survey. In *New Research on women and sex roles,* ed. D. McGuigan. Ann Arbor: Center for the Continuing Education of Women, University of Michigan.

Zimbalist, A., ed. 1979. *Case studies on the labor process.* New York: Monthly Review Press.

Zimmerman, J. 1979. Women's need for high technology. In *Conference proceedings, women and technology: Deciding what's appropriate,* ed. Judy Smith, 19–23. Missoula: Women's Resource Center.

Contested Terrain Revisited: Technology and Gender Definitions of Work in the Printing Industry, 1850–1920

Ava Baron

This article examines the controversies over gender and skill definitions of work in newspaper composing rooms before and after the introduction of typesetting machines in the late nineteenth century. Printing is an ideal focus for the study of gender and work because it was much discussed in nineteenth-century public debates over what occupations were appropriate for women—a question that was part of the broader issues of class and gender relations. Different answers to the "woman question" were put forth by employers and workers, middle-class reformers and machine manufacturers. Its resolution was viewed by workers and by employers as critical in the development of social relations in the printing industry. Although women represented a minority in the printing industry throughout the period of my study, the intense debates over whether printing constituted woman's work highlight the significance of gender for the organization of printing.

In this article, I first discuss the research on the social relations of the workplace and its failure to examine how gender shapes the transformation of work. Second, I explore the relationship between masculinity and work in the newspaper printing industry from the 1850s to the 1880s. Third, I discuss the development of technology in the printing industry and the introduction of the Linotype in the late 1880s. Fourth, I explore the crisis of masculinity created by the transformation of work and class relations when the Linotype was introduced. Finally, I discuss how men's efforts to resolve this crisis were embedded in conflicts between workers and employers over such issues as establishing production norms, determining competence, and controlling training, hiring, and firing.

Gender and the Workplace

Older historical and sociological studies of work have inquired into the consequences of technological change for the nature of work, the divi-

sion of labor, workers' experience of work, and working-class organization. But the dominant tendency in these studies has been to focus on
occupational roles and structures separated from the social and economic forces that created a particular division of labor. This kind of
research takes occupational structure as a given and expects technological change to upgrade skill requirements in the labor force.

The best-known challenge to this tradition came from Harry Braverman in *Labor and Monopoly Capital* (1974). Braverman's thesis is essentially the following: Capitalists desire to control the labor process in
order to realize the most profit from purchased labor power. To this
end, capital reorganizes production to separate mental from manual
labor; or more accurately, conception from execution. Once conception
is removed from production to management, the production worker can
carry out the work without judgment or skill. Work is redesigned and
subdivided into its constituent elements to minimize the need for workers' knowledge of the work process, thus cheapening the value of labor
power. By reducing workers as much as possible to merely the technical
means of production, management enhances its control. This process,
called deskilling, is enhanced by scientific management: workers are
told exactly how to perform each detail of the job.

Deskilling results from the drive for capital accumulation and control rather than from the imperatives of technology and efficiency. Technology is merely one means that capitalists can employ to eliminate
worker judgment in carrying out the work and to enhance management's control over work (Noble 1984).

Braverman's theory inspired studies of the deskilling of work in the
nineteenth and twentieth centuries in fields as diverse as coal mining,
carpentry, tailoring, office work, computer programming, law, and medicine (Carter and Carter 1981; Kraft 1977; Baron 1983; Baron and Klepp
1984; Davies 1982; Zimbalist 1979a; Crompton and Jones 1984). But
Braverman's work has been criticized for underestimating the significance of workers' responses: in his text capitalists seem capable of always getting their way. Research has increasingly shown, however, that
the workplace is a contested terrain. Workers actively resist transformations of production that remove their control over work; in this process
of resistance, they shape the organization of work (Montgomery 1979).
Richard Edwards' well-known book *Contested Terrain* (1979), for example, described how new management strategies are developed, new technologies employed, and new job structures created in the dynamic response and counterresponse between workers and capitalists.

Most research on the historical transformation of work has focused
on the role of class antagonisms and portrays men as active agents, if not

controlling their work, then at least shaping it through resistance. Indeed, labor historians have considered virtually everything men workers did at the workplace a form of resistance or an indication of men's control over the production process. They have paid far less attention to the ways men workers acquiesced to capital or participated in the reproduction of the very class relations that operated to subordinate them (for an exception see Burawoy 1979).

Gender has not been considered integral to the study of the contested terrain. Under the rubric of gender-neutral analysis, labor historians placed men's work and experience at the center. Women have barely been visible in their narratives of workplace struggle. Instead, the focus of research on women was to explain their lack of resistance to capital. As Alice Kessler-Harris (1975) noted, women workers were considered unorganized and unorganizable. Only in the past few years has research on women workers begun to document a different version of women's labor activism. Such research has discovered that women engaged in collective, and at times militant, labor activity (Tilly 1978; Lamphere 1979; Shapiro-Perls 1979; Dublin 1979; Strom 1983; Turbin 1985; Blewett 1987).

Some recent studies of women's work—clerical and in the microcomputer industry, for example—indicate the importance of gender for understanding the nature of work and the development of forms of industrial supervision (Lown 1983; Cavendish 1982; Kanter 1979; Grossman 1980; Barker and Downing 1980). If gender is important for women's work, then why not for men's work as well?

Nevertheless, most analyses of the work process relegate gender to women workers or to footnotes. For example, Edwards (1979) provides little discussion of gender and sex divisions in the labor market (Thompson 1983, 187). As a result, gender has remained ghettoized in a new subspecialty, "women's labor history." Yet an understanding of the sexual division of labor is an integral part of the analysis of the labor process *even when* the occupation being examined is and has been considered male. A gender analysis must begin with a recognition that men are gendered beings, too.

Enormous shifts have occurred in men's and women's work over the past century. There has been relatively little direct substitution of one sex for the other in the same job; rather, the shifts were concurrent with substantial changes in the character and status of the jobs concerned (Kanter 1979; Carter and Carter 1981). Labor process analysis reinforces the view that the feminization of jobs is synonomous with deskilling, while the displacement of women by men means upgrading. Because men's experience of work and of women workers was the starting point of most investigations, the idea that women embody deskilling—that they are tools used by capital to deskill work—remains unchallenged.[1] Skill is conceptualized as something men have, and which women lack. In fact, whatever women lack in relation to men becomes the defining feature of the woman worker (Alexander 1984, 145). When men are the standard by which women are judged, women are kept marginal to skilled jobs and what women do bring to work is undervalued. This point has eluded us because the analysis of the ideological construction of skill has been severed from an understanding of the development of occupational categories.

Braverman (1974) contributed to the understanding of women's work indirectly by highlighting the artificiality of skill categories. Feminists took his idea further by exploring the extent to which divisions of male and female workers into skilled and less skilled jobs are artificial (Phillips and Taylor 1980).

As my research shows, gender is embedded in the division of labor: it affects the status and wages of jobs, the way work is organized, and the forms of authority and supervision in the workplace. Definitions of masculinity and femininity enter into the way work is structured, technology developed and implemented, and skills defined. However, gender has been largely invisible for two reasons. First, the categories we use to study workplace conflicts, whether class relations or impersonal market forces, are considered gender-neutral. Second, the presence of gender is difficult to study because we have learned to ignore it when it is there (Cockburn 1983, 194).

Recent labor history's focus on the transformation of work and men's responses as workers has ignored the crisis this transformation posed for men not as workers in gender-neutral terms, but specifically as men workers. The study of the separation of mental from manual labor—as exemplified in the division of *craft* work—is concerned with explaining quintessentially *male* work (Montgomery 1979; Dawley 1976; Hirsch 1978; *Social Science History* 1980; Bensman 1984; Wilentz 1981). In other words, the study of deskilling actually is a study of the demasculinization of work. Deskilling represents a crisis of masculinity, a crisis for men workers both as men and as workers.

The anguished confusion that men experience about their masculinity and that sociologists are exploring today was evident historically (Komarovsky 1976; Pleck 1981). If we rethought our conceptualization of masculinity we would move away from its reified form. In contrast to the complexity of class analysis, gender has been oversimplified. Gender is not a static structure or concept but a complex and dynamic social process. We need to examine conditions that heighten the idiom of sexual difference (Alexander 1984, 127). We need to look at how gender difference is socially constructed and how it changes.

The view that men shape work to protect their gender interests assumes that gender is monolithic rather than multidimensional and internally inconsistent. It also assumes that men are omnipotent—that they know what their gender interests are and have power to construct the world the way they want. Feminist research needs both to question male power rather than assume its existence and to examine what its limitations are.

Most importantly, we need to scrutinize how class and gender are constructed simultaneously. Efforts to enhance women's position in waged labor have ever been torn between demands for equality (to be like men) and claims of difference. But the meanings of equality and of difference have themselves been the stuff of struggle, as the case of U.S. newspaper printing exemplifies.

Hand Typesetting and Masculinity in the Newspaper Industry, 1850s–1880s

The printer, often called the compositor or typesetter, read manuscripts, selected typefaces, justified lines, set up pages, distributed types, proofread, and prepared types for the press.[2] This work required literacy, knowledge of orthography and grammar, artistic sensibility, familiarity with typefaces, and good eye-hand coordination. The men of the typographical union considered themselves skilled craft workers; they were proud of their work and its traditions (Baron 1981).

These printers viewed their work as masculine in two ways. First, waged work itself was a measure of manliness, essential to men's roles as family providers. Second, the particular nature of the work involved in printing and its occupational culture were considered masculine.

The ideal of the family wage and the concept of the male breadwinner developed in the nineteenth century. Men gained masculine stature by winning wages in the public sphere. The measure of manliness was not only the fact of wage earning but the amount of the wage. The degree of a male worker's manliness could be gauged by the size of his wage packet (Willis 1979; Matthaei 1982; Tolson 1979). The "woman question"—the appropriateness of women workers in the printing industry—therefore provoked extensive discussion and debate among union printers (Stevens 1913, 421–40).

Women printers threatened men's high wages and their role as family providers. Women printers, men claimed, increased the available labor supply and reduced men's bargaining position with capital, making men "impotent" in their warfare against capital (Lynch 1925, 24; Stevens 1913, 427). In turn, a reduction in men's wages jeopardized their positions as family providers and threatened men with a loss of manliness (Stevens 1913, 423). Men printers perceived efforts to introduce women into the printshop as an attack by capitalists, not by women. Women's entry into "masculine employments" made women "tools of employers who desire to use them as instruments of robbing their husbands, fathers and brothers. . . ." Union men advised women to

> pause and reflect upon the sad results of this last attempt to make them accessory to their degradation . . . for without their aid, the effort will fail—and then husbands, fathers and brothers will still be enabled to maintain the dignity of labor, and to hold the position of providers and protectors. . . . (*Finchers'* 1864, Oct. 1)

While men printers claimed that typesetting was masculine, employers viewed it as distinctly "woman's work." During the second half of the nineteenth century, newspaper publishers had increasingly employed women to do hand composition of straight matter—typesetting of columns of text with no headings or advertisement work (Herron 1905, 18; Abbott 1910, 255). Straight composition constituted over two-thirds of the work for newspapers. In the 1850s and 1860s publishers recruited women from the textile and clothing industries, gave them a six-week training program, and set them to work as typesetters (Baron 1982). As one publisher explained:

> We are completing our arrangement to avail ourselves of the labor of female printers and we are quite confident that typesetting is to become one of the regular employments of women, . . . to the very necessary help of the most oppressed and most needful of all working people, the feeble seamstresses. (Munsell 1860, 9:93)

According to one estimate in 1864, thousands of women were being instructed as printers in New York City, Philadelphia, and New England. One publisher concluded, "by the first of next year the female compositors will be crowding their male brethren to the wall and will monopolize the entire work" ("A chapter on printers: Revolution in the trade," *Chicago Post* 1864, Apr. 10).

During the 1850s and 1860s, employers and middle-class women reformers such as Susan B. Anthony made two different claims about the relationship between gender and the work of printing.[3] First, they claimed that the work *was* gendered, i.e., feminine, particularly in its intellectual aspects. Intellectual work was feminine because it was light, clean, and easy, they claimed, while manual work was masculine (Penny 1863). "The labor is light and pleasant, the hours not long and confining, and the operatives are usually of a higher order of intelligence" ("Woman's work and wages," *Harper's* 1868, June–Nov., 530).

Second, employers and reformers claimed that the work required particular aptitudes or characteristics. They considered printing "peculiarly adapted" to the inherent aptitudes of women. From the publishers' vantage point, women were "admirably suited for the work, having a nicety of touch which would enable them to manipulate type with greater facility than men" ("Women in printing offices," *IP* 1886, May, 470).

Men printers, on the other hand, thought printing conferred masculinity on those who worked in it. Men considered printing a "manly art" because it combined intellectual and manual labor (*PC* 1867, Feb. 1, 161, Nov., 328).[4] Although men conceded that women could do typesetting and even cited examples of women who could compose with rapidity and exactness, they still argued that women *should not* be printers (*PC* 1868, Dec., 293). Men argued that women printers would become "unsexed" by engaging in typesetting (*Finchers'* 1864, Oct. 1). Men pointed to the dangers to women's morals of reading the texts being typeset, especially medical and scientific material, "which contain matter eminently unfitted and highly improper for the perusal of modest young women" (Stevens 1913, 423). Further, the work culture was considered masculine and unfit for women. Men printers argued that women would lose their femininity by working alongside men, by hearing the language men used on the shop floor, and by contact with the aggressive, masculine nature of shop floor culture (*IP* 1884–85, Oct.–Sept., 109–10.).[5] The tramping and substitute systems, the tradition of applying for work at houses of call, the social drinking while waiting for work, and a host of other rituals enhanced the masculine features of the work culture (Baron 1981; Cockburn 1983).

Men printers described the "awful consequences" for women themselves and for society that would result from placing women workers in newspaper composing rooms (Munsell 1860, 9:96). As they put it: "For our part we should be loth to see a daughter or sister of ours confined to the atmosphere of a morning paper office. . . . We should be loth, too, . . . [for her to be in a workroom] where she is apt to associate, or come in contact with, men and youth of every grade of morals . . ." (*Finchers'* 1864, Oct. 1). Contact with the world "in the same method that man finds necessary would have a pernicious effect upon her morals" (Stevens 1913, 427).

Despite the union men's claims about the potential threat to women's morale, in the 1860s the International Typographical Union (ITU) established a policy of equal pay for equal work regardless of sex and admitted women into the union on the same terms with men (Stevens 1913, 428–29). Admitting women into the union was viewed as an extension of men's roles as protectors and providers. Union men considered equal pay for equal work "chivalrous and generous to the women" (*Printer* 1864, Aug.). The union would protect women from being used as the tools of unscrupulous capitalists. As some union men argued: "The men of our local unions . . . should throw around their sisters the protecting power of their organizations, and tell unscrupulous capitalists who thus use the female to degrade the male, that it can be no longer . . ." (Stevens 1913, 428–29). Thus gender was an issue for printers even before the Linotype heightened the salience of the "woman question."

Introduction of the Linotype, 1885–1905

The speed and output of printing presses increased dramatically during the nineteenth century.[6] As a result, bottlenecks developed in the composing room, where type was set by hand just as in Gutenberg's day—a slow and tedious process. Since the beginning of the century many typesetting machines had been invented, but none of them were widely adopted, despite their speed.[7] The high capital outlay required for most typesetting machines, generally three to five thousand dollars each, was a major deterrent (Dumas 1931). Employers had to weigh the potential for expanded productivity against enormously increased capital investment.

The tremendous growth of the newspaper industry in the 1880s changed this picture. Newspaper circulation increased from 3.5 million to 15 million (Emery 1950, 13). Chains and mergers were common, and so the industry became increasingly concentrated (Lee 1937, 165–209; Lee 1923). These large papers sought the capabilities of typesetting machines and had sufficient capital to afford them (Barnett 1926).

The Linotype, patented in 1885, became the standard mechanical typesetting system for newspaper composition by the early twentieth century.[8] Like other machines, the Linotype utilized a keyboard resembling a typewriter. But instead of the key releasing a type character, it released a small brass matrix, which was a mold for *casting* the type character. When enough matrices collected in the assembler to form a line, margins were justified. Then the operator pushed a lever to start the casting mechanism, which poured molten metal into the molds, thus creating a "line o' type" called a slug. After casting, the used matrices were mechanically distributed back to their appropriate channel to await reuse. After the slug was used it was melted for future recasting.

The success of the Linotype was not assured at the outset. Many options were available to publishers in the 1880s; even in the 1890s publishers debated the merits of the different typesetting machines (*Newspaperdom* 1892–93, 16–21). Nor was efficiency the reason for its success. When the American Newspaper Publishers' Association (ANPA) studied the various machines available in 1891, it concluded that other models were either cheaper or faster than the Linotype (ANPA 1892). According to the test committee's "Report on Machine Compositors," the Linotype "fell far short in the general result of accomplishing what had been claimed for it by its owners and others" (*Newspaperdom* 1892–93, 21).

The early Linotypes were extremely crude and constantly broke down. Sometimes newspapers that had adopted the machines found them so unreliable that they discarded them and reverted to hand composition (*IP* 1888, Oct.). Extra machines and expert mechanics had to be kept on hand in case of breakdown (Kjaer 1929, 45).[9] Therefore only the large metropolitan dailies could afford to experiment with the Linotype (Barnett 1926, 4). It was not until significant changes were made in the Linotype after 1900 that it became practical and was adopted on a wider scale (Byrn 1970, 167).

Nor can the Linotype's success be attributed to its revolutionary technical ideas. The Linotype was not the first to combine composing and casting, but earlier machines remained undeveloped due to lack of financial backing (Moran 1965). The Linotype received financial support from the publishers of the *New York Tribune, Chicago Daily News,* and *Louisville Courier-Journal* (Lee 1937, 122). The *New York Tribune* installed its first Linotype in 1886. Others began to install Linotypes in 1889, following an extended strike over publishers' unilateral reduction of wages (U.S. Congress 1904, 35).

To promote the machine in the 1890s, the Mergenthaler Company (the Linotype manufacturer) set up schools to train operators. These trainees were sent as strikebreakers to help publishers during strikes and lockouts (Dumas 1931, 247). The company made it clear to the ITU that it "intended to install the machines at all hazards and to fight if necessary to do so" (U.S. Congress 1904, 35). But eventually the ITU and the Mergenthaler Company negotiated an agreement. The company agreed to remain neutral in disputes between the union and employers and to refrain from training operators to be used as strikebreakers. The ITU agreed to encourage its members to learn to operate the machine and not to interfere with its introduction. When affiliated locals struck to oppose the introduction of the Linotype, the ITU interceded and in at least one case sent in union men from other locals to break the strike (Loft 1944, 49; U.S. Congress 1904, 35–36).

Controversies over Gender and Skill Definitions of Linotype Work

The union's acceptance of the Linotype caused conflicts between employers and printers over the machine's implications. The ITU sought to secure Linotype operation for union members, to replace per-piece rates with a per-hour wage system, to obtain wages equivalent to those paid for hand composition, to reduce the workday to eight hours, and to retain control over hiring and firing. The union also fought to retain its right to set the production norm and its certification of competence (Dumas 1931, 244; Loft 1944, 48).

Central to the union's strategy was its effort to define use of the Linotype as a skilled, masculine process. But in this effort it met significant resistance from employers.

Both employers and men printers made claims about the specific, inherent characteristics of men and women and the work they were capable of, but they articulated different versions of what was properly masculine or feminine. The union claimed that the work was intrinsically masculine, and that women did not have the necessary abilities to do the job. Employers, however, claimed that women were ideal linotypists because the work required typically feminine characteristics such as steadiness and dexterity. For over thirty years following the introduction of the Linotype, the typographical union and employers battled over the gender and skill definitions of the new occupation.

Linotype as Women's Work: The Employer's View

The Linotype, like most of the automatic typesetting machines of the period, was created to do straight composition only (Baker 1933, 117).[10] As far back as the 1870s, publishers expressed a strong interest in automatic typesetting machinery especially suited for use by women operators. The *Typographic Journal* stated in 1870:

> The composing machine is now an accomplished fact. Its precise construction is at present not definitely settled, but as certainly as the next dozen years will come and pass away is it that a composing machine will be used in every printing office. We cannot foresee the effect of this invention, but we

> may say that it cannot fail to exert a very important influence upon the question of the employment of women as compositors. The machine is specially suitable for female use. (1870, June)

Even before automatic typesetting technology was developed, employers viewed it as a logical extension of women's work as hand compositors. To the publishers, all typesetting machines were suitable for female use.

Use of the keyboard appeared to open up the work of printing to educated women. Unlike publishers' recruitment efforts of the 1860s, which mainly focused on uneducated, foreign-born women from the clothing and textile industries (Baron 1982), publishers in the 1890s sought to recruit literate, native-born American women trained in stenography and typewriting (Barnett 1926, 26).

Many of the typesetting machines were marketed as suitable for women with little training (*Printer* 1865, July, 88; *IP* 1889, Apr., 580; *Newspaperdom* 1894, Sept., 122; 1894, Mar., 425). Linotype advertisements showed women operating the machines (*IP* 1888, Mar., 442); to emphasize the ease with which the machines could be operated, advertisements and articles in the *Linotype Bulletin* portrayed monkeys, blind people, deaf mutes, and one-handed people as expert, efficient operators.[11] Employers and the Linotype manufacturer claimed that women typists and stenographers could efficiently operate the machine with little or no training on the machine itself. As one publisher put it, "There is apparently no reason why women can not operate typesetting machines quite as well as can men. They are especially apt at the work if they have already acquired proficiency at the typewriter . . ." ("Typewriters as typesetters," *EP* 1905, Sept. 30). In testimony before an arbitration board, a publisher exhibited a Linotype keyboard. He then showed an uncorrected galley proof, claiming his stenographer had produced it on the Linotype after less than ten days' experience (ANPA 1904, Bulletin no. 1249, Jan. 25).

Employers built on their earlier claims that typesetting was respectable work for women because it was intellectual. An article entitled "Woman's Work and Wages," considered the position of typesetter or compositor to be "one of the most pleasant, respectable, and profitable occupations" for women (*Harper's* 1868, June–Nov.). These claims were bolstered in the 1890s by contemporary changes in clerical work, particularly the introduction of the typewriter and the growing feminization of office work (Davies 1982; Srole in this volume).

Because publishers identified keyboard work on the Linotype as essentially the same as on the typewriter, they claimed that both required the same worker abilities and characteristics ("Women and the Linotype: The machine offers a new employment for the fair sex," *FE* 1907, Jan. 26, 7). They then tried to establish that Linotype work was unskilled because it did not require extensive special training of stenographers and typists. Women linotypists, recruited from the pool of available typists, received no recognition for the keyboard training they already had and so could be paid less because the work did not require "skill": typing skills were assumed to be natural feminine abilities that women automatically brought to the work ("Women and the Linotype: The machine offers a new employment for the fair sex," *FE* 1907, Jan. 26, 7; "The woman compositor," *Newspaperdom* 1893–94, 241).[12]

Linotype as Men's Work: The Union's View

Linotype work heightened existing dilemmas for male printers. The bases of their definition of masculinity through work were progressively disintegrating. The physical strength requirements of printing eroded during the nineteenth century through division of labor and advancing technology. The physically demanding presswork was accomplished by specialized pressworkers and steam-powered presses with hoists. The mental aspects of their work were either threatened by increased supervision and management control or increasingly defined as analogous to clerical work and therefore as feminine. How could men printers maintain the integrity of printing as distinctly masculine work and also as skilled craft work? Male printers' responses to the Linotype attempted to resolve these dilemmas.

Men may have accepted the Linotype in part because it diminished rather than increased opportunities for women printers (Abbott 1910, 258). The percentage of women in machine typesetting was lower than of those in hand composition. In 1884, just a few years prior to the Linotype, one quarter of Boston's compositors were women ("Of interest to the craft," *IP* 1884, Oct., 43). By 1900, women made up only 15 percent of printers and compositors, and by 1904 only 520 women operated typesetting machines, about 5 percent of the total number in the United States and Canada (Barnett 1926, 28). It was the typesetter who specialized in straight matter, not the all-around craft printer, who was displaced by typesetting technology; 95 percent of the unemployed printers in 1899 had specialized in straight composition (Tracy 1913, 577).

The men supported the Linotype over other machines precisely because it posed less of a threat to their class and gender positions. While other machines separated the setting of type from the justification of lines and from the distribution of type, the Linotype made typesetting a single integrated operation. The Linotype could be viewed as enhancing craft respectability because it did not subdivide the work and because it made typesetting a more masculine process by adding type casting to the typesetter's job. At the same time (unlike machines that used type characters or kept type casting as a separate mechanism and so kept the operator free from the heat, dust, and discomfort created by the casting) the Linotype required the operator to contend with "a trying heat and offensive gases" produced by its pot of molten metal. Men embraced the Linotype because its dirty work made it less respectable for women (New York State Bureau of Labor Statistics 1906, xciii).

Printers disagreed with employers' and machine manufacturers' claims about the skills and characteristics needed for proficiency in Linotype operation. Lee Reilly, a printer-operator, called the Mergenthaler Company's assertions about the ease of operating the linotype "a hoax." According to him, "to be rapid and competent requires training as a printer. The assumption that [women] typewriters—or typewritists—as a rule made efficient operators of composing machines is a delusion." He claimed that women could not grasp "office style," which is "too perplexing" for them, therefore requiring the resetting of considerable portions of their output ("About machine composition," *Newspaperdom* 1894, Mar., 425).

In an effort to deal with the crisis of masculinity posed by the new job process, men began to redefine the source of their masculinity. Earlier, men had claimed that the work itself was masculine; after the Linotype, in contrast, they claimed that there was "no sex in labor." *Work* did not embody gender; only *workers* did, and some workers could do work that others could not. "In some varieties of work strength of a man is required, or endurance which is too exacting for the female frame. In others, the greater delicacy of manipulation which women can give is demanded" (*Unionist* 1901, Feb. 14, 26). Further, men held on to the belief that they possessed both skill and masculinity, even if the job did not.[13] Inherent masculine characteristics, not just acquired skills, were needed for machine proficiency. Therefore men made better operators than women.

Sexual differences between men and women workers were redefined and heightened. Women, men printers argued, could not do the work because women were physically inferior and lacked the necessary mental abilities and natural temperament. Men also pointed to their ability to lift heavy forms and to change the machine magazines. Although the operator rarely actually did these tasks, they claimed it was important that they had the necessary physical strength. But most significantly, men printers claimed that the work required endurance that women lacked.

For the men, endurance was important because it symbolized their intellectual and physical superiority to women. It was used to distinguish hand composition, which they had formerly acknowledged women could do, from machine composition, which they claimed women were not capable of doing. They argued that "The higher speed attained on machines makes the work more exhausting than hand composition, and thus both mental retention and physical endurance are required of the operator" (U.S. Department of Labor 1906, 742).

Men printers were forced to emphasize the physical attributes necessary for the job because keyboard work—where the definition of the work as intellectual resided—was increasingly associated with natural female attributes. As a New York City printer described the work in composing rooms in 1903:

> Typesetting is exhaustive work. Standing hour by hour brings on backache and in some men varicose veins and swollen feet. Sitting on the high printing office stool doubles the typesetter up, constraining his arm motions and interfering with his digestion. (New York State Bureau of Labor Statistics 1906, xciii)

Gender, Productivity, and Worker Competence

In the conflicts over gender and skill definitions of the new job created by the introduction of the Linotype, new standards of worker competence and measurements of worker performance developed. Prior to the Linotype, a completed apprenticeship certified competence and was a prerequisite for ITU membership. As a printer explained before the U.S. Industrial Commission in 1900, "We hold, and believe we can safely maintain, that a card of the International Typographical Union is prima facie evidence of a man's competence" (U.S. Industrial Commission 1901, 583).

The introduction of the Linotype intensified conflicts over wages and the pace of work. Rather than workers' competence being established upon entrance into the union, publishers required workers to prove their competence on a daily basis at work by meeting a production standard in order to obtain and maintain their jobs. The union, concerned over potential wage reductions and work speedups as early as 1891, sought to replace the piece wage system with an hourly system (Loft 1944, 45; Barnett 1926, 10). Employers, recognizing the problem of establishing production norms for new machinery, agreed to a time system. By 1909 piece-rate provisions were virtually obsolete (Loft 1944, 45).[14] But hourly wages further exacerbated conflicts over the pace of work and the production norm.

With the time system, employers became increasingly concerned with controlling and measuring the output of each individual employee. As one employer expressed it:

> To run a printing office properly it is necessary to know what each man can do, and what he does do, and see to it that he keeps up to a reasonable schedule of production. If this is not done systematically there will be paying of wages to those who do not earn them, which will have to be made up by overcrowding the willing workers, which is obviously unfair. (Francis 1917, 300)

Elimination of the piece system compelled publishers to seek other means to control output. In the early days of the machine, employers and the Mergenthaler Company encouraged speed contests (*EP* 1901, Nov. 2, 8; "A record broken," *FE* 1894, Mar. 22, 9; U.S. Congress 1904, 38). Some employers also adopted bonus systems; some measured the output and speed of each employee with a linometer attached to the machine (*EP* 1901, Nov. 2, 8; U.S. Congress 1904, 43). The president of the ANPA encouraged publishers to adopt the techniques of scientific management to improve production and to reduce workers' control (ANPA 1911, 25–26).

Men's efforts to resolve the crisis of masculinity led them to redefine competence in terms that heightened the demands on them both as men and as workers. In earlier decades they stressed the difference between men and women printers in terms of morality and training. In the 1890s, by contrast, men viewed competence as derived from particular biological traits, which women lacked, that enabled men to work faster and for longer periods. These definitions of masculinity in terms of speed and endurance, however, meant that men workers had to prove themselves as men on an ongoing basis. As the U.S. Bureau of Labor Statistics stated in 1906, "the effect of new processes and machinery in modern industry has been to enhance quantitative skill while decreasing the relative importance of qualitative skill" (U.S. Department of Labor 1906, 707). In other words, quantitative skill—worker speed and productivity—required endurance (which men purportedly had) and became more important than qualitative skills such as manual dexterity and intellectual ability (which women supposedly had). By cooperating in publishers' construction of the new technology as requiring endurance and speed, men printers locked themselves into the new standards of masculinity, as well as into speeding up production.

Thus men's desire to prevent their work from being defined as analogous to that of typists enmeshed them in speed contests for greater productivity. As the U.S. Bureau of Labor Statistics explained:

> The high average speed maintained by linotype operators is the foremost factor in preventing the displacement of men by women in this line of work. When the machines first came into use there was a great fear among the printers that female stenographers would work the machines, a fear arising from the close resemblance of the keyboard of the linotype to that of the typewriter. While it is true that women learn to operate the machine readily they have not the endurance to maintain continually the speed which men maintain. (U.S. Department of Labor 1906, 721)

Social Relations and Deskilling

While men printers articulated the requirements of the machine in terms of endurance, publishers focused on characteristics of workers that would transform the social relations of the workplace. Publishers sought to enhance managerial authority by seeking out and rewarding workers who had the "proper" behavior traits and personality characteristics along with technical skills (Edwards 1976).

A focus on deskilling diverts attention from the construction of the social relations of production and from the role gender plays in identifying what characteristics are considered important and are rewarded. For publishers, traditional notions of craft worker manliness interfered with production and with management's control. The masculine work culture of the pre-Linotype years enhanced printers' control over the work process. They set the work standards and the union was the arbitrator of labor-employer disputes. Even in the initial years of the Linotype, the union set the "dead line" or minimum standards of competency (U.S. Congress 1904, 54).

In the 1850s and 1860s, men's work culture had been consistent with the characteristics of hand composition. The old method, particularly on newspapers, required a good deal of "standing time" followed by rush periods. There was little pressure to be a steady worker and to work consistently because extra workers were taken on during the busy periods. This work schedule was compatible not only with drinking and gambling, but also with tramping (traveling from town to town in search of work), and with a less disciplined attitude toward work time and dependability. The ANPA complained of problems disciplining printers who were "incompetent, insubordinate, and intoxicated" (ANPA 1911, Labor Bulletin no. 358, July 1). Employers found men printers to be "supremely offensive in their manners; uncleanly in their personal habits; filthy in their language" (*IP* 1885, Sept., 439).

Publishers' efforts to change the work were simultaneously an effort to transform authority relations and to redefine masculinity. Publishers used the Linotype as leverage to make this transformation. They emphasized that the machine required work styles and worker characteristics that were distinctly different from those needed for hand composition. Because the Linotype lessened the rush before press time, employers argued that work required more consistent rates of speed over longer periods of time. The Linotype reduced the need for temporary substitutes, and the tramping system virtually went out of existence. Optimal production on the machines, publishers claimed, required sobriety, which they made a condition of employment (McCann 1901, 81; *FE* 1895, May 16, 9). Typesetting with the machine, according to management at the *New York Herald,* changed the nature and pace of work, and as a result, "the great magician Progress has summoned the new printer to the helm, and the old printer in consequence passes from the scene of his former usefulness, perhaps to death, surely to oblivion" (*FE* 1895, May 16, 9).

As publishers established the speed capability of the machine, they became more concerned with continued steady operation and they increasingly sought workers "of steady, moderate speed who can be relied upon rather than 'record breakers,' who are too nervous, irritable, and prone to 'lay off' " (U.S. Congress 1904, 76). A "good operator" was not one who could "set a word, or two or three words, very rapidly," but one who could "maintain an evenness of speed" (*LB* 1905, June–July, 123). The change in work styles and characteristics was reflected in changes in attire:

> The contrast between the careless attire and prodigal habits of the old-timer and the garb and deportment of the machine operator is marked. The latter are neatly dressed, bright, active, and of steady habits, and their general appearance would suggest a large class of students rather than newspaper compositors. (*FE* 1895, May 16, 9)

Women, publishers claimed, had the right work habits and proper characteristics for work on the Linotype: dexterity, sobriety, and dependability (Massachusetts Bureau of Labor Statistics 1895, 41–45). Employers preferred women clerical workers as linotypists because they considered these women neater, quicker, more industrious, more loyal, more trust-worthy than men printers (Massachusetts Bureau of Labor Statistics 1895, 29, 41, 45; *IP* 1884, Oct., 33; U.S. Department of Labor 1897, 255). Women's lower wages were justified because the characteristics that made them ideal workers were not considered skills but part of women's natural temperament.

Publishers' efforts to transform printing into women's work following the Linotype ultimately failed. An article in *Editor and Publisher* in 1913 (July 19, 97) accepted the ITU's claims about the need for workers capable of physical endurance: "Standing at case handling type is no fit employment for a delicate or impaired physique, but demands strength of body as well as clearness of brain power."

There were many reasons for this failure, chief among them publishers' inability to recruit female typists. The demand for clerical workers expanded rapidly in this period, and the relatively higher wages for women in clerical work, combined with perceptions of office work as more respectable for women, made typesetting less attractive to educated women.[15]

Nevertheless, publishers were successful in transforming the social relations of the workplace into forms they found more acceptable, through a complex process that included redefinitions of masculinity and shifts in the relationship between gender and work. Men printers, for their part, could only successfully maintain their craft and manly respectability by redefining the meaning of masculinity and work. The idiom of sexual difference at work was transformed in conjunction with changes in their job and control in the workplace.

In conclusion, my aim here has been to show how gender was incorporated into the organization of work and technology in printing, and how it shaped workplace conflicts and their resolutions. Like class, gender is not fixed or settled, but is continuously transformed. This points to the need to examine the changing power relations that affect gender transformations.

The gender constructions discussed here are only a part of the process. I have not discussed women's participation in these processes. What I have said does not imply that women necessarily accepted the gender terms of the work or the arguments and claims made by men printers and employers. In fact, the protest of women printers against night work legislation in the first two decades of the twentieth century and their success in getting some legislation repealed indicate otherwise (Baker 1925). Further study should explore the limitations on men's and capital's power to construct gender by examining women's resistance, reinterpretation, and negation of their construction as "other."

NOTES

Research for this project was supported by a fellowship from the National Endowment for the Humanities. An earlier version of this article was presented at the Bunting Institute of Radcliffe College, Mar. 25, 1986. The author would like to thank Robert Asher, Mary Blewett, Richard Butsch, Rosalyn Feldberg, Myra Marx Ferree, Maurine Greenwald, Sara Kuhn, Helen Marchant, David Noble, and Lise Vogel for their help.

1. Braverman did not develop an explanation for the relationship between deskilling and the feminization of the labor market. He simply attributed it to women being an ideal reserve army of labor (Beechey 1982).
2. Presswork and typesetting became distinct operations by the 1850s. Although the National Typographical Union, formed in 1852, included both compositors and typesetters, there was often conflict between the two groups. By 1889 the pressmen seceded and formed their own union, the International Printing Pressmen's Union (Baker 1957).
3. Publishers of women's reform papers such as the *Una,* the *Lily,* the *Literary Journal,* and the *Revolution* advocated making typesetting women's work and often hired women, but at lower than union wages (Baron 1981).
4. "Clean," "intellectual," delicate work not involving physical labor was considered feminine (Eisenstein 1983, 79). Willis (1977) found that working-class boys in England in the current period defined manual work as masculine and desirable and mental work as effeminate. Cockburn found that contemporary British printers believe white-collar work makes a boy's masculinity suspect (1983, 139).
5. Rubin (1975) explains that women are "the subject of a traffic among men" that enhances men's solidarity with each other. Cockburn (1983) develops this idea in her discussion of contemporary British printers.
6. Steam-powered cylinder presses were introduced in the 1830s and 1840s and web rotary presses in the 1860s; stereotyping was available for newspaper use in the 1860s.
7. The first patent for a typesetting machine was granted in England in 1822. Thompson (1904) lists over seventy different typesetting machines developed before 1904.
8. Most typesetting machines were used in newspaper offices, and most of these were Linotypes: in 1904 there were 5,491 machines in newspaper offices, and 1,638 in book and job offices (Barnett 1926; U.S. Department of Labor 1906, 743n).
9. In smaller plants (with less than four machines) the linotypist became responsible for these tasks (Kjaer 1929, 45). The new function, directly connected to the Linotype, with machinist-operators representing both functions, created a conflict between two interested international unions—the ITU and the International Association of Machinists, who both claimed jurisdiction over the Linotype machinists and machinist-operators (Tracy 1913).

10. Other machines such as the Ludlow Typograph and the Monotype were later introduced into newspaper composing rooms to do more complicated composition for display and headlines (Mott 1941, 603).
11. "Monkey operates a Linotype" (*LB* 1910, Sept., 66); "A blind Linotype operator" (*LB,* 1913, Nov., 183); "Operating the Linotype with the left hand" (*LB,* 1917, Sept.); "Deaf mutes made good Linotype operators" (*LB* 1917, July, 179).
12. Prior to introduction of the Linotype, women compositors earned less than copyists; in Boston, in 1884, women in printing and publishing earned an average weekly wage of $6.61 while women copyists earned $7.00 (Wright 1969, 83). Assuming a woman printer worked fifty weeks in 1884 she would have earned $330.00. By contrast, the average yearly wage of women printers nationwide in 1900 was only $310.00. Men printers in 1900, however, earned $610.97, considerably more than women (calculated from figures in Herron 1905, 15). Most women printers remained hand compositors, while men became linotypists.
13. Cockburn (1983, 1981) discusses how skill gives men leverage both as workers *and* as men.
14. According to Edwards (1979), management cannot maintain control over output with the piece wage system since workers retain the ability to resist.
15. In 1901–2 women printers' average yearly earnings were $316.35, while stenographers' and typists' were $535.39 (U.S. Department of Commerce 1903, 912).

REFERENCES

Newspapers and Periodicals

Chicago Post. 1864.
EP (*Editor and Publisher*). 1901–14.
FE (*Fourth Estate: A Weekly Newspaper for the Makers of Newspapers*). 1894–1920.
Finchers' (*Finchers' Trades Review*). 1864.
Harper's (*Harper's New Monthly Magazine*). 1868.
IP (Inland Printer). 1884–1920.
LB (*Linotype Bulletin*). 1902–20.
Newspaperdom: A Trade Journal for the Makers of Newspapers. 1892–1920.
New York Tribune. 1854.
PC (*Printers' Circular and Stationers' and Publishers' Gazette*). 1866–90.
Printer. 1858–75.
Typographical Journal. 1889–1920.
Typographic Journal: The Southern Quarterly Magazine. 1870.
Unionist. 1899–1907.

Manuscripts and Reports

ANPA (American Newspaper Publishers' Association). 1892. *Report by the committee in charge of Type Composition Machines Tournament held in Chicago, Ill., Oct. 12–17, 1891.* New Haven: Tuttle, Morehouse and Taylor.
———. 1902–20. Bulletins and Labor Bulletins.
———. 1903–14. Reports on proceedings, annual conventions.
———. 1911. Report of the Twenty-fifth Annual Meeting, New York City, Apr. 26.
Columbia Typographical Union, ITU Local 101. 1899–1902. Yearbooks, vols. 1–4. Washington, D.C.
International Typographical Union. 1871. *Report of the corresponding secretary.* Proceedings of the Nineteenth Annual Session of the ITU, Baltimore, Md., June 5–9. Philadelphia: Cooperative Printing.
McCann, J. W. 1901. Linotypes in newspaper offices: Comment on changed conditions. In 1901 Columbia Typographical Union Yearbook.
Munsell, Joel, comp. 1860. Printers' scraps. Vol. 9, Biographical sketches of printers and editors, strikes and conventions of journeymen, state of the trade, etc. Typographic Library, Manuscript Division, Columbia University.

Government Documents

Andrews, John B., and W. D. P. Bliss. 1910. *History of women in the trade unions.* Vol. 10 of *Report on the condition of woman and child wage-earners in the United States.* Hearing, 61st Cong., 2d Sess., S. Doc. 645. Washington, D.C.: GPO.
Kjaer, Swen. 1929. *Productivity of labor in newspaper printing.* U.S. Department of Labor, Bureau of Labor Statistics Bulletin no. 475. Washington, D.C.: GPO.
Massachusetts Bureau of Statistics of Labor. 1895. Compensation in certain occupations of graduates of colleges for women. Part 1 of *Twenty-fifth annual report.*
New York State Bureau of Labor Statistics. 1886. *Fourth annual report.*
———. 1906. *Twenty-fourth annual report.*
Stevens, George A. 1913. *New York Typographical Union no. 6: Study of a modern trade union and its predecessors.* New York State Department of Labor, Bureau of Labor Statistics, Annual Report, 1911. Albany: J. B. Lyon.
Sumner, Helen L. 1910. *History of women in industry in the United States.* Vol. 9 of *Report on the condition of woman and child wage-earners in the United States.* Hearing, 61st Cong., 2d Sess., S. Doc. 645. Washington, D.C.: GPO.

U.S. Congress. House. 1904. *Regulation and restriction of output* Eleventh Special Report of the Commissioner of Labor. 58th Cong., 2d Sess., H. Doc. 734.
U.S. Department of Commerce. 1903. Bureau of Labor Bulletin no. 8.
U.S. Department of Labor. 1897. Bulletin no. 2.
———. 1906. Bureau of Labor Statistics Bulletin 13, no. 67 (Nov.).
U.S. Industrial Commission. 1901. *Report of the Industrial Commission on the relations and conditions of capital and labor.* Vol. 7, *Manufactures and general business and testimony taken November 1, 1899.* Washington, D.C.: GPO.
Wright, Carroll D. 1969. *The working girls of Boston.* New York: Arno Press. Reprint of Massachusetts Bureau of Statistics of Labor, *Fifteenth annual report* (for 1884).

Books and Articles

Abbott, Edith. 1910. *Women in industry: A study in American economic history.* New York: D. Appleton and Co.
Alexander, Sally. 1984. Women, class and sexual differences in the 1830s and 1840s: Some reflections on the writing of a feminist history. *History Workshop Journal* 17 (Spring): 125–49.
Baker, Elizabeth Faulkner. [1925] 1969. *Protective labor legislation with special reference to women in the state of New York.* Reprint. New York: AMS Press.
———. 1933. *Displacement of men by machines: Effects of technological change in commercial printing.* New York: Columbia University Press.
———. 1957. *Printers and technology.* New York: Columbia University Press.
———. 1964. *Technology and woman's work.* New York: Columbia University Press.
Barker, J., and H. Downing. 1980. Word processing and the transformation of the patriarchal relations of control in the office. *Capital and Class* 10:64–99.
Barnett, George E. 1909. *The printers: A study in American trade unionism.* Cambridge, Mass.: American Economic Association.
———. 1926. *Chapters on machinery and labor.* Cambridge, Mass.: Harvard University Press.
Baron, Ava. 1981. Woman's "place" in capitalist production: A study of class relations in the nineteenth century newspaper production. Ph.D. diss., New York University.
———. 1982. Women and the making of the American working class: A study of the proletarianization of printers. *Review of Radical Political Economics* 14, no. 3 (Fall): 23–42.
———. 1983. The feminization of legal work: Progress or proletarianization? *Legal Studies Forum* 7, nos. 2–3: 330–57.
Baron, Ava, and Susan Klepp. 1984. "If I didn't have my sewing machine":

Women and sewing machine technology. In *A needle, a bobbin, a strike: Women needleworkers in America,* ed. Jane Jensen and Sue Davidson, 20–59. Philadelphia: Temple University Press.

Beechey, Veronica. 1982. The sexual division of labour and the labour press. In *The degradation of work,* 54–73. *See* Wood 1982.

Bensman, David. 1984. *The practice of solidarity: American hat finishers in the nineteenth century.* Urbana: University of Illinois Press.

Biggs, Mary. 1980. Neither printers' wife nor widow: American women in typesetting, 1830–1950. *Library Quarterly* 50, no. 4:431–52.

Blewett, Mary. 1987. *Men, women, and work: A study of class, gender and protest in the nineteenth century shoe industry.* Urbana: University of Illinois Press.

Braverman, Harry. 1974. *Labor and monopoly capital: The degradation of work in the twentieth century.* New York: Monthly Review Press.

Burawoy, Michael. 1979. *Manufacturing consent: Changes in the labor process under monopoly capitalism.* Chicago: University of Chicago Press.

Byrn, Edward W. 1970. *The progress of invention in the nineteenth century.* New York: Russell and Russell.

Carter, Michael, and Susan Boslego Carter. 1981. Women's recent progress in the professions, or women get a ticket to ride after the gravy train has left the station. *Feminist Studies* 7, no. 3 (Fall): 477–504.

Cavendish, Ruth. 1982. *Women on the line.* London and Boston: Routledge and Kegan Paul.

Cockburn, Cynthia. 1981. The material of male power. *Feminist Review* 9 (Oct.): 41–58.

———. 1983. *Brothers: Male dominance and technological change.* London: Pluto Press.

Commons, John R., David J. Saposs, Helen L. Sumner, et al. 1918. *History of labour in the United States.* Vols. 1–2. New York: Macmillan.

Cott, Nancy. 1983. Afterword to *Give us bread, but give us roses. See* Eisenstein 1983.

Crompton, Rosemary, and Gareth Jones. 1984. *White-collar proletariat: Deskilling and gender in clerical work.* Philadelphia: Temple University Press.

Crompton, Rosemary, and Stuart Reid. 1982. The de-skilling of clerical work. In *The degradation of work,* 163–78. *See* Wood 1982.

Davies, Margery. 1982. *Woman's place is at the typewriter.* Philadelphia: Temple University Press.

Dawley, Alan. 1976. *Class and community: The industrial revolution in Lynn.* Cambridge, Mass.: Harvard University Press.

Douglas, Paul H. 1921. *American apprenticeship and industrial education.* New York: Columbia University and Longmans, Green and Co.

Dublin, Thomas. 1979. *The transformation of work and community in Lowell, Massachusetts, 1826–1860.* New York: Columbia University Press.

Dumas, Charles J. 1931. When the Linotype came: How the craft was stirred by the appearance of the first successful composing machine forty years ago. *Typographical Journal* 79 (Sept.): 242–48.

Edwards, Richard. 1976. Individual traits and organizational incentives: What makes a "good" worker? *Journal of Human Resources* 11 (Winter): 51–68.

——. 1979. *Contested terrain: The transformation of the workplace in the twentieth century.* New York: Basic Books.

Eisenstein, Sara. 1983. *Give us bread, but give us roses: Working women's consciousness in the United States, 1890 to the First World War.* Boston: Routledge and Kegan Paul.

Emery, Edwin. 1950. *History of the American Newspaper Publishers' Association.* Minneapolis: University of Minnesota Press.

Francis, Charles. 1917. *Printing for profit.* New York: Bobbs Merrill.

Franklin, Clyde W. 1984 *The changing definition of masculinity.* New York: Plenum Press.

Grossman, Rachael. 1980. Women's place in the integrated circuit. *Radical America* 14, no. 1:29–50.

Hartmann, Heidi. 1979. The unhappy marriage of Marxism and feminism: Toward a more progressive union. *Capital and Class* 8 (Summer): 1–33.

Herron, Belva Mary. 1905. *The progress of labor organizations among women; together with some considerations concerning their place in industry.* Urbana: University of Illinois Press.

Hirsch, Susan. 1978. *Roots of the American working class: The industrialization of crafts in Newark, 1800–1860.* Philadelphia: University of Pennsylvania Press.

Kanter, Rosabeth. 1979. *Men and women of the corporation.* New York: Basic Books.

Kelber, Harry, and Carl Schlesinger. 1967. *Union printers and controlled automation.* New York: Free Press.

Kessler-Harris, Alice. 1975. Where are the organized women workers? *Feminist Studies* 3 (Fall): 92–110.

Komarovsky, Mirra. 1976. *Dilemmas of masculinity: A study of college youth.* New York: W. W. Norton.

Kraft, Phillip. 1977. *Programmers and managers: The routinization of computer programming in the United States.* New York: Springer-Verlag.

Kusterer, Ken C. 1978. *Know-how on the job: The important working knowledge of "unskilled" workers.* Boulder: Westview Press.

Lamphere, Louise. 1979. Fighting the piece-rate system: New dimensions of an old struggle in the apparel industry. In *Case studies on the labor process,* 257–76. *See* Zimbalist 1979a.

Lee, Alfred McClung. 1937. *The daily newspaper in America: A history of newspapers in the United States through 250 years, 1690–1940.* New York: Macmillan.

Lee, James Melvin. 1923. *History of American journalism.* Garden City, N.Y.: Garden City Publishing.

Lipset, Seymour M., Martin A. Trow, and James S. Coleman. 1956. *Union*

democracy: *The internal politics of the International Typographical Union.*
Glencoe, Ill.: Free Press.

Loft, Jacob. 1944. *The printing trades.* New York: Farrar and Rinehart.

Lown, Judith. 1983. Not so much a factory, more a form of patriarchy: Gender and class during industrialization. In *Gender, class, and work,* ed. Eva Gamirnokow et al., 28–45. London: Heinemann.

Lynch, James M. 1925. *Epochal history of the International Typographical Union.* Indianapolis: ITU.

Matthaei, Julie. 1982. *An economic history of women in America: Women's work, the sexual division of labor and the development of capitalism.* New York: Schocken.

Montgomery, David. 1979. *Worker's control in America: Studies in the history of work, technology, and labor struggles.* Cambridge: Cambridge University Press.

Moran, James. 1965. An assessment of Mackie's steam type-composing machine. *Journal of the Printing Historical Society* 1:57–65.

Mott, Frank Luther. 1941. *American journalism: A history of newspapers in the United States through 250 years, 1690–1940.* New York: Macmillan.

Noble, David F. 1984. *Forces of production: A social history of industrial automation.* New York: Knopf.

Oswald, John Clyde. 1928. *A history of printing.* New York: D. Appleton and Co.

Penn, Roger. 1982. Skilled manual workers in the labour process, 1856–1964. In *The degradation of work,* 90–108. *See* Wood 1982.

Penny, Virginia. 1863. *The employments of women: A cyclopedia of woman's work.* Boston: Walker, Wise and Co.

———. 1869. *Think and act: A series of articles pertaining to men and women, work and wages.* Philadelphia: Claxton, Remsen and Haffelfinger.

Phillips, Anne, and Barbara Taylor. 1980. Sex and skill in the capitalist labour process. *Feminist Review* 6 (Oct.): 79–88.

Pleck, Elizabeth H., and Joseph H. Pleck, eds. 1980. *The American man.* Englewood Cliffs, N.J.: Prentice-Hall.

Pleck, Joseph H. 1981. *The myth of masculinity.* Cambridge, Mass.: MIT Press.

Porter, Arthur R., Jr. 1954. *Job property rights: A study of job controls of the International Typographical Union.* New York: King's Crown Press.

Pugh, David G. 1983. *Sons of liberty: The masculine mind in nineteenth century America.* Westport, Conn.: Greenwood.

Roberts, Wayne. 1976. The last artisans: Toronto printers, 1896–1914. In *Essays in Canadian history,* ed. Gregory S. Kealey and Peter Warrian, 125–42. Toronto: McClelland and Stewart, Ltd.

Rothschild, Joan, ed. 1983. *Machina ex dea: Feminist perspectives on technology.* New York: Pergamon Press.

Rubin, Gayle. 1975. The traffic in women. In *Towards an anthropology of women,* ed. Rayna Reiter, 157–210. New York: Monthly Review Press.

Shapiro-Perls, Nina. 1979. The piece rate: Class struggle on the shop floor:

Evidence from the costume jewelry industry in Providence, Rhode Island. In *Case studies on the labor process*, 277–298. *See* Zimbalist 1979a.

Social Science History. 1980. Special issue, The skilled worker and working class protest. (Winter).

Stearns, Peter N. 1979. *Be a man! Males in modern society.* New York: Holms and Meier.

Strom, Sharon Hartman. 1983. Challenging "woman's place": Feminism, the left and industrial unionism in the 1930's. *Feminist Studies* 9 (Summer): 359–86.

Thompson, John S. [1904] 1972. *History of composing machines.* Chicago: Inland Printer Co. Reprint. New York: Arno Press

Thompson, Paul. 1983. *The nature of work: An introduction to debate on the labor process.* London: Macmillan.

Tilly, Louise. 1978. Paths of proletarianization: Organization of production, sexual division of labor, and women's collective action. *Signs* 7:400–417.

Tolson, Andrew. 1979. *The limits of masculinity.* New York: Harper and Row.

Tracy, George A. 1913. *History of the typographical union, its beginnings, progress, and development.* Indianapolis: International Typographical Union.

Turbin, Carole. 1985. Reconceptualizing family, work and labor organizing: Working women in Troy, 1860–1890. *Review of Radical Political Economics* 16:1–16.

Turpain, A. 1908. The development of mechanical composition in printing. Smithsonian Report for 1907. Washington, DC: GPO, 13–129.

Wilentz, Sean. 1981. Artisan origins of the American working class." *International Labor and Working Class History* 19 (Spring): 1–22.

Willis, Paul E. 1977. *Learning to labor: How working class kids get working class jobs.* Westmead, U.K.: Saxon House.

———. 1979. Shop-floor culture, masculinity, and the wage form." In *Working-class culture: Studies in history and theory,* ed. John Clarke, Charles Critcher, and Richard Johnson, 185–98. New York: St. Martin's.

Wood, Stephen, ed. 1982. *The degradation of work? Skill, deskilling and the labour process.* London: Hutchinson.

Zeitlin, Jonathan. 1985. Engineers and compositors: A comparison. In *Divisions of labour,* ed. Royden Harrison and Jonathan Zeitlin. Urbana: University of Illinois Press.

Zimbalist, Andrew, ed. 1979a. *Case studies on the labor process.* New York: Monthly Review Press.

———. 1979b. Technology and the labor process in the printing industry. In *Case studies on the labor process,* 103–26. *See* Zimbalist 1979a.

"A Blessing to Mankind, and Especially to Womankind": The Typewriter and the Feminization of Clerical Work, Boston, 1860–1920

Carole Srole

Until the second half of the nineteenth century, clerical workers in the United States were young men preparing for careers as merchants or manufacturers. By 1920, however, "the new woman," young, single, pert, and efficient, had replaced the male office worker of Charles Dickens's day. Although the most prominent explanations for the feminization of the office include regimentation and deskilling of the work, low female wages, a rise in the supply of educated women, and the introduction of the typewriter, the role of the typewriter has been minimized in recent years.

The historiography of the typewriter has followed the twists and turns of the historiography of technology in general. Until the 1960s, the typewriter was generally seen as the critical innovation introducing women to the office (e.g., U.S. Department of Labor 1947, 74). In the last twenty years, however, historians have minimized the revolutionary quality of the typewriter, placing greater emphasis on the influence of the socioeconomic conditions that preceded the technological changes and maintaining that the typewriter was merely a by-product of those changes. For example, Margery Davies pointed out that women had already entered the office, and that the office structure had begun to change with the routinization of work in the U.S. Treasury Department, well before the invention of the typewriter. Thus, the typewriter merely filled a technological gap, extending rather than introducing the process of regimentation and specialization of office work (Davies 1982, 37–38; Sandler 1979, 155–67; Braverman 1974, chap. 15).

But technology and socioeconomic conditions do not always coincide. Sometimes the needed technology is slow to develop (Musoke 1976, chaps. 1–2). At other times, its impact accelerates and transforms a process already underway. Obviously, the so-called computer revolution reinforces the current emphasis on the power of technology and, as a result, demands a new evaluation of the typewriter. Today, no one would deny the role of the typewriter in the expansion of women into the clerical office force. Yet how women came to predominate as typists and the role of technology in the feminization of clerical work remain clouded (Rapone 1981, 223–25; Rotella 1981, 74–75).[1] They can be clarified, however, by demonstrating first how copying provided women's entry into typing, then how typing influenced the concentration of women in business stenography, and finally how the two became critical factors in the expansion of women into the office in the 1880s and into the male clerical preserves in the early 1900s. Once typing and stenography had become female occupations, the image of clerical workers changed from male to female. This female image modified the perception of the skills needed for the job, thereby further excluding men.

Women's Entry into the Office

Women entered the office long before the typewriter was patented or introduced into the office in the late 1870s. Prior to the Civil War, a few women worked in the offices of family businesses, wrote letters for invalids and the infirm, and copied letters for the government and other businesses at home. In Boston, the 114 female clerks, bookkeepers, and accountants comprised only 2 percent of all clerical workers.[2] During the Civil War, there was a dramatic surge in the number and proportion of female clerical workers. As in all modern wars, federal, state, and local governments expanded their functions and so required additional office workers. Although the federal government had no difficulty finding men to work as clerks, it faced the problem of undermining its own propaganda that encouraged men to serve as soldiers. In order to save money and probably to avoid political embarrassment, a bold step was taken to fill the vacancies: both the United States and the Confederacy hired women as full-time clerks and copyists.[3]

U.S. Treasurer General Francis Spinner first employed women in 1862 to cut, sort, and clip treasury notes. Their employment saved the Treasury Department from 600 to 800 dollars a year for each woman hired (Aron 1987, 84–85).[4] Because this job entailed counting money, women could not be trusted to work at home as they had done with copying. Federal branch offices in Boston also began to hire women, especially as postal clerks. After the war, these government employees did not move back into traditionally female jobs but were retained because of the continuously expanding bureaucracy and the critical shortage of funds (National Archives 1869, 737–39; Aron 1987, 70–71).

During those same years, nearly every major industry in Boston hired a few women office workers. Women were hired by professionals, publishers, railroads, utilities, insurance companies, manufacturers, and banks. Department stores employed the most women office clerks, as bookkeepers and accountants. By 1870, there were 277 female clerical workers in Boston, 9.0 percent of the city's clerical work force. In addition, of course, was the unrecorded number of women who worked in family businesses (U.S. Bureau of the Census 1870).

The critical phase in the feminization of clerical work began during the Civil War and continued into the 1870s. After the war, women were not fired; nor were they let go when mass unemployment occurred in the 1872–77 depression. By 1880, the 524 women office workers in Boston comprised 10.6 percent of the clerical population (National Archives 1878, 2:383–86).

Clearly, women's permanent entry in the clerical work force occurred before the introduction of the typewriter in the 1870s. However, the number and proportion of women in Boston's office force skyrocketed from 10.6 percent (524) in 1880 to 17.5 percent (1,975) in 1885 to 25.2 percent (4,217) in 1890 (U.S. Bureau of the Census 1890, 638). It is during these years that the typewriter made its impact on the expansion of women in clerical work.

Women Become Typists

The typewriter was not patented until 1868, six years after the federal government first hired women as office clerks. Problems with marketing delayed the machine's entrance into the office even further. In 1873 the inventor, Christopher Latham Sholes, and his partner, promoter James Densmore, finally negotiated a contract with E. Remington and Sons to manufacture one thousand machines. Although these machines were completed in 1874, only four hundred were sold (Current 1954, 34; Foulke 1961, 12, 65, 73; Hatch 1950, 175).[5]

It took the rest of the decade for typewriters to gain a foothold in the office. Between 1874 and 1878, four thousand more were manufactured. In those early years, a few stenographers reported using the new typewriters for their work, but generally the typewriter remained a novelty. In 1875, Dun, Barlow & Co., (the predecessor of Dun & Bradstreet) revitalized the faltering typewriter industry by equipping its main and branch offices with typewriters. In the next few years, sales of typewriters began to improve and advertisements for typewriter ribbons and copying by machine appeared. By the end of the decade, its success seemed certain. In 1881 alone, nearly twelve hundred typewriters were manufactured and sold. In 1890, over thirty-six thousand were produced (Current 1954, 38, 71, 87, 105, 117; *Munson's Phonographic News and Teacher* 1884a, 47; Hatch 1950, 175).

Current scholarship holds that typing quickly and easily became a woman's job because the typewriter was a new machine, and therefore gender-neutral. And since women who typed were paid less, they displaced male hand copyists (Davies 1982, 58; Rapone 1981, 225). However, this was not the case. Well before the successful distribution of the typewriter, women outnumbered men as copyists. Margery Davies found that as early as the 1840s and 1850s, before women officially entered into offices, some offices subdivided clerical work into discrete, rationalized jobs with workers ranging from the lowest paid and least skilled copyists to middle ranked clerks to the few skilled and highly paid bookkeepers (Davies 1982, 12–15). My data on Boston show that women were employed in the least skilled of these jobs, copying. They worked at home copying letters for individuals, small businesses, and even for the federal government (Massachusetts Bureau of Statistics of Labor 1903b, 619; Deutrich 1971, 67; Rayne 1888, 95). In Boston, women predominated in copying, holding 85.4 percent of the jobs as early as 1870, before distribution of the typewriter.[6] By then, some worked in offices, others still at home. Their early predominance in this occupation occurred because it was the least skilled, demanded the least pay and smallest number of employees, and could be done in the home (*Munson's Phonographic News and Teacher* 1879, 98; 1884b, 142; Davies 1982, 12–14).

From the very beginning, the typewriter was not gender-neutral: female copyists were expected to be the primary users of this new machine. As Richard Current noted, its design—a cross between a piano and a sewing machine—appeared to cater to the female market. As early as 1872, inventor Sholes's daughter learned to type and posed at one of her father's machines for an article in *Scientific American*. Two years later, when Mark Twain purchased one of the early machines from a Boston store, his demonstrator was a "type girl." By 1875, advertisements pictured female operators (Current 1954, 54–55, 69–71; Davies 1982, 54). It appears that advertisers were well aware of the female presence in copying and aimed their product at a female market.

Men were not barred from using the typewriter, either by practice or public opinion. Some male stenographers learned to type, praising its usefulness. Government men continued to use the typewriter throughout the nineteenth and early twentieth centuries (Aron 1987, 87). Nonetheless, the concentration of women in copying and the advertising directed at them enabled their early and easy consolidation of this occupation. The low pay of $1.60 per week in the late 1880s discouraged male competitors and reinforced female predominance (U.S. Commissioner of Labor 1900, 2:1535). By the mid-1880s, typing was recognized as women's work (*Pho-*

nographic World 1886b, 34; *Munson's Phonographic News and Teacher* 1887, 73). By 1900, over 90 percent of Boston's typewriters (the nineteenth-century term for a typist) were female.[7]

Since women comprised an overwhelming majority of copyists and typewriters, they had a base from which to advance and eventually outnumber men in other clerical occupations. True, before the boom in typing women had already made strong inroads in the office. In 1880, 15.8 percent of bookkeepers and accountants and 5.9 percent of clerks and copyists in Boston were female (U.S. Bureau of the Census 1880b, 864).[8] Still, it was the typewriter that gave women the solid base to (1) create the job of business stenography and predominate in it, (2) replace the general clerk, and (3) alter the image of office work and the office worker. It is in these three areas that the typewriter played its major role.

Women Move into Business Stenography

Until the advent of business stenography in the late 1870s and early 1880s, stenographers primarily found employment in the courts, government legislative bodies, newspapers, and with individuals. Most were men and few worked in business (Rider 1966, 52, 73–74, 121; *Standard Phonographic Visitor* 1867, 268–69). A few women were involved in stenography from its early years, partly because of stenography's association with antebellum reform and partly because of the increasing numbers of women in teaching, especially on the eastern seaboard.

Modern shorthand was "invented" by the Englishman Sir Isaac Pitman. Stephen Pearl Andrews, one of the earliest proponents of stenography in the United States, first became acquainted with it at the 1840 World Anti-Slavery Convention in England, where he related that:

> Somebody . . . pressed into my hand a package of books and pamphlets, and whispered to me an earnest request that I would examine them and use my influence to get the subject of what they treated introduced to the American republic. On my return to my lodgings I partially examined the package, and for the first time saw the name of Isaac Pitman, and the words phonography. . . . Years before . . . I had discovered the irregularities of English orthography, and resolved sometime to devote myself to reforming it. There I found the same idea, before wholly my own, already under way; and it interested me profoundly. It was the spelling reform branch, and only in a very secondary way, at first, phonography, which fixed my attention. I made the study of the two, however, my main business of the voyage. (*Phonographic Magazine* 1893, 26)

Phonography, as shorthand was often called, was viewed as a means of language reform to improve English, as well as of international communication, like Esperanto (*American Shorthand Writer* 1880, 7; *Kirografer and Stenografer* 1878; *Phonographic Magazine* 1887, 2).

A few women who participated in the antebellum reform movements, such as Eliza Boardman Burnz, became acquainted with and learned phonography. Others, such as Clara A. Tissington, learned phonography as a skill for cultured women to use in copying religious sermons. A larger group were women who married men active in promoting stenography. One such significant stenographer, Jane Pitman, came to the United States from England in 1853 with her promoter husband, Benn, brother of Isaac. Here she taught classes in phonography as her husband's assistant. Margaret Vater (Mrs. Elias) Longley, began studying in 1849 after her marriage. From 1850 to 1851 she taught reading using the phonetic alphabet. When the Civil War broke out, she and her husband worked as reporters. Later, they taught phonography. Her husband wrote one of the earliest stenography textbooks, and she wrote an early textbook on typing fingering (*Phonographic World* 1886a, 167; *Browne's Phonographic Monthly and Reporters' Journal* 1883b, 334; *Browne's Phonographic Monthly* 1878b, 220–21; *Phonographic Magazine* 1897, 106–8; *Standard Phonographic Visitor* 1863, 12–13; *Phonographic Magazine* 1894, 236–37).

Eliza Boardman Burnz, the most prominent female stenographer, went beyond the limitations of a family business and was more than her husband's assistant. In 1844, as a twenty-one-year-old widow with an infant to support, she became a teacher and later the director of the Bolivar Female Seminary. After reading about phonography, she began to correspond with Stephen Pearl Andrews and later with Isaac Pitman. In 1847, she remarried, and both she and her husband, a minister, became spelling reform and phonography enthusiasts, preaching and teaching about it. She taught school, including stenography, while her husband attended medical school. In 1868 she opened a phonography school in Cincinnati. In 1869, when they moved to New York, she took charge of shorthand classes at the Mercantile Library on Astor Place. She offered free evening classes at Cooper Union beginning in 1872 and published *The Phonetic Shorthand*. Even before her husband's death in 1874, she was recognized as a phonography leader in her own right (*Phonographic World* 1886a, 167). Like other women in the field, she worked with her husband or father; unlike them, she transcended her male relative's interest, making the field her own specialty.

Only a few women actually earned their livings as phonographers rather than as teachers. Annie E. H. Lemon became a stenographer in the late 1860s, and Mrs. J. R. Palmer became an official stenographer of Chenango County, New York, in 1873 (*Phonographic Magazine,* 1891, 233–34; 1890, 284; 1896, 13). Even so, phonography promoters were anxious to attract anyone to their schools and to sell them books and magazines. Thus they encouraged women to learn stenography either as a refinement or as insurance in case they needed to support themselves (Weiss 1981, 411; *Students Journal* 1873, 5; 1876, 10; *Barnes' Shorthand Magazine* 1890, 89–90). At this time, women were clamoring for jobs, especially middle-class women whose only respectable option was teaching.

The number of people learning stenography remained modest. In 1870, no stenographers were listed in the federal census of Boston, though undoubtedly there were some, because periodically men wrote of their stenographic exploits in Boston. A few more were employed in 1880. Their number grew to 113 in 1885. By 1900, about 2,500 stenographers were employed in Boston (Massachusetts Bureau of Statistics of Labor 1885, 1:338, 342; U.S. Bureau of the Census, 1870, 1880a, 1900; *Browne's Phonographic Monthly and Reporters' Journal* 1882, 326).

Most of these new stenographers worked in business, thus creating a new job category, the business stenographer. And most were women: in Boston in 1885, over half; by 1900, five-sixths (Massachusetts Bureau of Statistics of Labor 1885, 1:342; U.S. Bureau of the Census 1880a, 1900). The typewriter contributed to this proliferation of women office stenographers.

The key area of change came in training. Women were encouraged to learn both typing and stenography, enabling them to offer employers both skills. The first male and female stenographers learned on their own from books or correspondence with leaders in the field. By the 1850s and 1860s, promoters of the various stenographic languages had established mail-order companies to teach their particular form of stenography. In the 1870s and especially in the 1880s, increasing numbers of these promoters set up private schools. And it was women who turned in great numbers to the private schools for their training.

The women went to school in order to learn typing. Unlike stenography, typing required an expensive tool; typewriters cost from twenty to over one hundred dollars. So it was difficult to learn the skill at home through mail-order catalogs or magazines, as was possible with stenography. As a result, women enrolled en masse in typing courses (Weiss 1981, 413; *Browne's Phonographic Monthly* 1878a, 226; *Browne's Phonographic Monthly and Reporters' Journal* 1883a, 37; 1887, 107; *Phonetic Educator* 1882, 110; Current 1954, 103, 106, 108; *Phonographic World* 1893b, 15).[9]

The YWCA and public evening schools offered some typing classes.

Business schools, often run by phonography promoters, offered the majority. Once in school, many women learned stenography, too, because it was a more skilled, higher-paying, and more prestigious job. Stenography schools encouraged this to lengthen student attendance. Recognizing the trend, they opened more schools specifically geared toward teaching women both stenography and typing. It is ironic that the women moved into stenography from typing, which cost more to learn, rather than the other way around.

The introduction of women typing students to the higher-paying skill of stenography also ended up creating a beneficial package deal for potential employers. Employers uncertain about women's business skills could retain total control over the contents of their letter, dictating quickly to much faster machine operators rather than delegating the composition of the letter to a skilled clerk.

Women were especially attracted to the schools because they offered legitimacy. Since many of the stenography students came from small towns, big-city employers lacked personal knowledge of their qualifications; the certificates of graduation offered tangible proof of their skills. It is conceivable that women in general sought out degrees as proof of their competence and were attracted to the schools' promises of job placement as a way to avoid scrambling for jobs (Srole 1984a, chap. 9; *Munson's Phonographic News and Teacher,* 1886, 120; *Phonographic World* 1891, 371). By 1900, over 60 percent of the total stenography enrollment nationwide was female, though the proportion was probably higher in some cities (Weiss 1981, 413).

The students' need to learn typing in school and the attraction of a diploma, combined with the schools' need to sustain enrollment and the employers' interest in a diploma that certified skill, set the stage for the rise in the proportion of female stenographers. Despite stenography's image as a male occupation, women were able to predominate in office stenography almost as quickly as they did in typing. Partially because of stenography's movement outside the courts and legislature into business, but also because the training in business schools helped unite the new occupation of business stenography with the female occupation of typing, women gained the upper hand. By 1900, over five-sixths of Boston's stenographers were female (Massachusetts Bureau of Statistics of Labor 1885, 342).[10]

Employers hired women stenographer-typewriters for varied reasons having to do with gender and status. Some employed them because they sought to acquire the personal attention that women appeared to offer. Women were expected to bring flowers, cheerfulness, and beauty to the office and hence confer higher social status on their employers.

Typical of the remarks made in the many magazines written by male stenographers were these in the *Phonographic World* (1893c, 65): "Female neat, clean, no bad habits, except talking. Less salary than male. She and her flowers brighten and give tone to office." Others employed stenographers and typists as symbols of authority. Hiring a stenographer meant that the employer was truly a boss, one who "dictated" and told others what to do. For small businessmen and professionals, the presence of a stenographer-typist validated their power. A female in the office was always the inferior; the male, the superior. So the presence of women underscored the power of the man in business for himself, and having a typist who took dictation was a status symbol even within larger firms. And finally, male employers found women appealing because they were not potential competitors. The fear that male stenographers were untrustworthy because they would leave to establish competing businesses was echoed repeatedly by employers: "wants early rise in salary. Shorthand merely stepping stone" (*Phonographic World* 1893c, 65). The lower pay women received was important, but in combination with the restricted options women faced in the labor market, it also meant that employers could expect increased skills without increasing pay.

Others hired stenographers for less gender-specific reasons. Some appreciated the time saved by dictating rather than writing. Still others were attracted to the typewriter because it represented the new, mechanical, and most important, modern office practice and proved that they were familiar with the latest business methods, techniques, and equipment. And finally, as the total numbers of office workers grew, some employers may have sought more control instead of entrusting composition to others, because of uncertainty about the general business skills of the new office workers, possibly because they were female, or because so many came from the working class (*Munson's Phonographic News and Teacher* 1885, 286; *Phonographic Magazine* 1892, 122–23; *Standard Stenographic Magazine* 1888, 2; Srole 1984b, 9).

The Changing Nature of Clerical Work

The employment of business stenographers and typists, not the typewriter alone, "revolutionized" the office. Before stenography entered the office, some employers wrote letters themselves, employing copyists to copy the letters neatly and legibly to be sent to the recipients and to make additional copies for office records. Many other employers left the exact wording of letters to clerks, who were expected to know how to write a general business letter. The clerk was expected to know the form of a business letter and to possess sufficient English and business vocabulary to construct a letter. Typing replaced the copyist, but office stenography reduced the number of clerks who actually wrote business letters. Instead, the employer who dictated to a stenographer-typist retained total control of the content and wording of the letter, reducing the clerk's job from a partially intellectual to a merely mechanical function.

The concentration of women in stenography and typewriting became critical in the period from 1890 to 1920. In 1890, women made up 25.2 percent of clerical workers in Boston. Their proportion grew to 35.4 percent in 1900; 47.4 percent in 1910; and 52.0 percent in 1920. It was in those years that women as typewriters and stenographers slowly began to replace male general clerks. Nationally, in 1870, 77.4 percent of office workers were clerks; this percentage fell to 61.3 percent in 1900 and to 50.4 percent in 1920; stenographers and typewriters grew from 2.8 percent of office workers in 1880 to 9.9 percent in 1900 to 20.8 percent in 1920 (Anderson and Davidson 1940, 584).

The predominance of women in typing and stenography during those years also introduced them into offices where employers preferred to retain men. Some industries, such as railroading and banking, were bastions of the male clerks. These industries maintained traditional forms of career mobility, that is, promoting clerks to higher management positions. They also required either travel or use of firearms, which justified keeping clerking in male hands (Morris 1973, 320–24; *Shorthand Review* 1890b, 58–59).[11] Still, women moved into railroads and banks as typewriters and stenographers because employers needed those skills and of necessity turned to women. For example, in 1903 in downtown Boston's railway terminals and steamboat companies, none of the thirty-seven clerks, bookkeepers, and stenographers were female, while five of the six typewriters were female (Massachusetts Bureau of Statistics of Labor 1903b, 17). Thus typing and stenography provided an important inroad into even those remaining strongholds of male clerks.

These years of growing female employment began to change the image of the clerical worker. It was through female predominance first in typing and then in stenography that the image of the office worker was altered. Once the image of clerical workers had become female, the work was assigned to women only and would henceforth carry the lower status characteristic of women and their work.

Feminization of the Image of Clerical Work

In a society where jobs were mainly gender-segregated, a job had to have male or female qualities. Everyone looked for distinctions between men and women. For example, one stenography promoter reported:

It is often asked "Which make the best shorthand students, ladies or gentlemen?" Our experience is that in learning the principles and applying them in slow miscellaneous writing, the ladies excel, because they are generally more careful and pains-taking [sic] in their studying and writing. But in the subsequent work—writing from dictation and attempting to write fast—they are not at first equal to the young men. This arises from ladies being generally more timid and nervous, and not as good long-hand writers as the other sex. . . . (*Munson's Phonographic News and Teacher* 1887, 73)

When office workers were male, employers portrayed clerical jobs as requiring skills and character traits that only men could offer. Men desired to learn a business, so they were seen as intellectual and less mechanical in their job performance. They studied on the job, trying to improve their skills and knowledge of the business world. Because men saw a clerical job as training for proprietorship, not just a source of income, they would work nights or travel distances. Also, it was safer for them to do so (*Shorthand World* 1896, 1–2; *Shorthand Review* 1890a, 30–33; *Practical Phonographer* 1884a, 213–14).

Conceptualizing gender as implying opposite traits meant that male strengths were also seen as female weaknesses. If men were independent, women were dependent. If men studied on the job, women read novels and took long lunches. If men were "original and progressive," women were "mechanical," even with better performance. If men could and would work nights, women could not because of unscrupulous, lecherous employers. If men took criticism in a businesslike manner, women took all criticism as a personal insult and were easily moved to tears. If men saw the job as a career, women wanted only marriage. They might spend hours primping themselves in front of mirrors or pining for men, rather than working. In such ways negative female stereotypes were adapted to a business context (*Shorthand Review* 1890a, 30–33; *Phonographic World* 1889d, 86; *Shorthand World* 1896, 1–2; *Phonographic World* 1889c, 216).

But the prevalence of women in typing and stenography forced employers to revise their image of women workers to include more positive views of feminine nature as well. Eventually these stereotypes were incorporated in the qualifications needed for those jobs. At first the image was sexual. Employers, male stenographers, and the general public alternately lauded, vilified, and teased typists as beauties, threats to wives, and flirts (*Phonographic World* 1889b, 253). Poems, songs, and sonnets were dedicated to them. Even the prose waxed rhapsodic:

She is a sweet-briar rose that has bloomed among the dull weeds of commercial life, and she thrives upon her own fragrance. (*Phonographic World* 1889a, 187)

But the typewriter, as she was called, was soon credited with bringing clean habits and a high moral tone to the office, cheerfully performing her duties and loyally guarding business secrets rather than leaving her employer to open up a competing business (*Phonographic World* 1893a, 307; *Shorthand Review* 1890a, 30–33; *Business Woman's Journal* 1889, 53–55; *Phonographic Journal* 1896, 315; *Practical Phonographer* 1884b, 244). By the end of the 1880s, females were considered more suited than men for typing: "Type-writing is essentially woman's work because women are nimbler, neater and steadier at it than men" (*Phonographic World* 1886b, 34). Others reported that women were preferable to men because they were:

more orderly, more quiet and more obliging. They carry with them an air of refinement and a sense of fidelity that is comforting to a busy, worried man. They seem to belong to the place somehow to fit in deficiencies [*sic*]. A girl, such as I have in mind, has her eyes about her, she is full of sympathy, constantly on the alert for unpleasant things which she may avert or turn to good account. She anticipates the wishes of her employer and gratifies them almost before he has them. She not only wins his favor by her faithfulness, she commands his respect by respecting herself. (*Phonographic World* 1890, 201)

These gender-linked traits and occupational requirements then carried over from typing and stenography to general clerking, bookkeeping, and secretarial positions:

young women are more contented with their lot as private secretaries, more cheerful, less restless, more to be depended [upon], more flexible than young men. [She is] more willing to do as asked, more teachable . . . than the young man. (*Pernin's Monthly Stenographer* 1883, 46–47)

With females now seen as inherently possessing superior traits for clerical work, employers were moved to hire women. Men were less likely to look for work in an occupation requiring female qualities. Thus image consolidated the feminization of clerical work.

Conclusion

The typewriter played a major role in the feminization of clerical work: not in instigating women's entry into offices, but in accelerating their numerical domination. Its successful marketing came as a response to changes already under way in the office. But it became the critical factor in the expansion of women in the office in the 1880s, in their proliferation within male clerical preserves such as banking and railroading, and in the final transformation of the image and skills of clerical workers.

Women's earlier gains in the office as copyists opened the way to their predominance as typewriters. Anxious to take advantage of women's lower pay scales and limited upward mobility, male employers did not balk at hiring women as typewriters. And conversely, women wanted these new, relatively high paid, clean, stable, and prestigious jobs. Once typing became a female occupation, women were able to enter into the new field of business stenography. The interests of schools, employers, and the women workers served to link these two occupations and the subordinated but skilled work they entailed soon made women preferred employees, thereby displacing men from this area of clerical work.

The final phase in the feminization of clerical work entailed a changing image of the office worker and of the skills necessary for clerical jobs. The large female presence in typing and stenography forced male employers to reevaluate the content of office jobs in general. These male employers combined with advertisers and the women office workers themselves to create a new feminized image of office workers and office work. This new definition drove many of the remaining men from clerical work in the twentieth century. By 1920, when my husband's immigrant grandfather, a bookkeeper, went looking for employment, he was told that bookkeeping was women's work and he was forced to turn elsewhere. By then, clerical work was no longer men's work, whether men wanted it or not.

NOTES

I would like to acknowledge the helpful criticisms and suggestions of Cindy S. Aron, Alan Freedman, and Lesley Kawaguchi. An earlier draft of this article was presented at the Western Association of Women Historians, Los Angeles, in the spring of 1984.

1. Rotella's graph shows that the rise in clerical employment and office machinery occurred simultaneously (1981, 76).
2. The total of male and female clerical workers in the following occupations

was tabulated from the manuscript censuses of 1860, 1870, and 1880: accountants, bookkeepers, copyists, unspecified clerks, clerks in offices, secretaries, stenographers, and typewriters. I excluded clerks in pharmacies, hotels, groceries, stores, and other clerks who appeared to be working in stores. I included clerks in manufacturing, wholesale trade, insurance companies, railroads, banks, societies, and offices of professionals, as well as others. For 1900, I did not include unspecified and specified female clerks.

Two-thirds of the women, as well as two-thirds of the men, were recorded as clerks without any designation specifying whether they worked in sales, offices, or both.
3. Thanks to Cindy Aron for pointing out that the federal government had no trouble finding male employees even during the war.
4. The men earned between $600 and $2,900 with the median at $1,400 and the mode at $1,200. The women earned $600.
5. Current noted that Sholes received a patent in 1869.
6. In 1870, there were forty-one female and seven male copyists.
7. Calculating from my data and the published census, 22 men and 248 women listed themselves as typewriters in 1900. From my data alone, which included fewer typists, there were 20 male and 219 female typists (9.1 percent). Others who typed but also listed themselves as stenographers, bookkeepers, or clerks were classified under those occupations.
8. The published census combined clerks, salesmen, and accountants in stores, where 16.7 percent (2,281 out of 13,636) were female. Among clerks and bookkeepers in manufacturing establishments, 3.4 percent (7 out of 207) were women.
9. The proportion of business students in stenography classes grew nationally from 12 percent in 1880 to 36 percent in 1900 (Weiss 1981, 413).
10. Calculating from my data and the published census of 1900, there were 333 male and 1,929 female stenographers (85.3 percent female). From my data alone, there were 310 male and 1,705 female stenographers (84.6 percent female).
11. Thanks to Gayle Gullett for information on her grandfather's use of firearms as a bank teller as late as World War II.

REFERENCES

American Shorthand Writer. 1880. 1 (Dec.): 7.
Anderson, Dewey H., and Percy E. Davidson. 1940. *Occupational trends in the United States.* Stanford: Stanford University Press.
Aron, Cindy Sondik. 1987. *Ladies and gentlemen of the civil service: Middle-class workers in Victorian America.* New York: Oxford University Press.
Barnes' Shorthand Magazine. 1890. 2 (Nov.): 89–90.
Braverman, Harry. 1974. *Labor and monopoly capital: The degradation of work in the twentieth century.* New York: Monthly Review Press.

Browne's Phonographic Monthly. 1878a. Personal: Brief sketch of Miss Alice C. Nute. 3 (Dec.): 226.

———. 1878b. Women to the front. 3 (Dec.): 220–21.

Browne's Phonographic Monthly and Reporters' Journal. 1882. Pioneer stenographers: Thomas Towndrow. 7 (Dec.): 326.

———. 1883a. Biographical sketch of Miss Mary S. McCalla of Philadelphia, Pa.: Stenographer to the Board of Extension of the M. E. Church. 8 (Feb.): 37.

———. 1883b. Mrs. Pruella Rheuama Fawcett. 8 (Dec.): 330, 334.

———. 1887. Biographical sketch of Mrs. Eldora J. Schofield of Providence, R.I.: Principal of the R.I. School of Phonography. 12 (Apr.): 106–7.

Business Woman's Journal. 1889. 1 (Apr.): 53–55.

Current, Richard N. 1954. *The typewriter and the men who made it.* Urbana: University of Illinois Press.

Davies, Margery M. 1982. *Woman's place is at the typewriter: Office work and office workers, 1870–1930.* Philadelphia: Temple University Press.

Deutrich, Bernice M. 1971. Property and pay. *Prologue: The Journal of the National Archives* 3:67–72.

Foulke, Arthur Toye. 1961. *Mr. Typewriter: A biography of Christopher Latham Sholes.* Boston: Christopher Publishing.

Hatch, Alden. 1950. *Remington Arms in American history.* New York: Rinehart and Co.

Kirografer and Stenografer. 1878. Shorthand and women. (Jan.).

Massachusetts Bureau of Statistics of Labor. 1885. *Census of Massachusetts: Population and social statistics.* Vol. 1. Washington, D.C.: GPO.

———. 1903a. Mercantile wages and salaries. In *Thirty-third annual report,* 117. Boston: Wright and Potter.

———. 1903b. Sex in industry. In *Thirty-third annual report.* Boston: Wright and Potter.

Morris, Stuart. 1973. Stalled professionalism: The recruitment of railway officials in the United States, 1885–1940. *Business History Review* 48:320–24.

Munson's Phonographic News and Teacher. 1879. Stenography and humbug. 2 (May): 98.

———. 1884a. Writing machines—their uses and abuses. 4 (Aug.): 45–48.

———. 1884b. Stenography, type-writing, etc. 4 (Nov.): 142.

———. 1885. How shorthand is used. 4 (June): 286.

———. 1886. Answers to correspondents—Miss Brown and others. 5 (Jan.): 120.

———. 1887. News and things. 6 (Aug.): 73.

Musoke, Moses S. 1976. Technical change in cotton production in the United States, 1925–1960. Ph.D. diss., University of Wisconsin-Madison.

National Archives. 1869. Register of officers and agents, civil, military, and naval in the service of the United States.

———. 1871. Register of officers and agents, civil, military, and naval in the service of the United States.

————. 1878. Official register of the United States: Containing a list of officers and employés in the civil, military, and naval service. 2 vols.

Pernin's Monthly Stenographer. 1883. 1 (June): 46–47.

Phonetic Educator. 1882. 3 (Jan.–Apr.): 110.

Phonographic Journal. 1896. Shorthand and women. 3 (Dec.): 315–16.

Phonographic Magazine. 1887. 1 (Jan.): 2.

————. 1890. 4 (Sept.): 284.

————. 1891. Mrs. Annie E. H. Lemon. 5 (Aug.): 233–34.

————. 1892. Modern methods of business correspondence. 6 (Mar.): 122–23.

————. 1893. Stephen Pearl Andrews. 7 (Feb.): 24–27.

————. 1894. Mrs. M. V. Longley. 8 (Aug.): 236–37.

————. 1896. M. Jeanette Ballantyne. Woman stenographers. 10 (May): 131.

————. 1897. Elias Longley and Margaret Vater. 11 (Apr.): 106–8.

Phonographic World. 1886a. A talk with Mrs. Burnz. 1 (May): 167.

————. 1886b. The typewriter vs. salesmen and governesses. 2 (Oct.): 34.

————. 1889a. The pretty type-writer. 4 (May): 187.

————. 1889b. Hattie A. Shinn. In defense of the "pretty type-writer." 4 (July): 253.

————. 1889c. S. S. Packard. Are girls a nuisance? 4 (Aug.): 216.

————. 1889d. The type-writer's qualifications. 5 (Nov.): 86.

————. 1890. S. S. Packard. The "pretty type-writer". 5 (Mar.):201.

————. 1891. Arthur A. Thomas. Comer's Commercial College at Boston, Mass. 6 (July): 371–73.

————. 1893a. Joseph Howard, Jr. 8 (July): 307.

————. 1893b. The typewriter companies and the schools. 9 (Sept.): 15.

————. 1893c. Frank Rutherford. What is the difference between a male and a female stenographer? 9 (Oct.): 65.

Practical Phonographer. 1884a. A New York type-writer office. 1 (Oct.): 213–14.

————. 1884b. The typewriter girl. 1 (Nov.): 244.

Rapone, Anita. 1981. Clerical labor force formation: The office woman in Albany, 1870–1930. Ph.D. diss., New York University.

Rayne, M. L. 1888. *What can a woman do, or her position in the business and literary world.* Detroit: F. B. Dickerson and Co.

Rider, John Allen. 1966. A history of male stenographers in the United States. Ed.D. diss., Teachers' College, University of Nebraska.

Rotella, Elyce J. 1981. *From home to office: U.S. women at work, 1870–1930.* Studies in American History and Culture, no. 25. Ann Arbor: UMI Research Press.

Sandler, Mark Stuart. 1979. Clerical proletarianization in capitalist development. Ph.D. diss., Michigan State University.

Shorthand Review. 1890a. Joseph Howard, Jr. Shorthand as a business: Its inducements and demands. 2 (Feb.): 30–33.

————. 1890b. George K. Stoddard. Shorthand in the railroad office. 2 (Apr.): 58–59.

Shorthand World. 1896. William Billings. A phase of the girl problem. 5 (May): 1–2.

Srole, Carole. 1984a. "A position that God has not particularly assigned to men": The feminization of clerical work, Boston, 1860–1915. Ph.D. diss., University of California, Los Angeles.

———. 1984b. The rise of the working class clerk. Paper presented at the seventy-seventh annual meeting of the Organization of American Historians, Los Angeles.

Standard Phonographic Visitor. 1863. Phonography as an accomplishment. 1 (Aug.): 12–13.

———. 1867. Phonography in courts of record. 2 (Apr.): 268–69.

Standard Stenographic Magazine. 1888. The typewriter: Its growth and uses. 1 (Aug.): 2.

Students Journal. 1873. If reverses take the study of phonography. 2 (Sept.): 5.

———. 1876. Dr. Alva Curtis. Phonography—its value in recording and communicating thoughts—should be taught in all schools. 5 (May): 10.

U.S. Bureau of the Census. 1870. Manuscript census, Boston.

———. 1880a. Manuscript census, Boston.

———. 1880b. *Tenth census of the United States.* Vol. 1, *Statistics of the population of the United States.* Washington, D.C.: GPO.

———. 1890. *Eleventh census of the United States.* Vol. 1, *Statistics of the population of the United States.* Washington, D.C.: GPO.

———. 1900. Manuscript census, Boston.

U.S. Commissioner of Labor. 1900. *Fifteenth annual report.* Washington, D.C.: GPO.

U.S. Department of Labor. 1947. Women's occupations through seven decades. Women's Bureau Bulletin no. 218. Washington, D.C.: GPO.

Weiss, Janice. 1981. Educating for clerical work: The nineteenth-century private commercial school. *Journal of Social History* 14:407–23.

"For the Good of the Race": Reproductive Hazards from Lead and the Persistence of Exclusionary Policies toward Women

Patricia Vawter Klein

Scientific and technological advances over the last one hundred years have contributed to a greatly increased understanding of workplace hazards to the reproductive system. We might assume that as science provided ever more sophisticated information on the dangers of toxic substances, and as technology allowed more precise measuring of levels of exposure in all workers, old policies excluding women workers based on more primitive methods (e.g., simply counting the number of stillbirths) would be modified to reflect this progress and to enhance the health and safety of all workers. Yet this has not been the case. In the two periods under study in this article, we find a persistence of exclusionary policies directed deliberately and one-sidedly at women but not men, evidence of the hazards to men notwithstanding.

In the earlier period under consideration here, from the late nineteenth to the early twentieth century, state governments, labor unions, and reform organizations led the way in establishing exclusionary policies. The social climate of the times supported a "protectionist" attitude toward women, but private industry followed this trend with reluctance. In the more recent period to be examined here, that following the establishment of the Federal Occupational Safety and Health Administration (OSHA) in 1970, it is private industry that has played the leading role in establishing or maintaining policies to exclude women workers. Increasingly available, more highly quantifiable data have been used selectively to justify such policies.

The three industries to be considered here—printing, pottery making and battery manufacturing—have in common the fact that they expose employees to lead, a substance long known to adversely affect the reproductive function in both sexes. For each of these three industries there are studies available that have related adverse reproductive effects to work in the industry, and in each of the three, information from studies was used to support an exclusionary policy toward women. This paper will discuss the selective use of such information by both government and industry to formulate exclusionary policies.

Women have been involved in both printing and pottery making in the United States from at least the 1700s. Battery manufacturing dates from the early 1900s as an employer of women. The following historical investigation of these three industries will show that: (1) both men and women suffered physical damage from exposure to lead; (2) policies toward women workers developed separately from those toward men, although reproductive and other hazards were shared by both; and (3) political considerations in excluding women from jobs functioned quite separately from the medical ones, with the result that available information on adverse effects was used selectively with regard to women more often than men.

Medical Hazards from Exposure to Lead

The hazards from exposure to lead have been known for a very long time. At least one thousand years before Christ, in pre-Athenian days, the effects of lead on miners were reported. Each subsequent generation probably witnessed health hazards for both men and women resulting from exposure to the substance (McCord 1953, 394). Interest in the effect of lead on humans may be noted in the eighteenth century, when Benjamin Franklin in America and George Baker in Devonshire, England, both associated the "dry gripes" with the presence of lead in rum and cider, respectively (395). Poisoning occurred from prolonged exposure to or ingestion of lead, and death could result.

In the mid-nineteenth century, the effect of lead specifically on women was noted by French scientists and reported in the literature soon after. Constantin Paul, in 1860, observed that lead had an abortive effect on women working in type foundries; however, it also had an abortifacient effect on the wives of French lead workers, and he found sterility occurring in men exposed to lead (Hamilton 1925, 111; Rom 1976, 542; Oliver 1902, 302). In 1905, French scientist H. Deneufbourg published additional observations on the adverse reproductive effects for women working with lead (Hamilton 1925, 112). In England, pregnant women exposed to lead were found to suffer a higher rate of miscarriages than those outside the lead industry. Medical officers reported that children born to women in the lead industry suffered from poor health, and they found a higher than average frequency of infant deaths (Oliver 1902, 301). In addition, however, lead was observed to diminish the virility of men and to cause "puny offspring" when both parents worked in lead (303).

By the late 1800s, the effects of lead on women had received attention in a variety of industries, including printing, pottery making and battery manufacturing. Adverse effects on women in the printing industry were noted in Austria, Germany, Italy, and the United States (Hamilton 1925, 11; Rom 1976, 543; Hamilton 1919b, 25); investigations into the pottery industry were carried out primarily in Great Britain (Legge and Goadby 1912, 36; Oliver 1902, 353). Clearly, hazards to men were also present, but these received far less attention. The special emphasis on lead hazards to women led to their early exclusion from battery manufacturing shortly after it originated in the late 1800s.

Printing

The unhealthiness of the printing trades was observed and commented on by Benjamin Franklin in 1724 when he was working as a printer at Palmer's in London. McCord has suggested (1953, 394) that Franklin may have been the first person to connect lead poisoning with the printing trades when he observed the limp, dangling hands of fellow workers who did not protect themselves from exposure to lead. This affliction was known as "the dangles" and became closely associated with lead poisoning. Franklin advised workers to cover their mouths and noses in order to avoid the dust and fumes. He followed his own advice.

Printing was known generally as an unhealthy trade in early America, although specific information on reproductive hazards was apparently absent. Adverse effects on women were described in Europe and in the United States during the late 1800s, and women were said to be more susceptible to the toxic effects of lead than men (Legge and Goadby 1912, 35; Oliver 1902, 303). It is interesting to note that this knowledge of printing as hazardous did not result in the exclusion of women from their jobs, even though specific dangers to women working with type were brought out in the United States at least by 1875.

At that time, Azel Ames examined typesetting as an occupation for women and found, according to physicians' reports, lead poisoning as well as "cases of menorrhagia and retarded menstruation" (Ames 1875, 83, 93). However, he seemed to attribute these irregularities in the reproductive system to standing rather than to lead exposure:

> The fact [is] . . . woman is badly constructed for the purposes of standing eight or ten hours upon her feet. I do not intend to bring into evidence the peculiar position and nature of the organs in the pelvis . . . [or] call attention to the peculiar structure of the knee. (56)

In 1904, a British government report found the occupation of printing to have "a special feature of unhealthiness" but concluded that "there is no special danger to life or health in these industries from which the coming generations may suffer . . ." (MacDonald 1904, 16, 112). It, too, viewed long periods of standing as particularly unhealthy for women.

From these examples, it appears that the unhealthiness of lead in the printing trade was generally recognized, but that the direct correlation with reproductive ill effects was not made. The high mortality rate and frequency of tuberculosis among workers in the trade were not viewed as sufficient reasons to exclude women.

In the United States as in Great Britain, there were efforts to exclude women from the printing trade during the 1800s, but inititally they were not based on health considerations at all; instead, these efforts focused on the threat women posed to male workers in the trade. Women were paid less than men and were used to break strikes and replace men at their jobs (U.S. Congress 1911, 104; Abbott 1926, 252). Male workers' fears were ameliorated somewhat by action taken in 1869 to admit women to membership in the International Typographical Union. This represented a marked shift from earlier union policy, which had called for expulsion of male union members who agreed to work with women (Abbott 1926). Incorporating women into the union served to protect men's interests by giving the union control over the women.

Introduction of the Linotype in the late 1880s reduced the danger of exposure to lead, since less handling of the lead type was required. Thomas Oliver, chief factory inspector of Great Britain, commented that "Compositors working the linotype machine run little risk of lead poisoning if they keep themselves and the workrooms clean" (Oliver 1902, 332). Ironically, however, exclusion of women increased with the introduction of the new, "safer" machine because subsequent union policy allowed "journeymen only" to operate the Linotype. Few women in the United States reached the status of journeyman, since apprenticeship programs were not generally open to them (Abbott 1926, 258). In Great Britain, Ramsay MacDonald concluded in his report *Women in the Printing Trades* (1904) that male hostility and competition expressed through unions were the most important factors limiting the employment of women. However, he seemed to agree with the position of the unions when he wrote, "to allow women unrestricted access to the composing rooms would probably lead in time not only to the reduction of men's wages but to the undermining of the trade itself" (173).

It was at the 1910 meeting of the International Association for Labor Legislation (IALL) that reproductive arguments came to the fore. On the basis of a 1909 report compiled by the Austrian Royal Commission, Austrian and Italian delegates urged the exclusion of women from printing "for the good of the race," since the effects of lead poisoning were "transmitted to their offspring" (Hamilton 1919a, 25). They buttressed their position with evidence from earlier German and Italian studies showing that spontaneous abortions among women printers had increased three to five times over those of unexposed women (Rom 1976, 543). British and American delegates criticized the evidence presented to demonstrate women's greater susceptibility to lead poisoning, and they questioned the need to exclude women from the trade. Instead, they argued in favor of ridding the industry of lead poisoning and making it safe for both male and female workers (Hamilton 1925, 11).

The United States in 1910 was a relative latecomer to occupational medicine and was not yet accorded respect in the field by the nations of Europe. Alice Hamilton, a medical doctor and one of the first U.S. delegates to attend an international conference on the subject, became a major contributor to early work in American industrial medicine and helped significantly to raise U.S. status in the field. Hamilton commented, in a 1919 Bureau of Labor Statistics report, on the exclusion of women in the printing trade. She pointed out that the typographical industry was not the only one to attempt to prohibit women, and she took the position that "The danger to health in this industry is avoidable and the logical thing to do is to institute such sanitary measures in printing shops as will make them safe for both sexes" (1919b, 25). This statement reinforced the position the United States had taken at the IALL meeting in 1910 and reflected Hamilton's awareness that health issues lent themselves only too easily to selective use against women. In her view, health issues could be more successfully and justly addressed by seeking policies to protect both men and women.

Pottery Making

Adverse effects to health in pottery making result from the lead used in the glazing process and have been recorded in the United States at least since the eighteenth century. In 1785, the *Philadelphia Mercury* described lead glaze as extremely unhealthy for all persons:

> The best of lead glazing is esteemed unwholesome by observing people . . . and mixing with drink and meats of the people becomes a slow but sure poison chiefly affecting the nerves . . . and produces paleness, tremors, gripes, palsies, etc. sometimes to whole families. (McCord 1953, 78)

British studies on reproductive hazards to both men and women in pottery and other lead industries strongly influenced the first Americans investigating industrial poisons. For example, the work done by Thomas Oliver in 1902 and published under the title *Dangerous Trades* had a tremendous impact and directly inspired Alice Hamilton to move into state and federal service in order to study the effects of lead and other industrial hazards on the American worker (Hamilton 1943, 115).

Oliver took particular pride in his contribution to the exclusion of women under British law from working with dangerous white lead on the basis that women were particularly "susceptible" to lead poisoning (1902, 353). However, following the June 1898 Home Office directive to replace women with men, 86.5 percent of lead-related illnesses reported afflicted men, as opposed to 22.3 percent before. Women registered 77.7 percent of lead-related illnesses before the directive and 13.5 percent after it (297). Replacing women with men simply passed the adverse effects along to men; the percentages did not speak for greater female susceptibility. Nevertheless, Oliver recommended that women be excluded from employment in four of the major pottery-making processes in which lead was used. He recognized that lead was hazardous to men as well, for he recommended periodic checkups for them (354); but he argued that women should be excluded altogether due to greater susceptibility. In another British medical opinion, T. M. Legge, medical inspector of factories, believed that the evidence of women's greater susceptibility to lead was largely a function of age: the average age of women employed was much lower than that of men, and sensitivity to lead was greater among the young (Legge and Goadby 1912, 35).

Alice Hamilton also found evidence to contradict the sex susceptibility thesis in her study of potteries and tile works for the U.S. Department of Labor. She pointed out that women more frequently than men were unorganized, underpaid, poorly housed, poorly fed, and often supported dependents on a low wage (1912, 57). She argued that differences in state of health were based on economics rather than sex. In the pottery and tile works, both men and women were nonunion and earned low wages. There, Hamilton noted, "no such disproportion is found between the two sexes in the matter of lead poisoning"; indeed, a smaller proportion of the women than the men suffered (57). The testimony of 216 physicians interviewed in Zanesville, Ohio, supported the observation that "poverty is very great, the workpeople are underfed and underclothed" (50). Women were often employed in the most hazardous positions as dippers' helpers and finishers, which directly resulted in poisoning from the lead glaze and dust (Hamilton 1919a, 36).

Even though Hamilton concluded that women were no more susceptible to lead than men, she ultimately agreed with Oliver and found it advisable to exclude all married women of childbearing age from employment in potteries (1919a, 37). Hamilton became pessimistic that the workplace could be made safe for all and wished at least to protect the women. However, her recommendation, emanating from the U.S. Department of Labor, suggested an acceptance of unhealthy working conditions at least for men, and it carried important policy implications for all workers exposed to reproductive hazards.

Not all medical evidence was in agreement with Oliver on the dangers of lead to childbearing, although his position dominated the literature. Oliver reported on data from two factory inspectors, who found in 1897 that among 77 married women in potteries, only 61 children remained alive from 212 pregnancies while 111 stillbirths or miscarriages had occurred (Oliver 1902, 302). In a contrasting study, another British physician, J. F. Arlidge, found that child deaths among women in the pottery industry remained about the same after employment (37.7 percent) as before (40.4 percent). Yet the Oliver position was not seriously challenged over the years until Anna Baetjer reviewed these early studies and found no conclusive evidence that women were more susceptible to lead than men. She pointed out that the position presented by Oliver had simply been reiterated without new proof over the years and accepted by others (Baetjer 1946, 149).

Storage Battery Manufacturing

The danger of lead exposure in storage battery making was recognized by every country in Europe and reflected in government regulation of the industry by 1919 (Hamilton 1925, 166). Germany had excluded women and minors from employment in storage battery factories in 1898 (Hamilton 1927, 346) and the International Labor Organization later joined this position (Hamilton 1925, 13).

According to a U.S. Bureau of Labor Statistics report, the U.S. government only became aware of the dangers to women in the trade following the 1918 study *Women in the Lead Industries* by Alice Hamilton. The 1918 study examined the possibility of substituting women for men during the war in any of the battery-making processes, and it recommended that "women should never be allowed" in the most dangerous jobs of mixing the paste and applying it to the plates (Hamilton 1919b, 33). The report went on to say that "because of the well-known danger to women in lead work," a factory that wished to employ women must separate relatively "safe" from dangerous processes, so that women employed in the "safe" processes would not be endangered by close proximity to the dangerous ones (Hamilton 1927, 350). As responsibility for exclusionary policies has shifted from the public to the private sector in recent years, women have been increasingly discouraged from seeking employment in this industry. For example, since 1952, General Motors Corporation has enforced a protective policy that excludes women from some areas of employment (Trebilcock 1978, 372).

Policy and Reproductive Hazards

The exclusion of women from printing in the United States followed two major paths. Introduction of the Linotype machine had a negative impact on the employment of women printers from 1900 onward, since according to the policy of the powerful International Typographical Union only journeymen printers could be assigned to the machines, and only males were apprenticed to become journeymen (U.S. Congress 1911, 189). Passage in some states of "protective" night work legislation during the early 1900s, which limited the hours of work for women, also had an adverse impact on women who worked at night. Between 1900 and 1940 the number of women employed in the printing industry dropped. The proportion of printers who were women reached 10.3 percent in 1900 and thereafter declined to 4.7 percent by 1940 (U.S. Bureau of the Census 1904, cxxxiv; U.S. Bureau of the Census 1943, 76). Since that time, the proportion has risen again.

Printing was known worldwide as an unhealthy trade for all workers and associated with a high rate of tuberculosis in workers (Aub et al. 1926, 235). However, the health hazards of the trade were not a major factor in the exclusion of women, nor was the printing industry treated in the United States as hazardous to reproductive health. It appears that women were excluded largely for economic reasons, and in this printing differs from the pottery and battery industries.

In pottery making, as noted above, adverse reproductive effects on both men and women were observed by the British in the late 1800s. The position that emphasized the greater "susceptibility" of women was most widely accepted. The contrasting position, documented by both British and American investigators, emphasized similarities between male and female susceptibility when both were exposed to similar lead hazards. The British showed that men and women reversed their proportion of symptoms when men replaced women in highly hazardous positions, and the American studies showed economic factors to be more important than sex. Pottery making was found to be a hazardous industry for all workers.

Thus the exclusion of women from lead-exposed work in potteries seems consistent with the information available at the time; the placement of men in the same lead-exposed positions, however, does not, since there was evidence of lead-induced male infertility and transfer of adverse effects from fathers to their offspring (Oliver 1902, 303). The course of action consistent with the findings would have been to exclude both men and women in their fertile years from lead-exposed jobs.

Storage battery manufacturing in the United States began prior to 1880. There is no mention of women employees in the industry until 1926, when a government survey indicated that "women have already entered and will probably enter in very considerable numbers in the near future" (Hamilton 1927, 366). The first U.S. survey, which was conducted in 1914, mentioned only male employees (346), as did an earlier study carried out on the lead industries for the state of Illinois in 1910 (State of Illinois 1911). A Department of Labor report in 1919, also written by Alice Hamilton, recommended that women of childbearing age be excluded from employment. By taking this position, Alice Hamilton, as a government official and a recognized expert on the hazards of lead, helped to establish public policy toward women that viewed them as especially susceptible to reproductive hazards. Thereafter women continued to be strongly discouraged from entering this industry.

An Update

Nowadays, references to adverse effects from lead in printing and pottery making appear much less frequently. Technology was used to free printers from the handling of lead type, while improved hygiene in the shop made the trade safer. Potteries were encouraged to use lead-free glazes, which eliminated the major source of poisoning. Of the three industries under study here, it is battery manufacturing that currently poses the highest risk to workers' health. Of all industries in the United States, battery manufacturing is the one that now uses the largest quantity of lead each year. Today, storage battery manufacturing continues to place the worker in danger from lead exposure, and the industry continues to exclude women of childbearing age (Chavkin 1979, 310).

Meanwhile, available information continues to provide evidence that both men and women face reproductive health hazards from lead, and there are clear indications that the unborn can be affected by lead exposure through either the mother or the father. Some of the effects identified in recent studies include infertility, miscarriage, stillbirth, chromosomal abnormalities, and mutagenic changes. Thus the policy of excluding only female workers of childbearing age from employment in the industry is not consistent with the information available.

The discovery that lead is transferred to the fetus through the placenta has become an important basis for exclusion of women today.

Although this is not a recent discovery, it has taken on increased importance. The earliest recorded studies that confirmed the placental transfer of lead were performed on animals during the 1930s by A. Baumann and his associates in Germany (Barltrop 1969, 136). The question of when the maternal-fetal lead transfer takes place during development was addressed in follow-up studies on both animals and humans.

In studies on humans, Barltrop showed that the distribution of lead to the fetus occurred by the fourteenth week of gestation (146). This suggests that the fetus may not be contaminated by the mother's exposure to lead during the first trimester, which is generally thought to be the most sensitive period for the fetus. This delay in the transfer of lead would weaken the underlying assumption of exclusionary policy, which is supposed to protect the woman during the earliest period of an often unknown pregnancy. Barltrop cautioned that "the significance of the quantities transferred for the foetus remains unknown at the present time and must await further work" (149).

In other human studies, however, there is evidence that a lead burden in the fetus is present whether or not the mother is exposed to lead in the workplace. The lead content in fetal membranes has been shown to be three to six times higher in both term deliveries with premature rupture and preterm deliveries than in normal term deliveries, regardless of the mother's exposure to lead (Fahim, Fahim, and Hall 1976, 309). In a study by Chaube of ghetto mothers, lead was found to be present during the first trimester in two-thirds of embryonic and fetal tissue without apparent undue exposure to lead on the part of the mother (Chaube, Swinyard, and Nishimura 1972, 253).

The concentration of lead in the fetus has been compared with the concentration found in the "average" child (Scanlon 1969, 145). The "average" child's lead concentration measures between 20 and 40 micrograms per 100 grams blood. A study by the U.S. Public Health Service and the National Academy of Sciences identified the hazardous blood lead level for unborn and newborn infants at 30 micrograms per 100 grams (40 Fed. Reg. 45,936 [1975]). Thus the "average" child, in some cases, contains a higher level of lead than is considered safe for newborns and for workers in the industrial setting. This suggests that exposure of the unborn to lead occurs largely outside the workplace and that company policies that exclude mothers and women of childbearing age are not addressing the problem.

The effect on the fetus of the lead-exposed male parent has also been studied further and ill effects to the fetus have been demonstrated. Malformed sperm (teratospermia) in humans has been correlated with a blood level of 53 micrograms per 100 grams; a decrease in the number of sperm (hypospermia) and a decrease in the motility of sperm (asthenospermia) have been correlated with a blood lead level of 41 micrograms per gram. Iona Lancranjan and her colleagues divided male workers into four groups with blood lead levels of 74, 53, 41, and 23 micrograms per 100 milliliters respectively (density of blood is close to grams per milliliter and these two measures are sometimes used interchangably). The fertility of the two groups with the highest lead absorption was decreased and the frequency of asthenospermia, hypospermia, and teratospermia was increased (Lancranjan et al. 1975, 396).

Animal studies have pointed to a possible link between sperm abnormality and genetic mutation. A study on mice showed reduced pregnancy rates in normal females mated with lead-exposed males. The pregnancy rate was 52.7 percent in the control group compared with 27.6 percent in the group with lead-exposed males. It was suggested in the study that the reduced fertility in males was the result of a genetically related mutagenic change in the spermatozoa (Varma, Joshi, and Adeyemi 1974, 486). Another study showed that in mice, sperm abnormalities may be induced by mutation of the genes that regulate spermatogenesis; such mutation has also been associated with specific chromosomal rearrangements (Hollander and deSerres 1978, 275). This study concluded that sperm abnormalities may be transmitted to male progeny, that inheritance of abnormalities follows Mendelian rules, and that abnormal sperm seem less capable of entering the Fallopian tubes and participating in fertlization. The question remains, apparently, whether such abnormal sperm represent an increased genetic hazard.

Two studies of lead workers in storage battery plants suggest that results found in animals are consistent with those in humans. Workmen in storage battery plants were compared with others working in a lead-free occupational environment. Of the storage battery workers, 24.7 percent had sterile marriages, compared with 14.8 percent of the control groups. Pregnancies among the wives of the storage battery workers ended in miscarriage or abortion 8.2 percent of the time compared with 0.2 percent for the control group (Hardy 1966, 713). Chromosomal abnormalities have also been found among male storage battery workers and other workers exposed to lead. One such study compared a group of workers in Lyon, France, with one in Nerem, Belgium, and found chromosomal aberrations in one of the groups (DeKnudt, Leonard, and Ivanov 1973; DeKnudt, Manuel, and Gerber 1977).

Jeanne Stellman, executive director of the Women's Occupational Health Resource Center and a member of the faculty of medicine at the School of Public Health, Columbia University, has criticized the assumption that natural selection protects humans from birth defects that origi-

nate from the male (1983, 76). Yet such an assumption apparently under-
lies policies that "protect" the female and fetus through exclusion from
the workplace while ignoring evidence that males who suffer exposure to
lead will transmit the effects to their offspring.

Political Considerations

In *Women in the Lead Industries* (1919a), Alice Hamilton clearly delin-
eated the political considerations in the use of "expert" testimony or
"scientific" evidence pointing to health hazards for women in the lead
industries. Hamilton understood only too well how health information
that stressed adverse effects on women while ignoring the dangers to
men had been used to exclude women from jobs. This selective use of
materials to support different treatment for male and female workers
can be traced from earlier times to the present.

One of the more important examples of this technique can be found
in the *Muller v. Oregon* (208 U.S. 412) case in 1908. This was the
landmark case in which state legislation limiting working hours for
women but not for men was upheld in the courts, and it became a
cornerstone case for "protective" labor legislation. Louis Brandeis, representing the state of Oregon, presented the case before the U.S. Supreme Court and won the decision partly on the basis of the vast amount
of supporting evidence from "experts" that he included in his brief.
Making selective use of "expert" testimony before the court, Brandeis
argued that women's health was more endangered by long working
hours than men's.

Brandeis had stipulated in his agreement with the National Consumers League, when it procured his services to defend the ten-hour work
day for women, that he must be provided overwhelming documentation
in order to argue the case effectively (Goldmark 1953, 155). The gathering of more than ninety reports from committees, commissions, bureaus, factory inspectors, and other sources was carried out by Josephine Goldmark; these data accounted for 111 pages of the 113-page
brief (Brandeis and Goldmark 1906). The Brandeis brief subsequently
became a model for future "protective" labor law cases in Illinois, California, Louisiana, Ohio, Michigan, Virginia, and Washington (163).

A careful examination of the brief reveals that (1) of the forty-three
documents cited, only twelve referred specifically to adverse effects on
women; (2) the opinions of medical "experts" were cited without supporting evidence; (3) much of the material stressed the reproductive
weakness of women and then argued their unfitness and undesirability
as workers; and (4) health hazards that applied to both men and women

were emphasized only for women. Though a present-day reader may be struck by the large component of hearsay evidence from questionable "experts" about women workers, the brief was lauded by the justices and the approach successfully emulated in a series of cases that moved beyond regulatory legislation into the prohibition of women from working during night hours and in certain types of jobs.

The selective use of "expert" testimony continues today in more recent cases. In 1978, the General Motors Corporation (GM) policy of forbidding women of childbearing age from working in jobs with a "possibility" of exposure to lead was challenged at a plant in Ohio. In its brief, GM presented "expert" testimony from studies dating from 1910 and 1912 to support the argument that exposure to lead directly increased the rate of miscarriages among women workers. The brief also cited studies from 1936 and 1949 that recommended the exclusion of women from lead-related jobs. The only post-1970 data offered came from two studies that demonstrated damage to the central nervous system from lead (Carson et al. 1974; Bridboard 1978). Presumably, such damage would afflict males as well as females; however, the brief only referred to the effects transmitted from mother to fetus (UAW and General Motors Corporation 1978b). None of the studies cited included both male and female subjects, although, as has been shown, such studies do exist. Umpire Arthur Stark, who functioned as arbitrator in the case, gently chided GM for ignoring the many available post-1970 studies, and he actually concluded that there was evidence that risk to the fetus was present whether the father or the mother was exposed to lead. However, he supported the corporation's policy, arguing that it was based on reasonable medical evidence.

As has been shown above, since 1860 a growing body of research has emerged demonstrating the harmful effects of lead exposure on *all* workers and transmission of these effects to offspring through *both* the male and the female. Repeatedly, however, it is the harmful effects to the fetus through the mother that are emphasized, while the role of the father is ignored or minimized. This tendency clearly parallels—and reinforces—the assumption in our society that childbearing and childrearing are essentially women's domain, and that it is therefore women who bear the major burden of responsibility for the well-being of children. In this way, now as in the past, scientific data and medical evidence continue to be used to suit the political and social climate of the times (Tataryn 1979).

The belief that women are more susceptible to reproductive ill effects from lead—and hence more responsible for passing those effects on to offspring—surfaced again during hearings by OSHA on a proposed reduction of the permissible level of lead in the workplace. Comments received on the proposed rules (42 Fed. Reg. 810 [1977]) expressed concern for proper protection of female lead workers "of childbearing age" (ibid.). Initially, OSHA proposed that women workers should be protected at a lower lead exposure level than men, since lead in pregnant women crossed the placental barrier (40 Fed. Reg. 45,936/2-3 [1975]). Evidence from the U.S. Public Health Service confirmed the danger to the fetus of blood lead levels over 30 micrograms per 100 grams (43 Fed. Reg. 54,934/2 [1978]). The Lead Industry Association, a major speaker for the lead industries, contended that since fertile women require such low blood lead levels, "no feasible lead standard could possibly protect them, and that any standard that did protect them would keep virtually all workers out of the workplace" (43 Fed. Reg. 54,424/1 [1978]).

The Lead Industry Association argued that the only way to protect fertile women was to exclude them from the workplace or counsel them to leave individually. OSHA decided to lower the lead standard to a level safe for women and fetuses, and its Final Lead Standard moved to a position more consistent with the available evidence. OSHA accepted the figures presented in the study by the U.S. Public Health Service and the National Academy of Sciences that identified the hazardous blood lead level for unborn and newborn infants at 30 micrograms per 100 grams (40 Fed. Reg. 45,936/2-3 [1975]). The key study used to support the OSHA position was that by Lancranjan, which showed that blood lead levels as low as 41 micrograms per 100 grams could result in malformed sperm.

The Lead Industry Association took serious objection to the lower lead standard and appealed the decision (United Steelworkers of America, AFL-CIO-CLC, v. Marshall, 647 F.2d 1189, 1980). The U.S. Supreme Court eventually upheld the OSHA position and agreed with the federal court that OSHA had statutory authority to protect the fetuses of lead-exposed workers, finding that harm to the fetus is a material impairment of the reproductive systems of the parents (647 F.2d 1256, 1980). This gave the fetus protection under the Occupational Safety and Health Act, sec. 6(b). The lead industries continue to challenge OSHA on this standard for lead, however. Women in lead industries who cannot show proof of sterilization still face the prospect of exclusion (Williams 1981).

Conclusions

Exclusionary policies toward women workers in lead industries have existed in public law during most of this century. Since the courts defined such laws as discriminatory in the 1970s, exclusion of women has been continued by companies as private policy. These exclusionary policies, both in public law and in private enterprise, stress the reproductive function of women.

Medical technology has played an important role by increasing our understanding of the ways workplace hazards adversely affect reproduction, and in particular by providing more information on the reproductive mechanisms that respond to lead exposure in both male and female workers. However, even today, much of this information is used as one-sidedly as the documents and reports included in the Brandeis brief. Available evidence is used selectively, and health hazards that apply to both men and women are stressed more strongly for women. Women are viewed as being more susceptible to workplace hazards than men, particularly to reproductive hazards, and thus as requiring different treatment.

The unspoken assumption underlying such exclusionary policies seems to be that reproduction is primarily women's responsibility—and women's primary responsibility. Thus more sophisticated information on the maternal-fetal relationship and the crossover of substances through the placenta has strengthened exclusionary policies toward women, whereas information on the male contribution to chromosomal and mutagenic changes has not resulted in the exclusion of men.

REFERENCES

Abbott, Edith. 1926. *Women in industry*. New York: D. Appleton and Co.
Ames, Azel, Jr. 1875. *Sex in industry: A plea for the working girl*. Boston: James R. Osgood.
Aub, Joseph Charles, Laurence T. Fairhall, A. S. Minot, and Paul Reznikoff. 1926. *Lead poisoning*. Baltimore: Williams and Wilkins Co.
Baetjer, Anna. 1946. *Women in industry*. Philadelphia: W. B. Saunders Co.
Barltrop, D. 1969. Transfer of lead to the human foetus. In *Mineral metabolism in pediatrics*, ed. D. Barltrop and W. L. Burland, 135–51. Philadelphia: F. A. Davis Co.
Brandeis, Louis D., and Josephine Goldmark. [1906] 1969. *Women in industry: Decision of the United States Supreme Court in* Curt Muller vs. State of Oregon *and brief for the state of Oregon*. Reprint. New York: Arno Press.
Bridboard, Kenneth. 1978. Occupational lead exposure and women. *Preventive Medicine* 76:665.
Carson, Thomas L., Gary A. Van Gelder, George G. Karas, and William B. Buck. 1974. Development of behavioral tests for the assessment of neurologic effects of lead in sheep. *Environmental Health Perspectives* 7:233.
Chaube, S., C. A. Swinyard, and H. Nishimura. 1972. A quantitative study of

human embryonic and fetal lead with considerations of maternal-fetal lead gradients and the effect of lead on human reproduction. *Teratology* 5, no. 2:253.

Chavkin, Wendy. 1979. Occupational hazards to reproduction: A review essay and annotated bibliography. *Feminist Studies* 5, no. 2:310–25.

Commons, John R. 1918. *History of labor in the United States.* New York: Macmillan.

DeKnudt, G., A. Leonard, and B. Ivanov. 1973. Chromosome aberrations observed in male workers occupationally exposed to lead. *Environmental Physiology and Biochemistry* 3:132–38.

DeKnudt, G., Y. Manuel, and G. B. Gerber. 1977. Chromosome aberrations in workers professionally exposed to lead. *Journal of Toxicology and Environmental Health* 3:885–91.

Fahim, M. S., Z. Fahim, and D. G. Hall. 1976. Effects of subtoxic lead levels on pregnant women in the state of Missouri. *Research Communication in Chemical Pathology and Pharmacology* 13:309.

Goldmark, Josephine. 1953. *Impatient crusader.* Urbana: University of Illinois Press.

Hamilton, Alice. 1908. Industrial diseases with special reference to the trades in which women are employed. *Charities and Commons* 20 (Sept. 5): 655–59. Reprinted in *Employment of women,* ed. Edna D. Bullock, 57–63. New York: H. W. Wilson Co., 1920.

———.1912. *Lead poisoning in potteries and tile workers.* U.S. Department of Labor, Bureau of Labor Statistics, Bulletin no. 104. Washington, D.C.: GPO.

———. 1917. *Hygiene of the printing trades.* U.S. Department of Labor, Bureau of Labor Statistics, Bulletin no. 209. Washington, D.C.: GPO.

———. 1919a. *Lead poisoning in the smelting and refining of lead.* U.S. Bureau of Labor, Industrial Accidents and Hygiene Series, Bulletin no. 9. Washington, D.C.: GPO.

———. 1919b. *Women in the lead industries.* U.S. Department of Labor, Bureau of Labor Statistics, Bulletin no. 253. Washington, D.C.: GPO.

———. 1925. *Industrial poisons in the United States.* New York: Macmillan.

———. 1927. Storage battery industry. *Journal of Industrial Hygiene* 9:346.

———. 1943. *Exploring the dangerous trades.* Boston: Little, Brown.

Hardy, H. L. 1966. What is the status of knowledge of the toxic effects of lead on identifiable groups in the population? *Clinical Pharmacology and Therapy* 7:713–33.

Hollander, A., and F. J. deSerres, eds. 1978. *Chemical mutagens.* New York: Plenum Press.

Lancranjan, Iona, H. Popeson, O. Gavanescu, I. Klepsch, and M. Serbanescu. 1975. *Archives of Environmental Health* 30:396.

Lane, R. E. 1949. The case of the lead worker. *British Journal of Industrial Medicine* 6:125.

Legge, Thomas M., and Kenneth W. Goadby. 1912. *Lead poisoning and lead absorption.* London: Edward Arnold.

McCord, Carey P. 1953. Benjamin Franklin and lead poisoning. *Industrial Medicine and Surgery* 22, no. 9 (Sept.): 393–99.

———. 1954. Lead and lead poisoning in early America: Lead compounds. *Industrial Medicine and Surgery* 23, no. 2 (Feb.): 75–80.

MacDonald, J. Ramsay, ed. 1904. *Women in the printing trades.* London: P. S. King and Son.

Oliver, Thomas, ed. 1902. *Dangerous trades.* London: John Murray.

———. 1911. *Industrial lead poisoning with descriptions of lead processes in certain industries in Great Britain and the western states of Europe.* Washington, D.C.: GPO.

Rom, William N. 1976. Effects of lead on the female and reproduction: A review. *Mount Sinai Journal of Medicine* 43, no. 5 (Sept.–Oct.): 542.

———. 1983. *Environmental and occupational medicine.* Boston: Little, Brown.

Scanlon, John. 1969. Fetal effects of lead exposure. *Pediatrics* 49:145.

State of Illinois. 1911. *Report of commission on occupational diseases.* Chicago: Warner Printing Co.

Stellman, Jeanne. 1983. The occupational environment and reproductive health. Cited in *Environmental and occupational medicine,* 76–89. *See* Rom 1983.

Tataryn, Lloyd. 1979. *Dying for a living.* Ottawa: Deneau and Greenberg.

Trebilcock, Anne M. 1978. OSHA and equal employment opportunity laws for women. *Preventive Medicine* 7 (Sept.): 372–84.

UAW (United Automobile, Aerospace and Agricultural Implement Workers of America) Local Union No. 674 and General Motors Corporation, GM Assembly Division, Norwood Plant, Norwood, Ohio. 1978a. Appeal case Q-160, decision Q-6, July 26.

———. 1978b. Appeal case Q-160, General Motors brief, April 4.

U.S. Bureau of the Census. 1904. *Special reports: Occupations at the twelfth census, 1900.* Washington, D.C.: GPO.

———. 1943. United States summary. Part 1 of *Sixteenth census of the United States, 1940: Population.* Vol. 3, *The labor force.* Washington, D.C.: GPO.

U.S. Congress. Senate. 1911. History of women in the trade unions. Vol. 10 of *Report on conditions of woman and child wage-earners in the United States.* 61st Cong., 2d Sess. S. Doc. 645. Washington, D.C.: GPO.

U.S. Department of Labor. 1928. *The effects of labor legislation on the employment opportunities of women.* Women's Bureau Bulletin no. 65. Washington, D.C.: GPO.

Varma, M. M., S. R. Joshi, and A. O. Adeyemi. 1974. Mutagenicity and infertility following administration of lead sub-acetate to Swiss male mice. *Experientia* 30:486.

Williams, Wendy L. 1981. Firing the woman to protect the fetus. *Georgetown Law Journal* 69:641–42.

The Patent Office Clerk as Conjurer: The Vanishing Lady Trick in a Nineteenth-Century Historical Source

Autumn Stanley

In a now-famous article called "The Invisible Woman," Dolores Barracano Schmidt likens historians to professional magicians. They are as adept, she points out, at making women disappear as any conjurer who ever lived. One college-level history text surveyed by Earl Schmidt in preparation for the article performs the seemingly impossible feat of omitting women altogether from the discussion of woman suffrage in the twentieth century, so that the Nineteenth Amendment seems to spring full-blown from the forehead of the body politic. Indeed, the authors of this *Survey of American History,* Leland D. Baldwin and Robert Kelley, could have rivaled the famed nineteenth-century magician Buatier De Kolta of the Maskelyne Company in his Vanishing Lady trick; for they also manage to discuss the reform of insane asylums in the early nineteenth century without mentioning Dorothea Dix, muckraking without mentioning Ida Tarbell, and the Montgomery bus boycott of the 1950s without mentioning Rosa Parks (Schmidt 1971, 95–96)!

Although it is no longer true, as it was when Schmidt wrote, that none of the major college-level American history texts is written by a woman, women's interests, issues, and achievements are still very imperfectly integrated into American history. The Vanishing Lady is still a popular trick. The history of American technology is not only no exception to this rule, it is one of the worst offenders. Voltaire's dictum that "there have been very learned women as there have been women warriors, but there have never been women inventors" still echoes through its pages, finding advocates as late as 1976; and even those who wish to correct him find no names on the tip of their tongue.

One of the reasons, of course, why historians seem to make women vanish from their texts is that earlier generations of conjurer-compilers have already spirited women out of many sources-to-be. In short, the sources are corrupt from the start. Only rarely do we have an opportunity to catch these Ur-magicians in the act—black-handed, as it were, with the ink still wet on their fingers. Such an opportunity is provided by the case I wish to discuss here: the compiling of the only important

source on nineteenth century American women inventors. I will describe the source, detail some of its omissions and restore some of the
Vanished Ladies to the stage, unmask the sleight of pen involved, and
suggest a possible explanation for it.

The Source

As the centennial of the U.S. Patent Office (1890) and the end of the
nineteenth century approached together, a women's rights activist
named Charlotte Smith[1] persuaded the patent commissioner to compile a list of women who had received American patents since the
opening of the office. Listing more than five thousand patents, it was
issued by the Government Printing Office as *Women Inventors to
Whom Patents Have Been Granted by the United States Government,
1790 to July 1, 1888* (hereafter cited as LWP). Two later installments,
of 1892 and 1895, brought the list up through the last day of February,
1895. Only five hundred copies were ever printed. The list sold for
what seems to us the trivial sum of fifty cents. In an era of weekly
wages ranging from three to six dollars, however, the price was not
low.

   LWP gives the following information for each invention: patent
number, name of inventor (with assignees or copatentees, if any), city of
residence, nature of invention, and patent date. The patents are listed in
numerical (and thus chronological) order.

   The significance of this source for the history of American technology can scarcely be overestimated. To my knowledge, it is the only
comprehensive list of American women patentees ever compiled.[2] (The
list includes some foreign women who got U.S. patents, but the main
purpose was to identify American women inventors.) Scholarly and non-
scholarly researchers from Ida Tarbell to H. J. Mozans and the Wom-
en's Bureau of the U.S. Department of Labor have relied on it as
gospel. In ten years of research on women inventors I have never seen it
criticized.

   My own research, however, shows that this crucial source is far
from perfect—indeed, it needs to be used with considerable care. LWP
purports to be a complete list of women patentees from Mary Kies in
1809 to the last woman granted a patent in February of 1895. It is not.
The conjurer-compilers have already been at work making the ladies
vanish.

   The significance of finding substantial numbers of errors in such an
important historical source should be obvious. But some further clarification of its importance may be in order for those not familiar with the

special difficulties of patents research or of researching women's contributions to technology. LWP is not just one of several sources on nineteenth-century American women inventors. It is the *only easily usable source* with any pretensions to completeness. The alternative to using it (and the only means of completely correcting it) is to slog through more than five hundred thousand patents granted during its period. Alphabetical name lists of each year's patents are not available until the 1870s, and systems of access to patents in general are quite naturally geared not to the historian but to the inventor, who merely wants to know what has already been invented.

Moreover, there is nothing even vaguely comparable to LWP for the twentieth century. The only decent study was done in the 1920s by the Women's Bureau of the Department of Labor. It covered only ten years of a sixteen-year period, and though it provides some extremely useful statistics for that limited period, *it contains not a single name.* Also, so far as I can tell, this Women's Bureau study (hereafter cited as WB) is little known and seldom used. The only other study I have located is so riddled with errors as to be almost useless (Lee 1975). And here the alternative is truly mind-boggling, as the universe of U.S. patents granted has expanded to nearly 5 million. The records are computerized but cannot be searched by gender (i.e., the researcher must know the name of her quarry in advance). Thus most of what is known or has been written to date about American women as inventors has depended—at best—on LWP.

But more is at stake here than corrective or compensatory history, vital as that is. Unique and important sources such as LWP are used to predict women's inventive and innovative *capacity* for the future as well as to document their past achievement. These predictions influence the occupations a young girl will let herself aspire to, and the occupations her parents and counsellors will guide her toward as well. They reinforce—or undermine—the stereotypes that now keep technology largely a male preserve. This all-male technological establishment may represent not merely an equity issue but a planetary survival issue. If, by omission, LWP diminishes American women's past contributions to technology to any significant degree, the resulting disservice to society could be considerable.

The Omissions

Omissions from LWP that I have discovered thus far[3] range in date from Charity Shaw Long's consumption remedy of 1812 (Lee 1975, 60) at least through 1894. They range in importance from *unknown and proba-*

bly minor (as with Bernice West's improved fastening for windows and shutters of 1822) to *unknown but noteworthy* if only as stereotype breakers (as with Junia Chittenden's 1823 improvement in machinery for propelling boats) to *undeniably important,* as judged by wide adoption, commercial success, social, economic, or political impact, mention in other sources, or some combination of these. The omissions also range over virtually all areas of invention, as becomes clear below.

Let us look at some examples of omissions in the "undeniably important" category. We should note that significance of inventions is largely in the eye of the beholder and changes with the times. Today, for example, we would never class a straw-weaving or bonnet-making invention as important. But such were the Anglo-American trade conflicts of the day, and such was the size of the straw headgear market, that these inventions were significant indeed in late Colonial and early post-Revolutionary times.

By reinventing a popular weave formerly kept secret abroad and by adapting to local materials rather than imported ones, Sophia Woodhouse Welles and her fellow inventors in effect created entire new American industries and altered the balance of trade. Welles's "Wethersfield hats," bonnets made from local redtop hay and spear grass, enabled women to follow the fashion for straw bonnets and still support President Madison's embargo on British goods during the War of 1812. The bonnets won a silver medal at the Society of Arts in London in 1821 and a U.S. patent the same year. This invention, then, was both economically and historically significant; it was technically rewarded and well known in its day (Sherr and Kazickas 1976; Tharp 1960, 6). Yet Welles and her patent do not appear in LWP.

A second omission in this category needs no defense of its significance, even for today's readers. One of the most important of nineteenth-century women's inventions, and an important naval invention by any lights, including traditional male-defined standards, is Martha Coston's realization and improvement of her husband's signaling devices for use at night, which were left unfinished at his death. These three-color pyrotechnic signals revolutionized naval communication and have continued in use into modern times. As of the late 1970s, the Coston Supply Company established by Mrs. Coston was still in business. Patented in 1859, the invention was famous during the years of LWP's three compilations (1888, 1892, and 1895), having been shown at the Philadelphia World Exhibition in 1876, at Paris in 1878, and at the Chicago World's Columbian Exposition in 1893 (Warner 1979, 105–6, 112). It had also, of course, received considerable publicity when the United States and other navies adopted it. Mrs. Coston patented a further improvement in 1871, which did appear in LWP, and her autobiography *A Signal Success* appeared just two years before the closing date of the first LWP installment. Ida Tarbell wrote of Coston's achievements in an article appearing before that first installment. Yet LWP omits the 1859 patent.

Other important or potentially important inventions omitted by LWP include Henrietta H. Cole's "pony" fluting machine (two patents), Mary P. Carpenter's self-setting needle for sewing machines, and Geneva Armstrong's improvement in livestock cars. Cole's machine (a device used in the intricate ironing demanded by nineteenth-century clothing) was exhibited at the 1876 World Exhibition in Philadelphia, receiving a Centennial Award; was pictured in *Iron Age* magazine the same year; and was shown at the American Institute in New York, receiving a diploma in 1873 and a bronze medal in 1874 (Berney 1977, 56; Logan 1912, 885; Warner 1979, 112). LWP also omits Cole's patent for a piston packing, which was important enough to rate a reissue (extension) in 1871. Only patents with considerable economic potential, not realized during the early years of their term, were granted extensions.

Mary P. Carpenter of Buffalo, San Francisco, and New York City was one of the most prolific of known nineteenth-century American women inventors. She had thirteen patents to her credit between 1862 and 1894, covering things as diverse as an ironing and fluting machine, a barrel-painting machine, and a sewing machine needle and arm. The needle and arm invention was considered sufficiently important to be featured in the *Scientific American* for September 10, 1870 (164). Carpenter exhibited a sewing machine, presumably incorporating this invention, at the 1876 World Exhibition (Warner 1979, 111–12), and the model can be seen today at the Smithsonian.

Geneva Armstrong was a farmer from western New York. After inventing and patenting a new feeding-watering trough for livestock cars in 1885, she offered her invention to the railroads, personally addressing a meeting of railway officials. She also took it to the World's Columbian Exposition of 1893 (Handy 1893). Charlotte Smith considered the invention important enough to mention in her periodical the *Woman Inventor*.

But the most shocking omission I have discovered to date—and the one that sparked the study reported here—is that of Mildred Blakey of Pennsylvania. Mildred Blakey, who obviously came from a whole family of inventors and might deserve a brief biography of her own, is noteworthy not only for the numbers of her inventions, but for their exclusively mechanical nature. Moreover, her machines were designed for heavy manufacturing industries. Between 1874 and 1905 she received at least fifteen patents, mostly covering machines used in the manufacture of metal pipe and tubing, but also including one gasoline engine. Twelve of the fifteen lie within the scope of LWP, but *only one of the twelve appears on the list*—her 1890 patent for a welding key or strip used in welding pipe seams. At first glance, this looked to me like her least important patent.

Such glaring and extensive error showed me the need for a closer look at LWP as a source. Just how numerous were the omissions? Possibly even more important, were they random, or was there some pattern or bias in them?

To answer these questions, I decided to look systematically at an entire year of patents as listed in the annual name lists published by the Patent Office, count all the women's names, and compare the total with that year's total on LWP. Then I would look at what *kinds* of inventions were omitted, and whether the distribution of omitted inventions differed significantly from that of the listed inventions.

How Many?

As a single year to examine systematically, I chose 1876, partly for its importance as the centennial year, when many inventors of both sexes were presumably inspired to come forward with their inventions, and partly as one of the first years for which a published name list is available. I looked at regular patents only, not design patents. A search of the 212 pages of the 1876 name list[4] revealed thirty-three unmistakable omissions from LWP; that is, there were thirty-three patentees with unmistakably female names that did not appear on LWP (see app. A). Since LWP lists only 124 patents for 1876, this means that its clerk-compilers omitted roughly one woman's invention for every four they recorded, and the total number of women's patents for 1876 should be almost 27 percent higher, or 157.[5]

If this significant, high omission rate prevailed for the entire compilation, LWP should contain just over 7,000 names (7,008 counting only years for which names are now recorded) instead of 5,535 as it does now. The ratio of women's patents to all patents would not be greatly altered, up from barely over 1.0 percent to just under 1.3 percent. But the absolute totals would certainly be significantly higher.

We must next ask whether such a high rate does indeed prevail throughout; that is, whether 1876 is representative. A very preliminary look at 1890 indicates that it may not be. In forty-six pages of the 1890 name list—about 10 percent by page length—I found only 2 unmistakably female names not appearing on LWP: Mathilda Busby and Isabel Cassidy. If these pages listing names from the end of the *b*'s through the

c's and into the early d's are representative—a risky assumption in view of the small numbers involved—this would mean a total of only twenty omissions for the entire year. Since LWP lists 258 names for 1890, the year's omission rate would be less than one in twelve, and the correct total of women patentees only about 8 percent higher than the LWP figure. Thus it is possible, though by no means certain, that LWP's overall omission rate may be lower than that for 1876 (or that later records are better).

What Kind?

In addition to the gross numbers omitted, it is important to look at what kinds of inventions were omitted. The thirty-three unmistakable omissions from 1876 can be classified as follows (my categories; see app. B):

Agricultural	4
Chemical/Metallurgical	2
Furnishings	2
Health/Medicine	5
Heating, Cooling, and Related	1
Labor Saving (domestic)	2
Manufacturing	4
Timekeeping, Measurement, and Related	2
Transportation	4
Wearing Apparel and Related	5
Miscellaneous	2
	33

The categories I have chosen here, though influenced by the specific composition of this small sample of inventions, generally follow those used by WB. Nine out of eleven of them match either a major category (first-level heading) or a large subcategory (second-level heading) of that study (WB, 14–15). More importantly, my categories also accord well with the major classes used by the Patent Office itself, both at the time LWP was compiled, i.e., the late nineteenth century, and later. Two noteworthy differences are that I classify culinary inventions as "food processing" and place them under Agricultural; and that I classify dress-reform inventions with a hygienic or preventive-medicine purpose as "medical" and place them under Health/Medicine (cf. Warner 1979, 115–16; Warner 1978, 29). The rationale for placing them thus, rather than in a Culinary/Kitchen Equipment category or in my Wearing Apparel and Related category, respectively, is that such categories have traditionally been ignored or devalued in discussions of contributions to technology. These choices do not materially affect the findings reported here.

At first glance it might seem that the ideal way to detect any nonrandomness in the LWP omissions for 1876 might be to classify the 124 inventions that *are* listed for that year according to the eleven categories just suggested, and then compare category sizes for the two lists. But the sample sizes are so small in the omitted-inventions list that the results would scarcely justify the considerable work involved (owing to LWP's cryptic descriptions of the inventions and the nature of the early Patent Office records). I hypothesized, however, that two quick and useful indicators of nonrandomness would be the absolute and relative frequencies of machines and wearing apparel in the listed and unlisted samples. Accordingly, I broke out a composite Machines/Mechanical category, including mechanical devices and improvements of a mechanical nature in ordinary items, and added it to the omissions list as follows (Wearing Apparel and Related was already a category; see app. B):

Agricultural	3
Chemical/Metallurgical	2
Furnishings	2
Health/Medicine	5
Heating, Cooling, and Related	1
Labor Saving	2
Machines/Mechanical	8
Manufacturing	1
Timekeeping, Measurement, and Related	0
Transportation	2
Wearing Apparel and Related	5
Miscellaneous	2
	33

Once isolated in this way, *machines turn out to be the largest single category of the omitted inventions,* accounting for eight of the total of thirty-three. By contrast, the twenty machines in LWP (see app. C) are not the largest single category among the 124 listed inventions for 1876, being outnumbered at least by Wearing Apparel and Related with twenty-nine items. Nor, we should note, are Machines the largest category among the 652 patents classified by LWP compilers from LWP listings for 1892–95. Indeed, the Machines category does not exist for that classification. When broken out, the eighty-nine machines and me-

TABLE 1.   A Comparison of Selected Indicators among Listed and Omitted Inventions of Women Patentees for 1876

Indicators	Ratio of Listed (124 total)	Ratio of Omitted (33 total)
Machines to total	20:124 (16.1%)[a]	8:33 (24.2%)
Wearing Apparel to total	29:124 (23.4%)	5:33 (15.1%)
Machines to Wearing Apparel	20:29 (68.9%)	8:5 (160.0%)
Nontraditional Machines[b] to total	4:124 (3.2%)	8:33 (24.2%)
Nontraditional to Traditional Machines	4:16 (25.0%)	8:0

[a]If two ashsifters and a musical top, originally classed otherwise, are included here, the total for machines among the 124 listed inventions rises to 23, and the respective figures for the listed column become 23:124 (18.5%) Machines to total; 23:29 (79.3%) Machines to Wearing Apparel; and 4:19 (21%) Nontraditional to Traditional Machines.

[b]Commercial, industrial, agricultural, or highly technical machines used in nondomestic environment and in endeavors not usually (stereotypically) connected with women's work.

chanical inventions of that sample become the third largest category, outnumbered by both Wearing Apparel and Culinary Utensils.

It is worth noting in passing, however, that the prevalence of machines among nineteenth-century American women's patented inventions is higher than might have been predicted, whichever of these figures we take: 24.2 percent for the omitted inventions of 1876, 16.1 percent for listed inventions for the same year (see table 1), and 13.6 percent for LWP's 1890s classified listing.

Perhaps more illuminating is the relative prevalence of inventions in the Machines/Mechanical and Wearing Apparel and Related categories. As table 1 shows, Machines outnumber Wearing Apparel 8 to 5 or 160 percent among the omitted inventions, but are outnumbered 29 to 20, constituting only 68.9 percent, among the listed inventions for 1876. Similarly, among the 652 inventions from the early 1890s in LWP's own classification, Wearing Apparel is the most numerous category, outnumbering my Machines category by 132 to 89.

But most illuminating of all is a more refined breakdown of machines into subcategories I have labeled Traditional (connected with stereotypically female domestic or service-oriented work) and Nontraditional (commercial, industrial, agricultural, or highly technical machines used in nondomestic environments and in endeavors incongruent with the nineteenth-century stereotype or ideal of women's work).

If we look more closely at the eight machines omitted by LWP for

1876 (app. B), we see that all eight are strikingly nondomestic or what might be called nontraditional inventions for women: three manufacturing machines, two of them used in metal fabrication; a clock and a clock movement; dredging machinery; an agricultural machine; and an improvement in ship propulsion. Of the twenty machines appearing on LWP for 1876, by contrast (see app. C), twelve were either sewing or laundry machines (the spinning attachment is for a sewing machine). Of the two manufacturing machines listed in appendix C (nos. 10 and 4), one was probably a candy-making machine, and the other was used in wig making. At least two of the sewing machines may have been for commercial use (Carpenter's and Barton's); the centrifugal sugar machine could have been used by confectioners, and the hair-heading machine would probably have been used in a business as well. But all these are connected with women's traditional endeavors. Of the machines listed, only Marie Ronat's plow, Lydie Renshaw's steam generator and Emily E. Tassey's apparatus for raising sunken vessels and her siphon propeller-pump can readily be compared to the eight omitted machines for incongruence with the stereotype. This stereotype, lest anyone be in doubt, is part of the general view of women as confined to a domestic sphere—utterly false for working women and achieving women of all classes, and crippling to all women—that prevailed throughout the nineteenth century and has not yet been totally destroyed. When applied to women's contributions to technology it maintains, in the face of all evidence, that women do not invent; or if they do, they invent only wearing apparel or kitchen equipment or new foods.

Looking again at table 1, where I have broken out Nontraditional Machines as a separate subcategory, we see that these machines accounted for 24.2 percent of the omitted inventions, as compared with only 3.2 percent of the listed inventions. Furthermore, these stereotype-breaking machines constituted all of the omitted machines, but only 25 percent of the listed machines. Thus it would seem that, if 1876 is typical of the LWP compilers' labors, omissions from the list are not quite random.

Conclusion, or the Conjurers Unmasked

To summarize, then, if 1876 is representative of the LWP compilers' labors, the major and only substantial secondary source on women's inventive achievement omits significant numbers of women's inventions. Women's mechanical inventions in general seem particularly likely to have been omitted. And women's nontraditional machines seem disproportionately likely to have been overlooked in the one year systematically studied. The overall effect, if prevalent thoughout, is to distort and diminish the picture LWP conveys of women's contribution to technology.

LWP is still an invaluable source. Considering the nature of the early records, it is probably reasonably complete. But it needs to be used with somewhat more caution than exercised heretofore.

It remains to suggest how and why the ladies disappeared. I do not suggest any form of male conspiracy or malice at work, even though Charlotte Smith had to badger several patent commissioners unmercifully—she visited one of them seventeen times—and even appear before a Congressional committee in order to get the compilation under way (Smith 1890–91). I do suggest that partly because they were working under pressure, perhaps from imperfect or difficult sources, but mostly because they operated from the prevailing assumption that women invent, if at all, mainly in so-called domestic areas, the LWP compilers created a listing and categorization of nineteenth-century American women's inventions that both reflects and reinforces this stereotype.

NOTES

I would like to thank my former research assistant, Tim Coshow, and my daughter, Iris Simmons, for help with the name list searches.

1. Smith (1843–1917) was a magazine editor and publisher, labor leader, Congressional lobbyist, reformer, iconoclast, and social gadfly—a sort of nineteenth-century Ralph Nader. As early as 1890 she planned a book on women inventors. I have dedicated my forthcoming book *Mothers of Invention* to her and am planning a brief biography to rescue her from oblivion.

2. Mary Logan's section on women inventors (1912, 882ff) in her book on women's role in American history refers to a list of "prominent" women inventors that is obviously not LWP since she mentions some names not found therein. I have never located this other list and thus do not know its date, compiler, scope, or format; but I speculate that it was compiled by Robert DuBois for his periodical *Inventive Age,* and that it continues beyond the end date of LWP into the early twentieth century.

3. Where no other source is given, information is from U.S. Patent Office records (weekly gazette or yearly name indexes) or from my forthcoming *Mothers of Invention.*

4. I am grateful to my research assistant, Tim Coshow, who did the necessary photocopying and slogged through the first scan of the pages.

5. The name lists, though apparently very good, are themselves not perfect. For example, the 1876 name list contains one Jessie Park of Marlborough, N.Y., Pat. no. 175,740 of April 4 for "Book-binding." The gazette for that

date, however, shows the name as *Jesse* Park. As this seems to be the correct spelling, I deleted this name from my tabulations. Further, LWP lists one name for 1876 that the name list omits.

REFERENCES

Berney, Esther S. 1977. *A collector's guide to pressing irons and trivets.* New York: Crown.

Carpenter self-threading and self-setting needle . . . . 1870. *Scientific American,* Sept., 164.

Coston, Martha. 1886. *A signal success: The work and travels of Mrs. Martha J. Coston.* Philadelphia: Lippincott.

Gordon, J. E. 1978. *Structures: Or why things don't fall down.* New York: Plenum.

Handy, M. P., ed. 1893. *World's Columbian Exposition, 1893, official catalog.* Pt. 1. Chicago: Conkey.

James, Edward T., and Janet Wilson James, eds. 1971. *Notable American women, 1607–1950: A biographical dictionary.* 3 vols. Cambridge, Mass.: Harvard University Press.

Lee Katherine E. 1975. Women and patents: A historical investigation. Master's thesis, San Jose State University.

Logan, Mary S. [1912] 1972. *The part taken by women in American history.* Wilmington, Del.: Perry-Nalle. Reprint. New York: Arno Press.

LWP. *See* U.S. Patent Office 1895.

Mozans, H. J. [1913] 1976. *Woman in science.* New York: D. Appleton. Reprint. Cambridge, Mass.: MIT Press.

Robertson, Patrick, ed. 1974. *The Shell book of firsts.* London: Ebury Press.

Schmidt, Dolores Barracano. 1971. The invisible woman: The historian as professional magician. Reprinted 1972 in *Women out of history,* ed. Ann Forfreedom. Los Angeles: Forfreedom.

Sherr, Lynn, and Jurate Kazickas. 1976. *American woman's gazetteer.* New York: Bantam.

Smith, Charlotte, ed. 1890–91. *Woman Inventor.* (Apr.).

Stanley, Autumn. n.d. *Mothers of invention: Women inventors and innovators through the ages.* Metuchen, N.J.: Scarecrow Press. Forthcoming.

Tarbell, Ida. 1887. Women as inventors. *Chautauquan* 7, no. 6 (Mar.): 355–57.

Tharp, Louise Hall. 1960. Bonnet girls. *New England Galaxy,* Winter, 3–10.

Trescott, Martha. 1979. *Dynamos and virgins revisited.* Metuchen, N.J.: Scarecrow Press.

U.S. Patent Office. 1895. *Women inventors to whom patents have been granted by the United States government, 1790 to July 1, 1888.* With appendixes to March 1, 1895. Washington, D.C.: GPO. Cited as LWP.

Warner, Deborah J. 1976. The women's pavilion. In *1876: A centennial exhibition,* ed. Robert C. Post. Washington, D.C.: Smithsonian Institution.

————. 1978. Fashion, emancipation, reform, and the rational undergarment. *Dress* 4:24–29.

————. 1979. Women inventors at the centennial. In *Dynamos and virgins revisited. See* Trescott 1979.

Warrior, Betsy. 1975. Necessity is the mother of invention. In *Houseworker's handbook,* ed. Betsy Warrior and Lisa Leghorn. 3d ed. Cambridge, Mass.: Women's Center.

WB. *See* Women's Bureau, U.S. Department of Labor, 1923.

Weimann, Jeanne M. 1981. *The fair women: The story of the Woman's Building, World's Columbian Exposition, Chicago, 1893.* Chicago: Academy Chicago.

Women's Bureau, U.S. Department of Labor. 1923. Women's contributions in the field of invention. Bulletin no. 28. Washington, D.C. Cited as WB.

APPENDIX A: THIRTY-THREE UNMISTAKABLE OMISSIONS
FROM LWP, 1876

No.	Patent No.	Name and Residence	Invention	Date
1.	180,822	Marie E. P. Audouin, Paris, France	Composition for lining puddling and other furnaces	8/8
2.	180,313	Julia D. Banfield Boston, Mass.	Corset	7/25
3.	175,015	Mildred Blakey, Etna, Pa.	Machine for forming hollow welded cylinders	3/21
4.	182,795	Mildred Blakey, Etna, Pa.	Roll for welding and finishing tubing	10/3
5.	174,477	Mary P. Carpenter, New York, N.Y.	Barrel-painting machine	3/7
6.	177,207	Vashti Chandler, Pontiac, Mich.	Labor-saving dish drainer	5/9
7.	176,297	Laura J. Gott, La Grange, Ohio	Cleaner for jugs, etc.	4/18
8.	178,848	Ellen A. Hale, Rockford, Ill.	Ornamental wall bracket	6/20
9.	177,333	Iris Hobson, Ft. Scott, Kans.	Potato digger	5/16
10.	173,124	Catharine Judson, Boston, Mass.	Corset spring	2/8
11.	7,034	Catharine Judson, Boston, Mass.	Corset spring (reissue)	4/4
12.	180,138	Florence Kroeber, Hoboken, N.J.	Clock	7/25
13.	184,972	Florence Kroeber, Hoboken, N.J.	Clock movement	12/5
14.	181,960	Harriet H. May, Birmingham, Conn.	Corset	9/5
15.	178,184	Carrie M. Newell, Boston, Mass.	Culinary steamer	5/30
16.	175,154	Emmeline W. Philbrook Boston, Mass.	Underwaist	3/21
17.	177,882	Emmeline W. Philbrook, Boston, Mass.	Spring clasp garment support	5/23
18.	184,545	Emmeline W. Philbrook, Boston, Mass.	Underwaist	11/21
19.	185,782	Ruth T. Reed, Rochester, Ind.	Abdominal supporter	12/26
20.	185,352	Ellen P. Rich, Boston, Mass.	Pattern for garments	12/12

(*Continued on next page*)

(APP. A—*Continued*)

No.	Patent No.	Name and Residence	Invention	Date
21.	185,184	Lacy W. Simmons, Darbyville, Fla.	Grater	12/12
22.	179,362	Charlotte L. Slade, New York, N.Y.	Drawing slate	6/27
23.	176,206	Jennie H. Spofford, Philadelphia, Pa.	Riding saddle	4/18
24.	176,370	Jennie H. Spofford, Philadelphia, Pa.	Mosquito net frame	4/18
25.	176,413	Jennie H. Spofford, Philadelphia, Pa.	Mattress supporter	4/18
26.	177,970	Anna B. Stapler, Wilmington, Del.	Tea and coffee urn	5/30
27.	178,813	Jane G. Swisshelm, Pittsburgh, Pa.	Hot-air chamber	6/13
28.	184,997	Emily E. Tassey, Pittsburgh, Pa.	Propulsion of vessels	12/5
29.	184,998	Emily E. Tassey, Pittsburgh, Pa.	Dredging machinery	12/5
30.	172,677	Abigail S. White, Chunchula, Ala.	Composition for preserving eggs	1/25
31.	177,085	M. Amanda Wilson, Baltimore, Md.	Abdominal supporter	5/9
32.	177,779	L. Frances Woodward, Woodstock, Vt.	Ladies' worktable	5/23
33.	182,984	Leonora E. Yates, Washington, D.C.	Railway tie	10/3

APPENDIX B: CATEGORIZED LISTING OF THE THIRTY-THREE
WOMEN'S INVENTIONS OMITTED IN LWP, 1876

Category	No.	Appendix A	Name	Invention
Agricultural				
Culinary devices,	1.	(15)	Carrie M. Newell	Culinary steamer
food preparation	2.	(21)	Lacy W. Simmons	Grater
	3.	(26)	Anna B. Stapler	Tea and coffee urn
Food preservation	See no. 2 (30) under Chemical/Metallurgical			
Implements/machines	See no. 4 (9) under Machines/Mechanical			
Chemical/Metallurgical				
	1.	(1)	Marie E. P. Audouin (Paris, France)	Composition for lining puddling and other furnaces
	2.	(30)	Abigail S. White	Composition for preserving eggs
Furnishings				
	1.	(25)	Jennie H. Spofford	Mattress supporter
	2.	(32)	L. Frances Woodward	Ladies' worktable
Health/Medicine				
	1.	(19)	Ruth T. Reed	Abdominal supporter
	2.	(31)	M. Amanda Wilson	Abdominal supporter
	3.	(24)	Jennie H. Spofford	Mosquito net frame
	4.	(16)	Emmeline W. Philbrook	Underwaist (reform garment)
	5.	(18)	Emmeline W. Philbrook	Underwaist (reform garment)
Heating, Cooling, and Related				
	1.	(27)	Jane G. Swisshelm	Hot-air chamber
Labor Saving (domestic)				
	1.	(6)	Vashti Chandler	Labor-saving dish drainer
	2.	(7)	Laura J. Gott	Cleaner for jugs, etc.
Machines/Mechanical				
	1.	(3)	Mildred Blakey	Machine for forming hollow welded cylinders
	2.	(4)	Mildred Blakey	Roll for welding and finishing tubing
	3.	(5)	Mary P. Carpenter	Barrel-painting machine
	4.	(9)	Iris Hobson	Potato digger
	5.	(12)	Florence Kroeber	Clock
	6.	(13)	Florence Kroeber	Clock movement
	7.	(28)	Emily E. Tassey	Propulsion of vessels
	8.	(29)	Emily E. Tassey	Dredging machinery

(*Continued on next page*)

(APP. B—*Continued*)

Category	No.	Appendix A	Name	Invention
Manufacturing (including home production)				
	1.	(20)	Ellen P. Rich	Pattern for garment
Machines	See nos. 1–3 (3, 4, 5) under Machines/Mechanical			
Timekeeping, Measurement, and Related				
	See nos. 5–6 (12, 13) under Machines/Mechanical			
Transportation				
	1.	(33)	Leonora E. Yates	Railway tie
	2.	(23)	Jennie H. Spofford	Riding saddle
	See also nos. 7–8 (28, 29) under Machines/Mechanical			
Wearing Apparel and Related				
	1.	(2)	Julia D. Banfield	Corset
	2.	(10)	Catharine Judson	Corset spring
	3.	(11)	Catharine Judson	Reissue of corset spring (see no. 2 [10])
	4.	(14)	Harriet H. May	Corset
	5.	(17)	Emmeline W. Philbrook	Spring clasp garment
	See also nos. 4–5 (16, 18) under Health/Medicine			
Miscellaneous				
	1.	(8)	Ellen A. Hale	Ornamental wall bracket
	2.	(22)	Charlotte L. Slade	Drawing slate

No.	Patent No.	Name and Residence	Invention	Date
1.	171,774	Mary P. Carpenter, New York, N.Y.	Machine for sewing straw braid	1/4
2.	172,966	Elizabeth Sloan, New York, N.Y.	Plaiting attachment for sewing machine	2/1
3.	173,674	Mary F. Sallade, Philadelphia, Pa.	Plaiting machine	2/15
4.	176,219	Ella J. Crosby, Sabula, Iowa	Hair-heading machine	4/18
5.	177,084	Georgiana L. Townsend, Philadelphia, Pa.	Device for operating sewing machine	5/9
6.	179,792	Rosa Heilmann, New York, N.Y.	Washing machine	7/11
7.	180,286	Emily E. Tassey, McKeesport, Pa.	Apparatus for raising sunken vessels	7/25
8.	180,337	Laura E. Haack, St. Louis, Mo.	Automatic fan	7/25
9.	180,387	Julia E. Snapp, Georgetown, Ill.	Spinning attachment for sewing machines	7/25
10.	181,203	Emily Rochow, Brooklyn, N.Y.	Centrifugal sugar machine	8/15
11.	181,353	Sarah Lindsley, Collins, N.Y.	Washing machine	8/22
12.	182,016	Jennie M. Boyce, Belvidere, Ill.	Plaiting machine	9/12
13.	182,096	Kate C. Barton, Philadelphia, Pa.	Sewing machine	9/12
14.	182,636	Lizzie J. Boyd, Coatesville, Pa.	Plaiting machine	9/26
15.	182,773	Lydie F. Renshaw, Cohasset, Mass.	Improvement in sectional steam generators	10/3
16.	183,213	Marie E. Ronat, Rochelle, Ill.	Plow	10/10
17.	183,799	Emily J. Cutter (Cutler?), Malden, Mass.	Fluting apparatus	10/31
18.	184,959	Mary Duff, Benton, Ill.	Hemmer for sewing machine	12/5
19.	184,996	Emily E. Tassey, Pittsburgh, Pa.	Siphon propeller-pump	12/5
20.	185,040	Hannah Milsom, Buffalo, N.Y.	Ozone machine	12/5

(*Continued on next page*)

(APP. C—*Continued*)

Categorized Listing of LWP Machines for 1876

Category	Total	Invention No.
Agricultural	1	16
Health/Medicine	1	20
Heating, Cooling, and Related	1	8
Manufacturing[a]	8	1, 2, 4, 5, 9, 10, 13, 18
Services[b]	6	3, 6, 11, 12, 14, 17
Transportation	2	7, 19
Other[c]	1	15

Traditional/Nontraditional Distribution		
Traditional[d]	16	
Sewing[e]	5	1, 2, 5, 13, 18
Spinning[e]	1	9[f]
Washing (laundry)[e]	2	6, 11
Ironing, pleating (laundry)[e]	4	3, 12, 14, 17
Health, medicine	1	20[g]
Heating, cooling	1	8
Food production	1	10
Grooming aids	1	4
Nontraditional[h]	4	
Apparatus for raising sunken vessels	1	7
Steam generator	1	15
Plow	1	16
Siphon propellor-pump	1	19

[a] This listing counts home manufacturing, and assumes that the centrifugal sugar machine is for candy making, probably for use by a confectioner.

[b] All have to do with laundry.

[c] This could belong with heating apparatus—not yet determined.

[d] Defined as connected with women's traditional work in the nineteenth century, whether done at home or in a factory, irrespective of technological significance.

[e] All are related to sewing or laundry.

[f] Attachment for a sewing machine.

[g] Some studies indicate more women healers than men in the nineteenth century.

[h] Defined as heavy or highly technical machines: machines used in endeavors not connected with women's traditional work or areas of responsibility in the nineteenth century.

Part 2
Transformations of the Work Process

Introduction

Myra Marx Ferree

There is little doubt that technology is dramatically changing the working conditions of women today. Some commentators have seen the transformations of the work process that microprocessors and computerization in general have introduced to be nothing less than a second industrial revolution. It is also clear that much of the impact of these dramatic changes will be felt in occupations in which women workers are concentrated, particularly in clerical and service occupations where half of all employed women work.

The significant presence of women in the labor force (43 of every 100 paid workers are women) can in part be attributed to earlier technological transformations of the economy that created particular jobs for which women were thought to be well suited. For example, the expansion of businesses from local family-owned firms to national corporations cannot be separated from the invention of the typewriter, the new division between managerial and clerical occupations, and the sex segregation that defined women by their relationship to these new machines. The continued growth in the size and complexity of business enterprises has brought more and more women into the labor force to handle the ever-expanding information such enterprises generate, until today one of every three employed women works in a clerical occupation. What will happen now to these and other occupations and to the women workers in them as technological innovations continue to change both the nature of the work available and the conditions under which it is done?

Important as this question is, it captures only part of the relationship between women and technology in the workplace. Technology changes power relations as well as working conditions, and not always in ways that were anticipated or that one-sidedly reinforce the position of the more powerful party. The consequences of technological innovations are so complex that even those who have the power to control the extent and nature of technological transformation are not always able to assess the probable outcomes of specific changes with any degree of accuracy. In many instances there may be new and unintended opportunities for women workers to increase their control over their own work conditions. Women are not merely passive recipients of altered conditions of employment; women can and do actively intervene to introduce changes that they perceive to be to their advantage and to resist innovations that they see as threatening. It is thus equally important to ask how women evaluate and respond to particular new technologies and to consider the social and political circumstances in which these technologies are introduced.

The articles in this section bring these concerns about both work conditions and power relationships together as they address several important dimensions of technological transformation. First, each connects technology to a broader picture of economic forces such as market transformations, industrial shifts, or changes in the division of labor. They thus avoid a simplistic technological determinism in which inventions and innovations appear as the only dynamic forces reshaping the world of work. Instead the authors consider the economic context in which certain kinds of inventions become useful and ask the intriguing and important question, to whom are they important and for what purposes?

The problem of determining whose interests are served by the introduction of new technologies rarely has one unambiguous solution, even for the individuals directly involved. This is closely related to Timm Triplett's point about the "valence" of particular technologies. He suggests that technologies have both positive and negative values inherent in them, though not necessarily in equal measure. His consideration of the transformation of work experienced by recent generations of women in the Hebrides Islands highlights this ambiguity and emphasizes the importance of incorporating the users' own ambivalence into theories of technological transformation. Triplett prompts us to think critically about the pro- and antitechnology positions articulated in the literature and invites consideration of important questions about women's role in creating culture under different technological conditions, although it is not his intent to answer these questions here.

Instead, he offers the case of Hebridean women as a way of considering the social implications of technologies and as a reflection on the values gained and lost in technological transformation. The women of the Hebrides Islands interviewed in the 1950s had actually lived through the process of industrialization and with it the loss of some traditional skills and activities (such as cloth making). Triplett shows how industrial technologies brought other related costs to women, particularly the loss of the cohesiveness of the work community, the comprehensibility of the work, and the distinctive cultural expression of women's work songs. But he also provides evidence of important gains for women. The women themselves point out that the old days were not so good. While they readily admit the losses, they also see advantages, particularly that women no longer have to work so hard as they once did. Triplett's exploration of this ambivalence in a concrete instance gives weight to his theoretical position that technological transformation is too complex a process to simply support or oppose across the board. At the same time he prompts us to wonder if there are now or ever will be work songs suited to the rhythms of the technology of today.

In some cases, however, the consequences of new technology seem to be unambiguously good for women, even if other social changes are not to their advantage at that point. Christine Kleinegger's study of the transformation of farm work for American women in the first half of this century makes clear how important running water in the home was for farm wives and how they struggled to obtain this simple but significant technology to help them in their work. But Kleinegger also shows how this struggle was situated in the overall transformation of American agriculture that increased the size of farms, centralized chicken raising and butter and cheese production, eliminated women's independent sources of income (the proverbial butter-and-egg money), and sharpened the division between male (outdoor, income-producing) and female (indoor, consumption-oriented) labor. Faced with both the loss of their traditional sources of power and a heightened conflict of interest along gender lines, farm wives had to struggle for a redefinition of their roles and recognition of their work in order to make their demands for indoor plumbing effective. It is also worth noting that Kleinegger's study avoids a simplistic reduction of women's work to that which earns an income.

Eileen Appelbaum's analysis is also sensitive to the nontechnological dimensions of change. She situates the transformations of computer technology in a wider context of change in the insurance industry. Inflation, unstable but rising interest rates, government deregulation, and heightened competition all gave insurance carriers a new interest in finding technological ways not only to control their labor costs but also to decentralize and speed decision making. This dual purpose produced ambiguous outcomes for women workers in the industry. On the one hand, the low-skill clerical and routine technical jobs in which women have predominated are often eliminated by the new computer and communications technologies, along with the career paths that led from these jobs to low-level professional positions, paths that affirmative action had only recently opened. Thus skill requirements for clerical jobs have increased, even though these jobs are increasingly dead-end.

On the other hand, the extreme division of functions that automation produced in the factory does not seem to be replicated in the office. The new clerical jobs that have emerged are often less fragmented as well as more skilled, managers have more direct access to more integrated data, and agents and underwriters in the field have more latitude in issuing policies. Employers have adjusted their personnel policies to these changed conditions of work. As the most highly skilled clerical positions—such as adjustors and examiners—have been feminized (from 9 percent female in 1962 to 58 percent in 1981) and the number of low-skill clerical jobs has declined, insurance companies have moved out to the suburbs to find more educated clerical workers. This has dramatically decreased employment opportunities for black and urban working-class white women, while offering once isolated, college-educated suburban housewives new chances to find interesting work.

Thus Appelbaum makes clear that the significance of new technology for women will depend in part on their race and class, and that improved opportunities for some white women may be created by company policies that reduce employment and mobility chances for others. The use of computerization by the employer may extend beyond such direct effects as streamlining operations and coordination of decision making to encompass such second-order effects as deepening racial segregation, obtaining a female labor force that is more likely to be married and thus able to work for sub-subsistence wages, and reinforcing the structural barriers between male and female jobs that affirmative action threatened to erode. These effects are not due to technology alone but reflect the social, economic, and political context in which it is implemented.

A second way in which these articles avoid a crude technological determinism is by their focus on how women themselves interpret the meaning of technology and actively integrate it into their work lives. While women themselves rarely have the power to choose or reject the implementation of technology in the workplace, they do evaluate its implications for their own jobs and determine their response accordingly. Here, too, these authors alert us to the diversity of women's experiences.

Valerie Carter's article examines the variety of women's responses to a high-technology environment and situates these different responses in the broader work conditions that surround the introduction of computerization in the office. The usual sociological claim that computers, especially those used for word processing, will degrade and deskill clerical occupations has frequently been seen as an adequate rejoinder to the self-interested arguments of managers about the joys all will find in the electronic office. But Carter finds unexpected complexity in the clerical workers' own evaluations of how computerization has affected their jobs. Rather than attribute the positive regard that some workers show for the computer to naïveté or "false consciousness" about their own exploitation on the job, she looks more closely at the conditions of control that women workers experience in the office and within which computerization takes place.

Distinguishing between patriarchal control in direct interpersonal relations on the one hand, and structural control in the bureaucratic rules and technical conditions of work on the other, Carter is able to analyze the effects as contingent upon existing conditions of control in particular workplaces and on the contradictions between these different types of control as women experience them. Unlike previous research, which has focused almost exclusively on large centralized settings where the issue of patriarchal control was virtually invisible, her sample of clerical workers spans a variety of work and authority relationships and reveals correspondingly diverse views of the technology used there. For clericals in some small offices, the monopoly on technical expertise and ability to eliminate some of the routine drudgery of the job that the computer provided could give them increased control and enjoyment in their work. In clerical settings where job fragmentation was already more extreme, computerization could eliminate some jobs entirely while increasing the specialization and supervision experienced by the remaining workers.

The third and final common element in these articles is their attention to what Carter calls "the dialectical nature of the relationship between new technology . . . and workplace control and worker autonomy" and in particular to the resources workers have and the strategies they develop for resisting management control. While the introduction of new technology may change these relationships in important ways, this may not happen in the way management anticipates or in a direction it desires. While Carter considers the possibility that workers will use technological innovations directly to increase their leverage in the workplace, Frieda Rozen's article expands this view to include the indirect contributions of technology to worker resistance.

Rozen looks specifically at how changes in airplane design have affected the occupation of flight attendant and the relative power of workers in this occupation. As larger airplanes were introduced, the ratio of cabin to flight crew changed along with the absolute number of flight attendants. The more intimate settings and lower crew-to-passenger ratios of the smaller aircraft and the airlines' emphasis on noneconomic forms of competition when fares were still regulated contributed to sexualizing the job in the 1950s and 1960s. New large-body aircraft intro-

duced in the 1970s made the work more physically demanding and required more flight attendants, thus resulting in unions large enough to
make their voices heard.

But technology alone did not usher in the age of more militance.
The women's movement also contributed an awareness of the discriminatory impact of age, marital status, and appearance requirements. Once
these were legally overthrown, the average job tenure of the flight attendants could and did rise, and the greater experience and job commitment that resulted increased their willingness to fight to improve their
jobs. Rozen thus situates the influence of technology in a complex social
and economic structure and suggests that strikes and walkouts may be a
consequence of the jet age that airline executives never intended.

In sum, despite the striking diversity of the technologies and
workplaces with which these articles deal, they share several more fundamental characteristics. They all address the technological transformations of women's workplaces without losing sight of the broader economic and political forces that affect the nature of work and women's
response to it. Rather than allowing the processes involved in technological transformations to appear as things that happen to women without
their knowledge or participation, all of these articles also provide a view
of women who relate to technology in diverse ways. Women struggle to
exercise more control over their work conditions, sometimes with the
help of technology and sometimes in the face of its demands. The articles avoid presenting women as a homogeneous group and highlight
several important differences among women workers that may have
significant consequences for how technology affects their jobs and how
they respond to its effects. Such factors range from the social (e.g., race
or education) to the organizational (e.g., size of workplace, control
structure) to the individual (e.g., job tenure, work commitment). As
these few studies already indicate, future research on women, technology, and the workplace will have to take factors at all these levels into
account if it wishes to be true to the multidimensionality of women's
lives and experiences evident here.

Hebrides Women: A Philosopher's View of Technology and Cultural Change

Timm Triplett

This chapter examines certain aspects of the work and lives of women in the Hebrides Islands of Scotland. Hebridean culture has only recently begun to shift from a traditional to a more modern technological base, and examination of this shift helps to shed light on current theoretical debates within both the philosophy of technology and feminist theory. These debates concern the effect of technology on culture and values and more particularly, the relationship between technological development and the status of women. As a philosopher, my interest in these theoretical debates has led me to empirical cultural studies which might have a bearing on the evaluation of the theories.

The first two sections of this article describe the current debates about technology in philosophy and in feminist theory respectively. The third section focuses on women in the Hebrides, while the fourth considers how this specific case raises issues relevant to the evaluation of the theories being debated. I will conclude that current absolutist theories of technological change simply do not square with the ambivalence that Hebrides women express regarding their experience of such change.

Technology and Philosophy

The debate in the philosophy of technology revolves around attempts to assess the meaning and value of technology in its highly developed industrial and postindustrial form. I use the phrase "modern technology" to refer to all technologies that have emerged from the beginning of the Industrial Revolution to the present. Opposing sides of this debate are epitomized by the views of "antitechnologist" Jacques Ellul and "protechnologist" Samuel Florman.

Ellul has presented what have become familiar criticisms of modern technology (Ellul 1954, 1962). In "The Technological Order," he contends that technology, far from freeing us, is leading to greater centralization and ultimately to totalitarianism. Technology does not provide us with intrinsically neutral tools useful for enhancing our comfort and expanding our horizons. Rather, it tends to destroy traditional values by imposing a methodology that sees all human problems in quantitative terms.

> The technical society is not, and cannot be, a genuinely humanist society since it puts in first place not man [*sic*] but material things. It can only act on man by lessening him and putting him in the way of the quantitative. . . . Human excellence, on the contrary, is of the domain of the qualitative and aims at what is not measurable. . . . In our times, technical growth monopolizes all human forces, passions, intelligences, and virtues in such a way that it is in practice nigh impossible to seek and find anywhere any distinctively human excellence. And if this search is impossible, there cannot be any civilization in the proper sense of the term. (Ellul 1962, 401)

Ellul also sees the increased power technology offers us as destructive of traditional values: "I must emphasize a great law which I believe to be essential to the comprehension of the world in which we live, viz., that when power becomes absolute, values disappear. When man is able to accomplish anything at all, there is no value which can be proposed to him" (402). Freedom too is threatened, for "the more technical actions increase in society, the more human autonomy and initiative diminish" (xx).

In sharp contrast to this, Florman's "In Praise of Technology" (1979) extolls technology for enhancing the very values of which Ellul claims we are being deprived.

> It does not violate our common sense to be told that certain people are taking advantage of other people. But is it logical to claim that exploitation increases as a result of the growth of technology? . . . In fact, the evidence is all the other way. In technologically advanced societies there is more freedom for the average citizen than there was in earlier ages. . . . In spite of all the newest electronic gadgetry, governments are scarcely able to prevent the antisocial actions of criminals, much less control every act of every citizen. . . . The rebellious individual is more than holding his own. . . . Those who were slaves are now free. Those who were disenfranchised can now vote. Rigid class structures are giving way to frenetic mobility. (26–27)

Florman acknowledges that modern technology is not an unmixed blessing, but he claims that there is a general preference for it over preindustrial technologies.

> The antitechnologists romanticize the work of earlier times in an attempt to make it seem more appealing than work in a technological age. But their idyllic descriptions do not ring true. Agricultural work, for all its appeal to

the intellectual in his armchair, is brutalizing in its demands. Factory and office work is not a bed of roses either. But given their choice, most people seem to prefer to escape from the drudgery of the farm. This fact fails to impress the antitechnologists, who prefer their sensibilities to the choices of real people. (1979, 25)

What is going on here? It is not just a debate about the "real people" that technology affects, whether for good or ill. Conceptual and definitional issues abound. For example, many so-called antitechnologists, Ellul among them, quite explicitly disavow any claim that our preindustrial past was preferable or that we can and should return to such a mode of life (Ellul 1962, 403). Thus Florman appears to be misconstruing the claims of at least some antitechnologists and errs when he claims that "the antitechnologists repeatedly contrast our abysmal technocracy with three cultures that they consider preferable: the primitive tribe, the peasant community, and medieval society" (Florman 1979, 23). For Ellul, it is far from clear that phrases such as "human autonomy" and "civilization" (in the proper sense) have clear and uncontroversial meanings. These are conceptual issues requiring clarification and evaluation rather than more fact gathering.

Nevertheless, the Ellul-Florman debate is empirical as well as conceptual. Each side professes to give the most adequate description of social reality. Since it is technology specifically that is, according to Ellul, responsible for the present unhappy state of affairs, an examination of preindustrial societies could be quite revealing. For if Ellul's claims are true, then the specific ills he attributes to modern technology could be expected not to appear in a preindustrial society. Since Ellul does not claim preindustrial society is to be preferred, his thesis would not be disconfirmed—though I believe its impact would be considerably weakened—if an overall comparison of the problems of the two societies revealed degrading or brutalizing conditions in the preindustrial society that clearly mark our society as the one to be preferred.

As for Florman's empirical claims, he frequently writes, "the evidence suggests," without actually citing the evidence in question. Some of Florman's claims seem, on the surface, to be nothing but common knowledge, or propositions readily confirmable by straightforward studies of population patterns. But they can actually raise important questions in the mind of the reflective skeptic. For example, the movement from farm to factory was based on broad social trends that the individual could not control. It is far from clear that it was individual preference on a mass scale that led to the urban migrations of the nineteenth and twentieth centuries. Small-scale farms were less and less economically viable. Farmers and peasants were sometimes forcibly evicted from their lands (Prebble 1969). Multitudes of new jobs were meanwhile opening up in the cities. Thus, the existence of urban migrations does not automatically suggest that people prefer factory jobs to farming jobs. Where people's preferences are at issue, empirical research must include oral histories and sophisticated work in human psychology, in addition to the study of urban migration patterns.

More recent work in the philosophy of technology expands the set of concepts and categories relevant to the debate. Borgmann (1984) in *Technology and the Character of Contemporary Life,* divides theories of modern technology into three basic categories. *Substantivism* is defined as the view that modern technology is "a force in its own right, one that shapes today's societies and values from the ground up and has no serious rivals" (Borgmann 1984, 9). The substantivist can be either protechnology or antitechnology depending on how the impact of this fundamental force on society is evaluated. *Instrumentalism* is the view that modern technology is only a value-neutral tool—a "mere means" that does not in itself impose any specific direction on society. *Pluralism* opposes substantivism by claiming that modern technology creates too many often counteracting effects to display the one dominant pattern the substantivist claims to see. Yet in opposition to the instrumentalist, the pluralist maintains that specific technologies or technological systems can be value-laden (Borgmann 1984, 10–11). The concept of value-laden technology is clarified and developed in "Women and the Assessment of Technology" (1983) by Corlann G. Bush in her discussion of "valenced" technology. Bush argues that:

> to believe that technologies are neutral tools subject only to the motives and morals of the user is to miss completely their collective significance. Tools and technologies have what I can only describe as valence, a bias or "charge" analogous to that of atoms that have lost or gained electrons through ionization. A particular technological system, even an individual tool, has a tendency to interact in similar situations in identifiable and predictable ways. In other words, particular tools or technologies tend to be favored in certain situations, tend to perform in a predictable manner in these situations, and tend to bend other interactions to them. Valence tends to seek out or fit in with certain social norms and to ignore or disturb others. (154–55)

Technology and Feminism

Within feminist studies there is also a striking diversity of attitudes toward modern technology. The debates in this arena are not simply reducible to other fundamental debates, e.g., the debate between radical and liberal feminism, but they do reflect the three attitudes toward technology described above. Three specific positions will be described that help to illustrate this point. All are part of the radical feminist framework, yet each has a markedly different attitude toward modern technology.

In *The Dialectic of Sex* (1970), Shulamith Firestone argues that technological development is a precondition for complete freedom for women. She calls for "the freeing of women from the tyranny of their reproductive biology by every means available" (206). She describes pregnancy as a "barbaric" condition and holds that freedom is wholly attainable only after technology has rendered pregnancy obsolete (198). Firestone's optimism about the liberating potential of breakthroughs in reproductive technology is matched by her optimism about technology in general.

> The misuse of scientific developments is very often confused with technology itself. . . . As was demonstrated in the case of the development of atomic energy, radicals, rather than breastbeating about the immorality of scientific research, could be much more effective by concentrating their *full* energies on demands for control of scientific discoveries by and for the people. For, like atomic energy, fertility control, artificial reproduction, cybernation, in themselves, are liberating—*unless* they are improperly used. (196)

In direct opposition to Firestone's optimism, Sally M. Gearhart "indicts" technology on the basis of "its inherent values and epistemology" (1983, 172). Her pessimistic conclusion is that we cannot justify the use of any tool because of modern technology's capacity for human alienation and planetary destruction. The only solution would be to "undo Western sciences" and it is seriously doubtful whether that can happen. Indeed, Gearhart holds that "from the point of view of our fellow species and the earth itself, the best that can happen is that human beings never conceive another child" (180–81).

Here we see a difference on the issue of whether technology has or lacks a valence, as Bush puts it. In Borgmann's terms, we have a debate between Firestone's instrumentalism and Gearhart's substantivism. Gearhart is similar to Firestone, however, in that she does not oppose male and female values and modes of thought. She does not draw on different and specifically female sets of values in order to entertain the more optimistic possibility that new social institutions informed by female values may one day begin to address the problems brought about by traditional science and technology with their implicit male perspectives and biases.

A third, more pluralist, position on technology within radical feminism is taken by Ynestra King (1983). Like Firestone, and unlike Gearhart, King sees science and technology as potentially fulfilling a positive role in helping to achieve a nonsexist society. But King implicitly rejects Firestone's instrumentalism, which sees the problem only in terms of the abuse of tools that we are free to use for good or ill. For King, the very nature of science and technology must be radically transformed before they can serve positive ends. This transformation can come about if feminists consciously choose not to join male culture with its dualistic assumptions about the split between nature (seen as feminine, mysterious, to be dominated or controlled) and culture (masculine, objective, scientific). King calls for the creation of "a different kind of culture and politics that would integrate intuitive/spiritual and rational forms of knowledge, embracing both science and magic insofar as they enable us to transform the nature/culture distinction itself and to envision and create a free, ecological society" (123). In her emphasis on a different kind of technology, King highlights the valence of existing technologies.

I use radical feminism only as an example here. One can readily imagine similar disagreements over the technology issue within other feminist frameworks. This suggests that there is disagreement over some fundamental issue that crosses standard conservative/liberal/radical boundaries. What this fundamental issue is, and how it leads to marked differences within a single feminist perspective, is brought out by Maggie McFadden (1984), who distinguishes between "maximizers" and "minimizers" in feminist theory. The maximizer emphasizes and insists on fundamental differences between women and men; the minimizer deemphasizes the differences that do exist, attributing them to particular social and historical conditions. Firestone envisions an androgynous society where even reproduction is not tied to women and traditionally "male" and "female" characteristics are shared more or less equally by individuals of both sexes. This view, which falls within the same minimizer category as the liberal feminist perspective, holds that the essential equality of men and women will become evident as soon as relatively minor political and social changes are effected: for example, equal legal rights, affirmative action, and men's participation in child care and housework.

Although King calls for an integration of science and magic, the rational and the intuitive, she would seem to be best classified as a maximizer because she sees this holism as a product of the recognition that "we can   consciously choose not to sever the woman nature connections by joining male culture" (1983, 123). She also advocates political actions that "draw on women's culture: embodying what is best in women's life-oriented socialization, building on women's differences, organizing antihierarchically in small groups in visually and emotionally imaginative ways" (127). Thus, men have developed a culture, a way of thinking, that women can and should challenge from their fundamentally different perspective. As radical as King's stance is, it shares maximizer assumptions with conservatives who view women's traditionally subservient roles as justified by the very nature of women and their fundamental differences from men.

Women's Work in the Hebrides

A word on the transition from the theoretical discussions above to the specific cultural focus that follows: I have presented these theoretical debates preparatory to discussing Hebrides culture because it is instructive to reflect on whether the aspects of Hebrides women's lives presented here help support absolutist pro- or antitechnology positions, the maximizers or the minimizers, in debates over sex differences. But I do not regard the Hebrides material as simply a convenient arena in which to allow theoretical battles to rage; the culture itself is intrinsically and independently interesting enough to warrant attention.

Women's Work, Women's Songs

The Outer Hebrides, seventy miles off the Scottish coast, are bleak, rocky islands at the mercy of ocean winds and storms. Little will grow there, even animals are scarce, but the islanders have sustained their own unique culture. Largely bypassed by the industrial revolution of the nineteenth century, the Hebrides Islands retained important aspects of feudal social and economic structures into the twentieth century. Geographical isolation and the difficulty of travel prevented new social, economic, and technological trends from easily taking hold on the islands and required the islanders to maintain themselves with a high degree of self-sufficiency.

These factors make Hebrides culture a particularly valuable one for insight into questions about the transition from a preindustrial to an industrial technology. We can evaluate the felt experience of this transition and uncover attitudes toward the old and new ways of life quite directly because the individuals who embodied these experiences and attitudes were contemporaneous with the tape recorder, film, and other tools of modern scholarship, as well as with a community of scholars willing and able to record their changing ways of life. This allows us an unusually direct opportunity to find empirical contact points for some of the theoretical questions discussed above.

In traditional Hebrides society, work, social relations, and cultural expression were intimately tied together. The focus in this section is on the music of the working women, because it was such a vigorous and dominant form of expression. Polly Hitchcock was in the Hebrides in the early 1950s to record the work songs as they were sung in their appropriate work contexts. She provides a specific description of the "waulking," a unique work/social/musical activity that was an important aspect of traditional Hebrides culture.

> In this self-contained unit music played a tremendous part. Not only were all the daily chores, i.e., reaping, waulking, spinning, etc., accompanied by song to relieve the monotony of their tasks, but entertainment consisted of telling tales or singing the heroic songs or the laments that were such an intimate part of their lives and their history. No newspapers, no radios, no amusements, with the result that they were forced to use their own imagination and ingenuity for pleasure.
>
> One of the never ending tasks of the island women was the making of woolen cloth for blankets and clothing. This involved many time-consuming processes. After a shearing, the wool had to be washed, dyed, teased, carded, spun, woven and shrunk, and each of these operations was performed by hand. The last operation, the shrinking of the cloth, was a gay social occasion called a "waulking" and used to occur at least once a week. Today [1952] it is less often. A long table is set up and the heavy wet cloth is spread or laid down one side round the end and up to the other side of the table. The thumping begins and they swing to the right picking up the cloth, then swing to the left passing their portion on to their neighbor with another thump on the table. The cloth is kept in constant circulation, the moisture gradually being beaten out of it. The rhythm of the workers is steadily maintained by singing. One song may go on for fifteen minutes, then there will be a pause and the cloth is measured. Seven times the length of the middle finger is the desired width and may take an hour and a half of songs and labor to achieve, with an occasional resoaking of the cloth. After a final tapping song when the cloth has at last been folded and piled on the table a party follows and the men and children who watch on the sidelines join in for the food and dance that follows. (Hitchcock 1952, 1–2)

The waulking is clearly a social occasion and a means of cultural expression as well as a purely economic activity. Particularly striking is the way in which the cultural expression—in this case the music—is made integral to the work and is not just an addendum to it. This is true of most if not all of the work songs sung by the women. Margaret Fay Shaw (1977) has published examples of waulking songs, spinning songs, milking songs, lullabies, and "clapping" songs (cf. Hitchcock's "tapping songs") which she encountered on the island of South Uist in the Outer Hebrides. All of these songs accompany traditional activities performed by women. In addition, Alan Lomax (1951) has recorded women of Barra, also in the Outer Hebrides, singing dandling songs—playful songs for the entertainment of children—as well as lullabies and spinning, milking, and waulking songs.

These songs were not just a means of relieving the tedium of the work—although many of them surely had that function. They were also essential to the work itself. The songs set the tempo of the work and coordinated collective work activities. Indeed, the islanders must have felt that the work could not be done without the singing. This is particularly clear in the case of the waulking songs. As Hitchcock notes, this is an activity of five to ten women, all handling the same piece of cloth at once. The song was their means of coordinating the rhythmic thumping of the cloth. The waulking song itself is strongly rhythmic and is led by one woman—the reciter—with the rest of the women joining in on the chorus. The reciter sets the tempo of the song and thus of the work. In one of Lomax's recordings, the reciter can be heard gradually increasing the tempo to drive out the last bit of moisture as a piece of cloth is finished up. As the song's tempo increases, the thumping of the cloth on the table can always be heard in perfect time to the music.

The spinning songs are sung by women working alone and would seem to be less integral to the work. The spinning song recorded by Lomax does not have the driving rhythm of the waulking songs sung by the Barra women. Yet there is a gentle and steady pulse to the music that complements the pulse of the work, matching the rhythmic rise and fall of the treadle and the turning of the wheel. One could not say of a spinning song, as one could of a waulking song, that it coordinates and makes the work possible. For the spinning gives rise to the song as much as the song coordinates the spinning. And yet the felt inseparability of work and song is evident from Shaw's description of a woman spinning: "the rhythm of her foot on the treadle brought forth the songs as naturally as her fingers turned the wool to yarn" (1977, 6).

With respect to the lullabies and dandling songs, it is clear how the songs are integral to child care. What is perhaps not so obvious is the integral and essential role these songs had to play in the Hebridean household. One of the Barra women recorded in conversation by Alan Lomax remarked when discussing the dandling songs that there were no toys during her own childhood (Lomax 1951). Consider what the lack of toys means for childrearing work. We are willing to debate whether the television should serve as child entertainment center and babysitter, but we take the existence and usefulness of toys utterly for granted. Without them, songs as well as other forms of direct self-generated entertainment were absolutely essential components of child care.

An entirely different sort of work—matchmaking—seems to play a role in the tapping or clapping songs performed at the end of the waulking. Hitchcock refers to the party and dance that follow the waulking, immediately after the tapping song. Shaw reports further on the context of what she calls the clapping song:

> When the tweed is shrunk sufficiently it is rolled up tightly and two women, facing each other, clap it hard in quick time. In this [clapping] song, sung for that occasion, they will pair off for fun the young folk that are attending the waulking.
> The words of (the clapping) songs are to a great extent extemporized and consist of witty and ribald remarks about the people present with reference to their actual or possible love affairs. (1977, 268, 7)

Cohesiveness, Comprehensibility, Closure

These descriptions suggest that songs, socializing, certain relatively direct forms of parent-child interaction, and direct relationships with neighbors were integral and essential features of Hebrides women's traditional work. The community and family were directly aware of women's work and their songs. Their music was the creative product of the culture itself, not an external or standardized product imposed from without.

The nature of work in the Hebrides makes clear that there was, indeed there had to be, a cohesive community spirit. Clearly, this community of women was much closer than that normally found in modern suburbia, where each housewife engages in chores essentially similar to those of her neighbors, yet most of her work is done in isolation from them. At a waulking, the women had to work together almost as a single unit, sensing one another's beat and together creating rhythmic and melodic patterns that uniquely identified their culture and even their particular village. How different the ensuing material product, the cloth, must have seemed from cloth or clothing bought at the local mall. Yet the cohesiveness of the Hebridean community involves even more than the unity of materially productive labor and cultural or aesthetic expression. Social expression also is involved. The waulking was an occasion for gossip, courtship, group entertainment, and other forms of social bonding. This unity of work, play, social bonding, and artistic expression engenders an especially rich sense of community.

Comprehensibility is another feature of such a culture. This can best be illustrated by considering the children of that culture. In the Hebrides culture, the children could watch their parents participate in a goal-directed, comprehensible process. The sheep are tended and sheared, the wool is carded, spun, woven, and shrunk. The children see their mothers and fathers engaged in these activities and are not puzzled about what their parents do for a living. The activities go on all around them, and they can themselves begin to take part at a relatively early age. Contrast this with our children, who often cannot really understand why mom or dad or both spend the bulk of their time at the office or what exactly one does there; or how clothing, food, and other commodities purchased ready-made in the store got there in the first place; or what was involved in their production.

Another aspect of comprehensibility is recognition and respect. The role of music in the culture can be directly recognized and appreciated. So, too, the role of women as bearers of their culture's musical traditions and as productive workers is acknowledged.

Related to these properties of cohesiveness and comprehensibility is the concept of what Corlann Bush has termed "closure." In "Women and the Assessment of Technology," Bush compares laundry work past and present. She recalls the weekly laundry days of her childhood, when mother, grandmother, and children met together for socializing and work:

> Having laundry and a day on which to do it was an organizing principle . . . around which women allocated their time and resources. . . . There was closure, a sense of completion and accomplishment impossible to achieve today when my sister washes, dries, folds and irons her family's clothes everyday or when I wash only because I have nothing to wear. (1983, 59)

In the Hebrides, too, there was closure. A task, by its community nature, took place at a specified time and usually ended with a finished product. It is helpful to overlay the concept of closure with the factory work younger women in the Hebrides eventually faced. Like modern laundering as described by Bush, factory work lacks a sense of closure. It consists of single operations endlessly repeated. There is no finished product from the worker's point of view, no end to the task except that dictated by the boss or the clock.

Creativity

The strong connection I have noted between women's work and cultural expression in the Hebrides tradition deserves notice not just as a means of rediscovering something that has been lost in our own culture. The Hebrides example challenges the common belief that men embody a creative principle or essence denied to women—a belief expressed in the oft-asked question, But why haven't there been any great women artists? Even Simone de Beauvoir seems to have accepted the idea that in traditional cultures women historically have been, as she puts it, "doomed to immanence," the condition of living only for others or for one's most immediate needs, in contrast to "transcendence," the creative principle that is at the root of both art and science. In *The Second Sex* she writes:

> Woman perpetuated [the existence of the male principle] in the flesh, but her role was only nourishing, never creative. In no domain whatever did she create; she maintained the life of the tribe by giving it children and bread, nothing more. She remained doomed to immanence, incarnating only the static aspect of society, closed in upon itself. Whereas the man went on monopolizing the function that threw open that society toward the rest of humanity. . . . The male remained alone the incarnation of transcendence. (1952, 67–68)

The Hebrides women can hardly be said to fill this description. The songs I have discussed, performed by women to accompany tasks that were also performed by women, were surely as much women's products as were the fabrics they produced. If we grant to the men their fishing songs, battle songs, and drinking songs, we must grant to the women their dandling songs, lullabies, spinning songs, and waulking songs.

Studies of other cultures have also challenged de Beauvoir's assumptions (MacCormack 1980, 16–17; Harris 1980, 15–34, 175–76). Perhaps we need to look at women not as historically absent from artistic and creative roles throughout the past, but as being deprived of these roles when cultures that encouraged and required women's creative expression gave way to other, more limiting cultures. Perhaps as societal institutions and economies became developed enough to allow the emergence of high art, the mastery of which required long years of specialized training, these institutions, by now fully male dominated, were able to control the extent to which women could participate in the required training.

Evaluations

In the foregoing discussion it may seem as though I am taking the side of the antitechnologist, and, on the creativity issue, the minimizer. I have indeed been emphasizing apparently valuable and humanizing aspects of Hebrides life and have noted a creative role for women that does not place them apart from men in regard to creative expression. I also want to insist that we be willing to critically compare the values of modern technological societies to the often quite different values of preindustrial societies and be prepared to rethink and transform our own values in light of such comparisons.

But this is only part of the story. Thinking of Los Angeles rush-hour traffic on a smoggy day or the toxic waste dump in our town, thinking too of the hectic, individuated, overstimulated ways in which so many of us lead our lives, unattached to any sustaining community or even (more and more frequently) to a family, we are naturally inclined to focus on the positive aspects of Hebrides life that are lost to us. But this may not at all be what the Hebrideans themselves focus on. So far, I have discussed the purely traditional aspects of Hebrides culture. It is time now to recall that this is a culture in transition. Many of the traditional ways of life are rapidly disappearing or have already disappeared. What do the Hebrideans think of this? Consider this conversation between Alan Lomax and the Barra women (Lomax 1951):

Alan Lomax: Do the people still make their own clothes here?
First Woman: No, no dear.
Second Woman: Very little weaving done here.
First: No, that's too late. You know, all that is done away [from here?].
Lomax: What's happened to replace all these old arts?
First: The mills! And all these new things.
Lomax: Do you think it's too bad?
First: No, no. I think it's a very good idea, cause twas too much for the women here.
Second: Oh yes, life was too hard, taking up a family besides that.
Third Woman: But listen! They lived longer than they [do now].
Fourth Woman: Yes. They lived longer. My mother was ninety-two. And she had a loom and all that, and a family to bring up. . . . Twasn't an easy thing. They wouldn't do it today, though.

There is here a certain nostalgia for the past, a pride in hard work, a concern about the effects of the new way of life on health, but there is also, quite strongly, a statement of preference for the new over the old. Even the mention of the allegedly more healthy life of old ends with the remark that people would not work that hard today (see also Cooper 1977, 178). This sort of ambivalence in the statements of the islanders appears throughout the literature on the Hebrides (Thompson 1970; Cooper 1977; Ennew 1980).

There are also negative sides to each of the particular features of Hebridean society I have discussed. Cohesiveness surely offers positive values: a unity of purpose and a sense of place too often lacking in our own culture. But a cohesive community can also be closed, xenophobic, and oppressive. The individual can lack privacy and find that relationships, while relatively stable, are stultifying or even hostile rather than supportive. And there may be no escape short of completely severing ties, which is often not a realistic possibility. Comprehensibility also implies limitation. The fact that a child can understand the productive basis of a culture indicates that the culture is a relatively simple one that may not offer opportunity and challenge. As for closure, having a day of the week designated as laundry day or the day for a waulking means that the laundry (or waulking) is going to get done on that day, like it or not! Many Americans prefer the flexibility and freedom offered by twenty-four-hour supermarkets and laundromats open on Sunday mornings. All this suggests that attempts to draw support for the antitechnology position from the data presented here will not succeed.

More detailed empirical studies, including those specifically conducted with an eye toward informing the theoretical debates discussed here, are certainly necessary. It is unlikely, however, that such studies will prove that a property like cohesiveness is unambiguously negative in a given cultural context. For the very factors that tend to produce the positive qualities we associate with cohesiveness tend also to produce the negative ones. The very factors that make a community cohesive or supportive—for example, its smallness or intimacy—also allow it to be suffocating. Indeed, it can be both at once. And just as there are negative aspects to typical features of preindustrial societies, so there are positive aspects to typical features of postindustrial societies—for example, the freedom and flexibility that come with giving up closure. Having stores open at all hours may seem a trivial gain for the values lost with closure, but it is an important and unresolved question just how gains and losses are to be measured when comparing different sets of values.

Ultimately, I believe that a strong pro- or antitechnology position cannot be sustained. Modern technology does not impose a single value on us. Social reality is something more complex and ambivalent than can be accommodated by these relatively unqualified positions. Both Ellul's condemnation and Florman's praise of technology seem to me to be based on selective and seriously incomplete pictures of this social reality. Florman is more moderate and willing to make concessions than Ellul, yet he still appears not to recognize the full force of some of the antitechnologist positions. The picture presented by both valuations taken together is probably more accurate than either picture in isolation.

I also believe, though I am not as certain, that the same conclusion can be made regarding maximizer and minimizer positions in feminist theory. The fact that Hebrides women have an important creative role does not necessarily mean they are like men, even with respect to creativity. The creativity of men and women may be of different types. It may be that cases like this do not allow us to decide in favor of maximizer or minimizer theories because they do not isolate biological from environmental causes of behaviors, attitudes, and social roles. But I suspect that, in addition, theories are indeterminate with respect to the data because, analogously with the pro- and antitechnology theories, neither the unqualified maximizer theory nor the unqualified minimizer theory can accommodate a full range of data.

If this is so, then the fact that empirical studies are unlikely to unequivocally support the theories of the pro- or antitechnologists, the maximizers or minimizers, is the fault of the theories and not of the empirical studies. These particular theories oversimplify the complex, whereas the empirical studies themselves can be richly suggestive.

We surely do not need to resign ourselves to skepticism regarding these debates in the philosophy of technology and feminist theory. I am confident that the "pure" and relatively unqualified theories that scholars are naturally inclined to formulate first will give way to more complex but more accurate ones. But this means that we need more sophisticated empirical studies, not that we should give up hope of understanding a too complex social reality. The debates include evaluative as well as purely empirical elements, but we need not conclude that evaluative issues are unresolvable. For example, my claim that both positive and negative values are inevitably embedded in social properties like cohesiveness or closure should not be taken to imply that the positive and the negative are always exactly balanced and that it is therefore hopeless to try to determine whether cohesiveness tends in a given cultural context to be beneficial, all things considered. I see no reason why we could not find that the advantages of cohesiveness outweigh its disadvantages and take steps to reincorporate this value into our social structure. Determining this, of course, could not be a purely empirical matter, but I believe that carefully thought out empirical studies are essential if we are to fully understand and resolve the evaluative components of the debates.

Finally, we can find value in empirical studies and comparisons quite apart from any help they provide us in theorizing. Even before we determine which theory is the most adequate, we can see differences, with respect to features such as cohesiveness and closure, between modern and preindustrial cultures. We can see values lost and values gained in the transition to modern cultures. For reasons suggested above, we can probably never achieve a society that incorporates all the positive and none of the negative values of past and present, preindustrial and industrialized cultures. But it could well happen that a society might lose sight of any values except those it currently holds. Such a failure of imagination and empathetic understanding would seriously hinder a society's ability to draw on the full range of human experience in resolving its own conflicts and setting its own goals. To prevent this, we must continue to look back to the Hebrides and other traditional cultures to remind us not only of what we have gained but also of what we once valued and have since lost.

NOTE

I would like to thank the editorial collective of this volume for suggestions that improved this article. I am also grateful to Steve Reyna of the University of New Hampshire Sociology and Anthropology Department for bibliographical suggestions.

REFERENCES

Borgmann, A. 1984. *Technology and the character of contemporary life: A philosophical inquiry.* Chicago: University of Chicago Press.
Bush, C. G. 1983. Women and the assessment of technology: To think, to be, to unthink, to free. In *Machina ex dea. See* Rothschild 1983.
Cooper, D. 1977. *Hebridean connection.* Boston: Routledge and Kegan Paul.
de Beauvoir, S. 1952. *The second sex.* New York: Bantam.
Ellul, J. [1954] 1964. *The technological society.* Reprint. New York: Vintage.
———. 1962. The technological order. *Technology and Culture* 3:394–421.
Ennew, J. 1980. *The Western Isles today.* New York: Cambridge University Press.
Firestone, S. 1970. *The dialectic of sex.* New York: Bantam.
Florman, S. 1979. In praise of technology. In *Technology and change,* ed. J. Burke and M. Eakin. San Francisco: Boyd and Fraser.

Gearhart, S. M. 1983. An end to technology: A modest proposal. In *Machina ex dea. See* Rothschild 1983.

Harris, O. 1980. The power of signs: Gender, culture and the wild in the Bolivian Andes. In *Nature, culture and gender,* ed. C. MacCormack and M. Strathern. Cambridge: Cambridge University Press.

Hitchcock, P. 1952. Introductory notes to *Songs and pipes of the Hebrides.* New York: Folkways Records.

King, Y. 1983. Toward an ecological feminism and a feminist ecology. In *Machina ex dea. See* Rothschild 1983.

Lomax, A. 1951. *Heather and glen.* Century City, Calif.: Tradition Records.

MacCormack, C. 1980. Nature, culture and gender: A critique. In *Nature, culture and gender,* ed. C. MacCormack and M. Strathern. Cambridge: Cambridge University Press.

McFadden, M. 1984. Anatomy of a difference: Toward a classification of feminist theory. *Women's Studies International Forum* 7, no. 6:495–504.

Prebble, J. 1969. *The highland clearances.* Harmondsworth: Penguin.

Rothschild, J. 1983. *Machina ex dea: Feminist perspectives on technology.* New York: Pergamon Press.

Sanday, P. 1981. *Female power and male dominance.* Cambridge: Cambridge University Press.

Shaw, M. F. 1977. *Folksongs and folklore of South Uist.* 2d ed. New York: Oxford University Press.

Thompson, F. 1970. *St. Kilda and other Hebridean outliers.* New York: Praeger.

Out of the Barns and into the Kitchens: Transformations in Farm Women's Work in the First Half of the Twentieth Century

Christine Kleinegger

In 1917 Susan Keating Glaspell published an extraordinary story called "A Jury of Her Peers" about the grim life of a farm woman. The story is both a psychological drama and a murder mystery about a farmer who has been strangled to death. The sheriff and deputy, accompanied by their wives, go to the isolated farm to investigate the murder. While the men search the barn and yard for clues, they leave the ladies to putter among "the insignificance of kitchen things," since the sheriff wonders, "would the women know a clue if they did come upon it?" Ironically, all the clues to who strangled the farmer (his wife) are in the kitchen, in the form of domestic irregularities that only the women detect—half-done chores, erratic sewing on a quilt—and the lack of labor-saving devices, which suggests the wife's motive in killing her husband. Gradually the two women perceive who committed the murder, and their horror turns to sympathy for the murderess. The sheriff's wife observes, "The law is the law—and a bad stove is a bad stove. . . . Think of what it would mean, year after year, to have that stove to wrestle with. The thought of Minnie Foster trying to bake in that oven!" Ultimately these law-abiding ladies destroy the evidence that points to the guilt of the farm wife. They clean up the kitchen and rip out the quilting, while the men continue their fruitless search for clues in all the wrong places. It is a remarkably subversive story in that it suggests that the lack of a good cooking stove justifies homicide. Glaspell powerfully illustrates the drudgery, isolation, and frustration of many farm women's lives.

The story also serves as a cautionary tale for historians, showing that the "insignificance of kitchen things"—so long ignored by historians—holds clues to the meaning of women's work and women's lives. The context of women's work must be examined with a critical eye, in much the same manner that the sheriff's wife scrutinized the farm kitchen—with "that look of seeing into things, of seeing through a thing to something else . . . as if seeing what that kitchen meant through all the years."[1]

What the kitchen, the barn, and the yard have meant for farm women through all the years—or, more accurately, during the first half of the twentieth century—is the main subject of this article. Our focus is the domestic labor of farm women in the first half of the twentieth century, with special attention given to the transition from household production to consumerism, the sexual division of labor on the farm, and the role of labor-saving devices as an oft-proffered panacea for the ills of farm women.

In the late nineteenth century there existed a traditional integration of women's household production in the farm economy. In the twentieth century much of this production was removed from the home and female supervision, as dairying, poultry, and truck farming were ultimately organized as agribusinesses. This can be viewed as a stage in the "masculinization of agriculture," a process that can be traced back to earliest times when primitive women were primarily responsible for agricultural production. In the twentieth century, "masculinization" consists of increased mechanization, specialization, capital outlay, and scientific expertise. To none of these did the average farm woman have direct access.

Before the mid-nineteenth century almost all cheese, in the United States as well as Europe, had been made at home by women. A common saying in Great Britain was, "What does a man know about cheese?" and in France all the principal cheeses were created by women.[2] Madame Harel developed Camembert in 1781 and passed the recipe on to her daughter. While a woman invented the sublime Camembert, it was a man who is responsible for "American" cheese as we know it today. J. L. Kraft "perfected" processed American cheese in the first decades of this century, and through mass production, heavy advertising, and mass selling he built his business up to a $30 million concern by 1925.[3]

Cheese was the first dairy product to leave the purview of women for the factory. The first cheese factory in the United States was founded in 1831; by 1869, two-thirds of all cheese in the United States was manufactured in factories.[4] By 1910, 99 percent of all cheese was made in factories.[5] Although in the late nineteenth century a few women served as head manufacturers in the factories at salaries as high as one hundred dollars per month, more commonly women were employed in subordinate positions at sixteen to twenty dollars a month. A man with only a year or more of experience might earn thirty-five to forty-five dollars.[6]

The extent to which women were no longer involved in dairy production can be discerned from a survey conducted in Wisconsin in 1918. Managers of creameries, condenseries, cheese factories, and milk plants were asked whether hiring women workers would be a feasible solution to war-related labor shortages in the dairy industry. That several establishments had "already demonstrated that women *can learn* to . . . make cheese" suggests that most women no longer possessed this skill.[7] Some of the obstacles in hiring women included: protective legislation setting maximum hours, the inability of women to lift ten- and twenty-gallon cans of cream, and cultural proscriptions such as "a woman is out of place working in a creamery as women were intended by the Creator to make a home for men. . . ."[8] On the other hand, one milk plant manager reported that "it is an advantage to use women in this work because more hands can be employed for the same amount of money."[9] Most women workers in dairy plants did office work, washed bottles and milk cans and performed other janitorial duties, wrapped butter, and ran laboratory tests on the milk and cream.

In 1863 the *Rural New Yorker,* a farm weekly, praised the establishment of cheese factories by noting, "They save labor, relieving the 'women folks' of nearly all the drudgery of cheese making . . . besides they increase the quantity and generally improve the quality."[10] The *Rural New Yorker*'s concern about the dubious quality of home-produced cheese is not an isolated remark. One finds ample evidence in the farm literature that challenges any nostalgic notions about the intrinsic wholesomeness of farm-produced dairy products. One historian of the dairy industry declared in 1926 that in the nineteenth century "sanitary methods were unknown; science, art or skill in connection with the handling of dairy products were unheard of."[11] While this is probably an unjust exaggeration, there is no reason to believe all farm women were equally skilled in the tricky tasks of making butter and cheese. The problem seemed not so much consistently bad cheese and butter but an unevenness of quality that gave farm products a bad reputation. Yet, surely, the farm wife was not entirely to blame, since the system of marketing in the nineteenth century consisted of selling a few pounds of butter at a time to the local storekeeper, who would lump all the butter of varying quality together in a tub. He then waited until he had enough butter to make it worth transporting to a city. No wonder it arrived a rancid mess.

Butter factories, or creameries, it was believed, would produce a more reliable product. The first creamery in the United States was established in 1856 in Orange County, New York.[12] Yet creameries did not monopolize butter making in the early twentieth century to the same degree that cheese factories monopolized the production of cheese. In 1925, when 1.3 billion pounds of butter were produced in factories, there were still 600 million pounds of butter produced on farms.[13] And farm periodicals such as the *Rural New Yorker* and the *Farmer's Wife* continued to publish advice directed to women on butter making for both home use and market sale.

It is possible that because of factory competition, many farm women no longer trained their daughters in the tasks of butter making. A 1925 farm novel, *The Trouble Maker,* by *American Agriculturist* editor E. R. Eastman, alludes to the decline of butter-making skills in the farm households around Binghamton, New York, in 1916. The story recounts the great New York milk strike of 1916 organized by the Dairymen's League. The manufacturers had refused to pay what farmers considered a fair price for raw milk. Dairy farmers struck by withholding all their milk from market, but because milk is very perishable, they hoped to cut their losses by converting the milk into less perishable butter and cheese. For this the women were called into service. One character observes:

> Do you know, I've been surprised to find out that right here in this cow country, there's few people left who really know how to make good butter. Butter-making on the farms is a lost art and it's kind of too bad. Some of the homemade butter I've bought in the store would drive a dog off a garbage wagon . . . when all this homemade rotten butter is put on the market as a result of this strike, I can see how a lot of people are going to be driven to eat oleomargarine.[14]

The author calculates that milk had been sold in fluid form to factories for "a generation," which was long enough for the skills of butter making to become obsolete.[15] Thus, this farm writer placed butter making as a thriving art prior to 1900. Similarly, a California farm woman reflected somewhat wistfully in a letter to the U.S. Department of Agriculture (USDA) in 1915, "Our modern creamery is fast displacing the golden butter churned by our *grandmothers*. . . ."[16]

Since all cheese and two-thirds of butter was made in the factory, what dairy work did remain for women to do in the early twentieth century? (See table 1.) The main function of dairy farms became the production of raw fluid milk, which was delivered to factories to be transformed into cheese, butter, or ice cream, or sold as a beverage. On the farms the cows still had to be milked, and although women still helped out with this, milking machines were increasingly utilized. One job that remained "women's work" was operating the cream separator on farms that supplied cream to "gathered cream" factories. Advertisements for cream separators almost always showed women (and sometimes children) operating the machine, to show how easy it was to operate. Before 1879, women had separated the cream by putting milk in a shallow pan (which was relatively easy to clean) and skimming the cream that floated to the top. Because this gravity method proved inefficient in collecting all the valuable cream, a centrifugal cream separator was developed. It was a more sophisticated piece of machinery and its daily cleaning fell to women. If advertisements are any indication, it was a chore that women did not particularly enjoy. That it had to be done each day made it monotonous, and rising standards of sanitation required that it always be performed thoroughly and not just given "a lick and a promise."

Several factors led to the greater mechanization of dairying. The rapidly increasing population in urban centers created a demand for milk far greater than immediately surrounding farm areas could meet. Developments in transportation and refrigeration in the late nineteenth century allowed outlying farm areas to supply the expanding markets. Increased demand required larger herds, which required either more labor, which was often too costly or in short supply, or more machines. Moreover, the development in 1890 of the Babcock test for measuring butterfat demonstrated the need for dairy farmers to specialize in superior breeds of cattle that produced milk with higher butterfat content, and thus greater profits.[17] Cattle breeding required a scientific expertise and an understanding of genetics that could be acquired at any agricultural college, but generally "book farming" was reserved for farmers' sons, not their daughters. The typical farm woman did not have access to the capital or education to compete with the producers for Borden or the contented cows of the Carnation Company.

On the other hand, poultry raising was not transferred to Frank Purdue–style factories until after World War II. (See the Appendix.) A 1910 farm census revealed that 88 percent of farms raised chickens, with an average of 80.4 chickens per farm.[18] An estimate for 1939 indicated that 70 percent of poultry production was still carried out by women.[19] Even so, big business principles had to be applied in order to meet the increasing demand for poultry and eggs. In 1927 the poultry column of the *Farmer's Wife* reported the case of a farm woman who sent a dozen eggs to a large buyer. The columnist concluded, "Imagine the lady's consternation when she received an order by telegraph for 30 cases each week for a year! Because she was producing them by the dozen instead of by the case, she was unable to take advantage of the order . . . she may have the quality, but not the quantity."[20] In 1930 in the same farm woman's magazine, a poultry expert advised that flock owners keep a *minimum* of five hundred hens for a profitable business; otherwise a small flock of fifty would suffice to supply the farm table.[21] Thus, while many women did continue to raise poultry, others found that their usual round of housework did not leave them enough time or energy to tend to such large flocks. The 1945 novel *The Egg and I* is a frantic account of one woman who tried. After the Second World War, a minimum of two thousand layers was necessary to support a family,[22] and vast "chicken ranches" dominated the market. In the late 1960s, twelve thousand hens would be considered "a very small flock."[23]

As in the dairy industry, advances in technology ultimately demanded specialization and high volume production. Some of the major innovations that transformed poultry raising from the housewife's sideline to an automated agribusiness include the development of incubators for hatching large numbers of chicks, trap-nests (which allowed the producer to identify the poor layers to be culled since the hens were "trapped" on the nest), advances in genetics to breed better layers, use of artificial light to increase laying, and the development of expensive commercial feeds and conveyor-belt feeders.

For those farm women who forsook the production of poultry and dairy products even for home use, it became easier to buy the food the family consumed. Yet there is evidence of tension between the farm woman's role as consumer and her role as the wife of a producer. This conflict is evident in a letter a New York State farm woman wrote to the USDA in 1915:

> I am convinced that the brain work I have expended [on buying household supplies] has done more than any other agency toward building up our farm business. It is so much more the woman's province to buy than to sell that it seems to me here lies her greatest opportunity. Now here is where I encounter the blank wall. I find in the current number of [a farm journal] when the best time is to sell wheat. . . . Where, tell me, shall I look for information as to the best time to buy flour?[24]

Obviously, the best time for farmers to sell wheat is when prices are high, and the best time for housewives to buy that wheat-milled-into-flour is when prices are low. The farmer's wife is caught in the middle—wanting low prices for the food she has to buy in the marketplace and high prices for the food her husband is producing for the same marketplace.

During the Depression overproduction, considered to have driven down agricultural prices, was a perennial problem for egg producers. Thus, in a 1930 editorial in the *Farmer's Wife,* farm women were encouraged not to *produce* more eggs but to *consume* more. The writer noted, "If . . . 6 million farm families ate a dozen or two eggs more per week, it would reduce the number of eggs taken to market by ten or twelve million dozen a week. . . . [That] would help to keep the egg supply down and prices up. . . ."[25]

This conflict between the interests of the producer and those of the consumer was highlighted by a new emphasis on sticking to budgets in a cash economy. Budget (and cholesterol) notwithstanding, one finds numerous editorials in the *Farmer's Wife* urging farm women to cook generously with butter, eggs, and cream. Readers were warned, "The eggless cake is just as big a mistake on the general farm as the butterless table. . . ."[26] A 1938 article admonished frugal housewives:

> The butter-saving woman is not as scientific or wise a planner as it might seem if she looks to a cream check for cash. Multiply butter-saving and butter-substituting country cooks many times and it does things to the national supply of butter. Folks must use butter a bit more freely if the surplus is to be reduced and the price of butter kept stable.[27]

The harshest indictment was reserved for the farm wife who bought margarine, a product seen as a great threat to the dairy industry. The *Farmer's Wife* asked rhetorically, "Why shouldn't farm folks save money by using cheaper butter substitutes instead of higher priced butter?" It answered its own question emphatically by stating that the few cents the farm wife saved per pound on purchased margarine could not possibly equal the loss her husband would sustain when he sold his milk and cream at a lower price.[28]

The producer-versus-consumer conflict over the use of margarine is graphically illustrated by a 1930s controversy that resulted when the Federal Bureau of Home Economics endorsed the use of margarine as economical. The Bureau of Home Economics was a subdivision of the USDA, and the National Cooperative Milk Producers were indignant that a federal agency devoted to farming interests should favor the dread ersatz. Similarly, when the Bureau of Home Economics distributed bulletins on the relative cost and nutritional value of various foods, wheat producers and millers protested that the bureau did not tout the virtues of wheat vigorously enough. The chairman of the House Agriculture Committee proposed an amendment "which would prohibit any employee of the Department from making any statement that gave the impression that it was harmful or undesirable to consume wheat or anything manufactured from wheat." This amendment passed in the House, but not in the Senate.[29]

Tension also existed in the academic disciplines of home economics and agriculture. At Cornell University, where the Department of Home Economics was part of the College of Agriculture, there existed "a fundamental conflict of interest between the constituency of home economics and agriculture . . . the former represented the interests of food and fiber consumers [and] the latter represented the interests of food and fiber producers."[30] Dairy farmers tried to obstruct the home economists' efforts to objectively evaluate oleomargarine.

Recipes can be viewed as directives to women regarding what products to use or buy; the *Farmer's Wife* made the claim that its "recipes . . . consistently boosted farm products."[31] Ironically, though, advertisements that appeared in this farm magazine did not consistently boost farm products. For instance, during the Depression advertisements for Junket rennet tablets told farmers' wives "How to make smoother ice cream with less cream," and numerous advertisements for Swan's Down cake flour promised that one could use "half as many eggs, half as much butter" for their one-egg cake. Swan's Down included a cartoon of two housewives bemoaning the high price of eggs and butter.[32] The presence of such conflicting messages about household economy within the pages of a farm women's magazine that counted a large dairy audience among its subscribers reflects the contradictions inherent in the farm women's *new* role as a consumer and her *old* role as the wife of a producer.

"Out of the Barns and into the Kitchens" can be understood not just as a metaphor for changes that occurred in the *nature* of women's work, but also as a literal description of a change—or rather a contraction—in the *site* of that work. In what may be called "the geography of gender," the male workplace had long been the fields and the female sphere the house,[33] with the yard and barn constituting more or less shared, androgynous zones. As the sexual division of labor on the farm became more sharply defined in the twentieth century, the outdoor/indoor dichotomy also became more defined and the barn and yard were seen by many women (and men) as obviously outdoors and outside of the female domain. Some women viewed this with regret or rebellion; others welcomed the diminished productive role. The following letter, written in 1915 to the USDA by a Kansas woman, indicates an astute appreciation of what today would be called the "double burden" and expresses very definite ideas about the geography of gender. She begins with the pronouncement, "I protest against the Hens," and goes on to ask:

> This is my question: When I have cooked, and swept, and washed, and ironed, and made beds for a family of five . . . and have done the necessary mending and some sewing, haven't I done enough? In any fair division of labor between the farmer and his wife the man would take the outdoors and the woman the indoors. That would drop the chickens on the man's side, with the probable result that on most farms there would be no chickens; on some there would be big flocks.[34]

The distance between men's and women's separate spheres was not only a matter of *how* the work was divided and *where* the work was conducted; there is evidence to suggest that distance between their work sites was increasing in terms of *physical* proximity as well. A study done in 1953 showed that on prosperous farms, farmers were choosing to build their barns farther away from the house.[35] Moreover, the trend was toward larger farms. It can be argued that farm families were experiencing to a lesser degree what the urban and suburban household had already experienced—a separation of home and work for men, with the husband leaving the home for his work site, in this case the barn or the field. To what extent did the farm family maintain the preindustrial integration of personal life and work if it was not as convenient for husbands, wives, and children to physically interact? It follows that if wives did not frequent the barns and the fields, they had less practical knowledge of the farm business, which in turn might hinder their participation as truly equal partners in the business. The 1928 *Farmer's Wife*'s claim that "The woman on the farm is in the very *center* of the farm business and knows the details of sowing and planting, of harvesting and marketing the crops *just as intimately as her husband*" is not entirely convincing.[36]

The early twentieth-century literature for, by, and about farm women was divided as to whether farm women were drudges or equal partners on the farm. Many farm women did consider themselves equal partners in the family farm. For instance, a Michigan woman described pitching in to help milk the cows one evening, a chore she indicated was ordinarily her husband's. A female neighbor dropped in and commented, "I wouldn't milk any man's cows." "Well," the farm woman replied, "I'm not milking 'any man's' cows; I'm milking *our* cows."[37]

Yet some women felt the need to protect themselves from being exploited by their husbands as unpaid hired hands. A farm wife from New York State who wrote a letter to the *Farmer's Wife* entitled "Don't Start" and simply signed "Overworked" had this to say about helping with outdoor work in emergencies: "Show me a man who won't take any amount of help if his wife is willing to give it. From my experience and that of friends and neighbors I have found the more you 'help out' the more you will have to."[38] Similar advice came from a woman calling herself "Go Slow" from Iowa, who cautioned women, in a letter entitled "Let Brides Beware," not to let emergencies occur too often since women had enough to do cooking, cleaning, and raising children.[39] That many women were reluctant to take on the double burden is reflected in other letters to the *Farmer's Wife,* such as one from "Out-of-Breath Betty," who asked, "Is it really worth while to try to do the work of two or three women in a day? It is two or three, isn't it, when a woman does all the necessary work in a home and then helps her hus-band in the field, and raises a hundred chickens?" "Betty" concluded by saying that she tried to do her share by saving, apparently quite satisfied with her consumer role, and added that she "wouldn't milk [a cow] on a bet."[40]

Of course, some farm women were not just resisting the double burden but were enthusiastically embracing a feminine mystique. In a letter dated 1940 an Oregon wife observed, "To me it seems that mamma in a pretty housecoat, putting the children to bed and making coffee to share with Daddy in the living room, is doing her part better than if she drags in from the barn in dirty overalls to a dull and disor-derly house and neglected children."[41]

Women today might have more sympathy with the farm woman who in 1938 resented the image of a rural "Superwoman" as portrayed in the prescriptive literature. She wrote, "I have read the Success Stories of money-making women. Some of them, it seemed to me, must have gotten in 48 hours in the 24 to accomplish what they did. Some I just couldn't believe accomplished it all."[42]

There is an important difference in strategy between women today and these earlier twentieth-century women in resisting the double bur-den: working wives today often attempt to equalize the domestic work load by trying to get men to take on some of the "women's work," whereas earlier farm women tried to equalize it by saying no to "men's work." Apparently it was not common (and arguably not even possible given agricultural conditions) for farmers to share in the housework, except occasionally in the arduous task of doing laundry. In 1914 the *Country Gentleman* columnist Nellie Kedzie Jones noted, "I wish it could be burnt into the consciousness of every man and every woman that washing under average farm conditions is man's work, not a wom-an's."[43] Such a "redivision" of the sexual division of labor did not come to pass. Instead, farm women in their consumer role turned to a techno-logical solution—the washing machine—rather than challenging the sex-ual division of labor.

Like their suburban and urban counterparts, most farm women looked to consumerism, in the form of privately owned labor-saving devices, as an individual solution to housework. Thus, while there ex-isted a few examples of cooperative laundries, such as the first one opened in 1912 in Chatfield, Minnesota, where the boiler system of the local creamery provided the power to clean fifty families' clothing at five cents a pound,[44] most farm wives aspired to purchase their own washing machines.

It is important to note that "labor-saving devices" in the context of rural America in the first half of the twentieth century included utilities such as running water and electricity as well as major appliances and small tools. In fact, to understand how primitive the work conditions were in some farm households we must view a sink with a drain (for instance) as a modern "convenience": the agricultural census of 1945 revealed that three out of five farm households did not have this fundamental equipment.[45] Obviously the lack of a drain meant that all the water carried *into* the house for cooking, washing dishes, laundry, bathing, and so on had also to be carried *out* of the house, a function of modern plumbing we probably take for granted. The rural sociologist Carl Taylor asked numerous farm women in the 1930s which modern convenience they would choose first and reported that they were "unanimous in saying they would take running water and a kitchen sink."[46] Only 17.8 percent of farm households had running water in 1940. By 1950 only 42.7 percent of farm households had running water, and as recently as 1960 only 74.8 percent of farm households had acquired running water.[47] By one estimate, a farm household of five persons needed 175 gallons of water a day for household use alone,[48] and much of this water was carried by farm women. In a 1919 survey of farm households conducted by the USDA, 61 percent of women reported that carrying water was one of their chores and that they hauled it an average distance of thirty-nine feet many times a day. (Out West farm women "fetched" water an average of sixty-five feet!)[49] (See table 1.) Electricity was also lacking on most farms. In 1930 only 10.6 percent of farm households had electricity; by 1940 only 32.6 percent of farm households were electrified.[50]

In some instances the lack of modern conveniences was a direct result of poverty, and *both* farm men and women made do with obsolete tools and labor-intensive, back-breaking methods of running farms and farm households. Yet over and over again farm women complained that they put up with antiquated equipment while their husbands enjoyed the latest in agricultural machinery.

The hard life of some farm women was summed up in a 1915 rural sociology textbook:

> Perhaps the sorest spot in the rural problem is the lot of the neglected farm wife and mother. Even where agricultural prosperity is indicated by great barns filled with plenty, often a dilapidated farm-house nearly devoid of beauty, comfort, or convenience, measures the utter disregard of the housewife's lot. Money is freely spent, when new machinery is needed on the farm, or another fifty-acre piece is added after a prosperous season, but seldom a thought to the needs of the kitchen. While the men of the farm

ride the sulky plough or the riding harrow of the twentieth century, the women have neither a washing-machine nor an indoor pump, to say nothing of running water, sanitary plumbing, or a bath-tub. Sometimes the drudgery of the farm is endured by the mother uncomplainingly, or even contentedly; but the daughter recoils from it with a growing discontent.[51]

The fear of discontented daughters was a real one, as the "woman question" for rural America became "How ya gonna keep 'em down on the farm?" The mass exodus from rural areas in the twentieth century was led by women, and in 1917 in New York State the sex ratio on farms was 120 men to every 100 women.[52] By 1984 the imbalance in the Farm Belt had grown to 134 men to every 100 women.[53]

In 1917 the *Farmer's Wife* informed fathers that they could stem this female out-migration and keep their daughters on the farms by providing them with labor-saving devices.[54] Even an advertisement aimed at men for Ford tractors appealed to farmers' concerns about their daughters, suggesting that a farmer who owned a Ford tractor would be a better dad to his daughter since he would be less tired. Furthermore, his daughter would have a more positive view of the farm and be more inclined to stick with it herself.[55] The implication of the "if not for your wife, then for your daughter" theme suggests that men may have been more responsive to egalitarian appeals on behalf of their daughters than on behalf of their wives, who may not have been as mobile.

A USDA survey of farm households conducted in 1919 found that 42 percent of the farms surveyed had power-driven farm machinery, while only 15 percent of the homes had power-driven appliances for household use.[56] To equalize this uneven distribution of modern equipment, a group of Nebraska farm women put forth this six-point technological agenda in 1923:

1. A power washing machine for the house for every tractor bought for the farm.
2. A bath tub in the house for every binder on the farm.
3. Running water in the kitchen for every riding plow for the fields.
4. A kerosene cook-stove for every auto truck.
5. A fireless cooker for every new mowing machine.
6. [Their] share of the farm income.[57]

This question of a fair share of the farm income is at the heart of the drudge-versus-equal-partner debate. While it is true that in the early twentieth century many women still earned money from marketing poultry and dairy products (generally butter) or selling garden produce, these women often did not get to keep their earnings for their own use.

TABLE 1. Farm Women's Work, 1919

	Eastern States	Central States	Western States	United States
Helps to milk cows	24%	45%	37%	36%
Makes butter	43%	66%	74%	60%
Sells butter	31%	33%	33%	33%
Keeps butter money	9%	9%	16%	11%
Cares for poultry	69%	89%	84%	81%
Average size flock	90 hens	102 hens	71 hens	90 hens
Keeps poultry money	13%	25%	21%	22%
Keeps egg money	16%	16%	17%	16%
Carries water	54%	68%	57%	61%
Distance water carried	23 ft.	41 ft.	65 ft.	39 ft.
Helps in fields[a]	27%	22%	23%	24%
Cares for garden	41%	67%	57%	56%

Source: Derived from Florence Ward, "The Farm Woman's Problems," U.S. Department of Agriculture Circular no. 148 (Washington, D.C.: GPO, 1920), a survey of 10,044 farm women conducted in 1919.

[a]An average of 6.7 weeks per year

As illustrated in table 1, the 1919 USDA survey discovered that only 11 percent of the farm women surveyed kept their butter money, 22 percent kept their poultry money, and 16 percent kept their egg money.[58] Farm women often commented that their work in running the household—which included raising much of the food for the table, preserving foods, feeding threshing crews and hired hands, caring for children, cleaning, and sewing—was not rewarded with an equal share of the family income or in decision making.

A common bit of nineteenth-century folk wisdom was that where the farm home was more imposing than the barn, "the woman is the boss."[59] This suggests that some rural people identified a "battle of the sexes" or at least tension between farmers and their wives over financial decisions, family resources, and competing priorities in the adoption of modern technology. The most famous fictional representation of this struggle is, of course, Mary Wilkins Freeman's 1891 short story "The Revolt of Mother." "Mother" moves her family out of the shack that has long been their home into the palatial new barn, a kind of "out of the barns and into the kitchens" in reverse.[60] For some reason Freeman later repudiated her own story. She wrote:

> all fiction ought to be true and "The Revolt of Mother" is not true. . . .
> There never was in New England a woman like Mother. If there had been
> she certainly would not have moved into the palatial barn. . . . She simply

would have lacked the nerve.   She would also have lacked the imagination. New England women . . . coincided with their husbands that the
sources of wealth should be better housed than the consumers. . . . Mother
would never have dreamed of putting herself ahead of Jersey cows which
meant good money. . . .[61]

That cows had better accommodations than people was a common
assertion. A Kansas farm woman wrote a sarcastic letter to *Farm Journal*
in 1948 charging that "It seems that the cows, calves, horses, sheep, hogs,
chickens, and turkeys must be made *comfortable* first, then if the machinery and house are paid for, if there's time and money left, the little woman
may get her sink and drain." She added that running water had recently
been put in for the chickens and turkeys on her farm, although she herself
still labored in a kitchen without piped-in water or a drain in her sink.[62]
That this letter hit a raw nerve in many other farm women is reflected by
the fact that it was voted the best letter to the editor by the (mostly female)
readers of *Farm Journal*'s women's section.

And yet there was a logic to providing fowl with running water first,
for elsewhere *Farm Journal* advised that running water could increase
the chicken's winter egg production by 19.5 percent and thus increase
profits.[63] In their quest for modern conveniences farm women had to
struggle against a compelling economic imperative requiring that limited
resources be reinvested in the farm in the form of more land, more
labor, or more machines, because that was were the income was. This
hardheaded reality was summed up in the aphorism, "A barn can build a
house sooner than a house can build a barn."[64] Unfortunately, many
farm women like "Mother" discovered that a barn only built another
barn.

It would be too simple to suggest that farmers were acting in an
economically "rational" way in their single-minded devotion to profit
while farmers' wives were "irrational" in valuing family comfort, leisure,
and health over profits. In fact, as capitalist expansion in the twentieth
century depended on consumer purchasing, I would suggest that farm
women, in their desire to buy major applicances, were every bit as
"modern" as their husbands in integrating farm households into the
consumer economy.

Farm women were encouraged in their roles as consumers on many
fronts: the USDA, agricultural colleges, extension services, and farm
journals all offered consumer information to farm women. A New York
State farm woman answered a 1915 USDA query as to what were the
needs of farm women by saying, "To my mind the Department can do
no better for the country woman than to help her buy intelligently."[65]

Naturally, farm women had their allies in the world of finance as well as in their desire to own labor-saving devices. A trade journal devoted to rural banking called the *Banker-Farmer,* published in the 1910s and 1920s, had a surprising number of articles devoted to women. The thrust of most of these articles was to urge the purchase of large appliances, preferably bought on credit or on the installment plan. To this end rural bankers advocated that farm women have their own checking and savings accounts, accompany their husbands when conferring with local bankers about loans, and generally be given a greater say in the financial decisions on the farm—in short, that farm wives be treated as genuine business partners. The *Banker-Farmer* put this on a sound financial basis by observing, "It pays to make the women happy. It pays to emancipate the slaves, and especially when those slaves are our wives, our mothers, our daughters. It pays in money, indirectly, if not directly, but whether or not it pays in money it must be done."[66] Bankers recognized that farm women as equal partners were bigger spenders than drudges were.

The *Farmer's Wife* is another source rich in information and messages to farm women about consumerism. With a circulation of 1.25 million readers by 1939, when it was absorbed by *Farm Journal,* the *Farmer's Wife* was the most popular women's magazine aimed at a rural audience. The magazine was established in 1896 and was originally more a primer for production with many columns on dairying, poultry, gardening, and the production of other marketable items. By the 1920s and 1930s the *Farmer's Wife* gradually put more emphasis on consumerism, including the establishment of a test kitchen and a *Farmer's Wife* seal of approval to endorse products and appliances. Articles that promoted brand names also demystified the new stoves, refrigerators, cleaning products, miracle fabrics, and convenience foods on the market. So engaging seemed consumer culture that an article on organizing community get-togethers went so far as to suggest an entertainment called "Advertise," in which teams matched up products and slogans.[67]

No surprise, then, that the advertisements in the magazine reinforced its consumer emphasis. For instance, an advertisement for overalls depicted a winsome farm wife in a feminine frock announcing, "I don't wear the pants, but I buy 'em. . . ."[68] Similarly, an advertisement for a new stove asked readers, "What makes a man brag about his wife? The answer you hear most often is that she knows how to buy wisely."[69] This emphasis on buying as opposed to producing (and selling) marked a departure from the traditional nineteenth-century integration of farm women's household production into the farm economy.

In 1917 the *Farmer's Wife* printed a virtual prose poem to self-actualization through labor-saving devices, entitled "I Resolve to Grow." The author conceded, "I am not developing as a woman should develop for the sake of herself and all whom she is associated." She observed that "Time is necessary for Growth and Development" and concluded, "I resolve to buy not less than one first-class time-and-strength saving tool every year. . . ." The resulting free time would be spent on leisure pursuits such as music, reading, outings, and establishing closer ties with family and the community.[70]

Compare this to a feature about another farm woman who we are told saved seven hours a week by trading in her old wood stove for an electric range in 1948.[71] She used her newly acquired "free" time to do all the family sewing, which she had previously hired someone else to do. The point of the article, of course, was that free time gained from a labor-saving device can translate into a cash saving, since in this case the wife was able to produce goods and services that she had formerly bought. But her story also illustrates the point that new tasks (or higher standards) rush in to fill the "free" time that labor-saving devices "save."

Not only did the *Farmer's Wife* urge the purchase of labor-saving devices, it addressed the problem of persuading reluctant husbands to agree to these investments. An article called "600 Ways to Get That Running Water" noted that a farm woman who has to lug water may have forgotten how to "manage" her husband. Earlier, the editors had suggested that lack of modern conveniences was not a matter of money but a "human relations problem." They solicited readers' suggestions on the "psychology" they had used on their husbands, which implies that many farm women did not have direct access to the purse strings and were actually less than equal partners.

The six hundred replies from readers ranged from the coy to the militant. Strategies included feigning illness, going on strike, placing the order for the pipes and installing them oneself (even bungling the job to secure male assistance), and calculating the net savings from the investment and presenting the figures to one's husband. Not infrequently farm women reported that all it took was to have their husbands tote the water for even a short while to convince them to pipe in water.[72] An inventive—if somewhat vindictive—strategy was organized by the We Want Water for Christmas Club: this group of Illinois farm wives published the names of their husbands in a public newsletter until one by one the recalcitrant husbands surrendered and installed running water.[73] Strategies such as this suggest that Mary Wilkins Freeman was shortsighted in repudiating "The Revolt of Mother": real-life farm women did exist who had the nerve and the imagination to revolt against a division of labor that assigned decision making and money spending to men. The method the *Farmer's Wife* endorsed over all others was the idea of partnership. It concluded, "If you can make your husband think of you as his partner, the rest is easy. . . ."[74]

The *Farmer's Wife* summed up its philosophy that the quality of life on the farm was as important as the profits in its motto, "A good life as well as a good living." Yet, as we've seen, messages abounded that "a good life" could be purchased—that in fact, it required "a good living" to afford "a good life."

Labor-saving devices failed to liberate women from housework; on the contrary, women spent at least as much time as before meeting higher standards, and the sexual division of labor in the home was reinforced. All of this has been well demonstrated by historians of technology such as Joann Vanek, Ruth Schwartz Cowan, and Charles Thrall. With disturbing prescience the *Rural New Yorker* reflected in 1900:

> So many labor-saving devices have been common that woman's work should now be simpler, but with these improvements, our standard of comfort has been so greatly raised that the present-day housewife seems more overworked. . . . It is indeed unfortunate if we permit labor-saving devices to increase our work, rather than to lessen it.[75]

The promise of "a good life" in the form of consumerism blended with domesticity was one that many farm women ultimately found to be elusive.

NOTES

1. Susan Keating Glaspell, "A Jury of Her Peers," in *American Voices, American Women,* ed. Lee R. Edwards and Arlyn Diamond (New York: Avon Books, 1973), 359–81.
2. T. R. Pirtle, *History of the Dairy Industry* (Chicago: Mojonnier Bros., 1926), 213, 327.
3. Pirtle, *History of the Dairy Industry,* 102.
4. Pirtle, *History of the Dairy Industry,* 110–12.
5. Elmer O. Fippin, *Rural New York* (New York: Macmillan Co., 1921), 279.
6. Eric Brunger, "New York State Dairy Industry, 1850–1900" (Ph.D. diss., Syracuse University, 1954), 72.
7. E. H. Farrington, "Women in Dairy Manufacturing," *American Produce Review,* July, 1918, 366. Emphasis mine.
8. Farrington, "Women in Dairy Manufacturing," 368.

9. Farrington, "Women in Dairy Manufacturing," 368.
10. *Rural New Yorker,* Dec., 1863, 398. Cited in Brunger, "New York State Dairy Industry," 64.
11. Pirtle, *History of the Dairy Industry,* 74.
12. Fippin, *Rural New York,* 278.
13. Pirtle, *History of the Dairy Industry,* 99, 101, 102.
14. E. R. Eastman, *The Trouble Maker* (New York: Macmillan Co., 1927), 125.
15. Eastman, *The Trouble Maker,* 189.
16. U.S. Department of Agriculture, *Domestic Needs of Farm Women,* Report no. 104 (Washington, D.C.: GPO, 1915), 73. Emphasis mine.
17. Pirtle, *History of the Dairy Industry,* 80.
18. Page Smith and Charles Daniel, *The Chicken Book* (Boston: Little, Brown, 1975), 232.
19. "We Honor the Hen," *Farm Journal,* Feb., 1939, 3. In 1939, when *Farm Journal* absorbed the *Farmer's Wife,* the latter continued as a "magazine within a magazine" with its own cover page and staff. Henceforth, notes cite the titles *Farmer's Wife* before 1939 and *Farm Journal* after 1939 for ease in locating quotations, but my text still refers to the *Farmer's Wife* even after 1939 if the citation refers to the women's section.
20. "Poultry and the City Market," *Farmer's Wife,* Oct., 1927, 56.
21. "Fifty Hens or Five Hundred?" *Farmer's Wife,* Feb., 1931, 52.
22. "How Many Chickens?" *Farm Journal,* Apr., 1946, 124.
23. Smith and Daniel, *Chicken Book,* 292.
24. U.S. Department of Agriculture, *Economic Needs of Farm Women,* Report no. 106 (Washington, D.C.: GPO, 1915), 64.
25. "Have Another Egg, Dear?" *Farmer's Wife,* Oct., 1930, 3.
26. "Better Prices for Better Eggs," *Farmer's Wife,* May, 1930, 60.
27. "Use Butter Generously," *Farm Journal,* Nov., 1938, 11.
28. "Is It True?" *Farmer's Wife,* Mar., 1930, 3.
29. Gladys Baker, "Women in the U.S.D.A.," *Agricultural History,* Jan., 1976, 197.
30. Gould P. Colman, *Education and Agriculture: A History of the New York State College of Agriculture at Cornell University* (Ithaca: Cornell University, 1963), 284.
31. "Frugal or Economical?" *Farm Journal,* Dec., 1938, 16. Which farm products to push was an occasional issue. A feature on the new "one-bowl" method of mixing cakes may have pleased the pork producers since it substituted lard for the usual vegetable shortening. This was hardly likely to please corn farmers or other producers for vegetable oil manufacturers.
32. See the *Farmer's Wife,* Jan., 1931, 21; Feb., 1936, 21; *Farm Journal,* Feb., 1937, 27; June, 1937, 30.
33. Mary P. Ryan, *Womanhood in America: From Colonial Times to the Present,* 2d ed. (New York: New Viewpoints, 1979), ix. See also Corlann G. Bush, "The Barn is His, the House is Mine: Agricultural Technology and

Sex Roles," in *Energy and Transport: Historical Perspectives on Policy Issues,* ed. George H. Daniels and Mark H. Rose (Beverly Hills: Sage Publications, 1982), 235–59.

34. U.S. Department of Agriculture, *Social and Labor Needs of Farm Women,* Report no. 103 (Washington, D.C.: GPO, 1915), 51.
35. James W. Green, "Distance as a Factor in Farmhouse Location," *Rural Sociology,* Sept., 1953, 261–62.
36. "A Portrait: The Typical Farm Homemaker," *Farmer's Wife,* July, 1928, 9. Emphasis mine.
37. "Are Wives Loyal?" *Farm Journal,* Feb., 1938, 10.
38. *Farmer's Wife,* Jan., 1936, 18.
39. *Farmer's Wife,* Nov., 1935, 13.
40. *Farmer's Wife,* Oct., 1929, 18.
41. *Farm Journal,* Dec., 1940, 52.
42. *Farm Journal,* Aug., 1938.
43. Jeanne Hunnicutt Delgado, "Nellie Kedzie Jones' Advice to Farm Women: Letters from Wisconsin, 1912–1916," *Wisconsin Magazine of History,* Autumn, 1973, 14.
44. E. B. Forney, "How Farmers Formed the World's First Cooperative Laundry," *Banker-Farmer,* Apr., 1916, 12.
45. "Are You Emancipated?" *Farm Journal,* Nov., 1947, 124.
46. Carl C. Taylor, "Address to the Associated Country Women of the World," in *Proceedings of the Third Triennial Conference, May 31–June 11, 1936,* U.S. Department of State Publication no. 1092, Conference Series 34 (Washington, D.C.: GPO, 1937), 198.
47. Joann Vanek, "Keeping Busy: Time Spent in Housework, United States, 1920–1970" (Ph.D. diss., University of Michigan, 1973), 2.
48. "Running Water Runs Up Profits," *Farm Journal,* Mar., 1946, 125.
49. Florence Ward, *The Farm Woman's Problems,* U.S. Department of Agriculture Circular no. 148 (Washington, D.C.: GPO, 1920), 8.
50. Vanek, "Keeping Busy," 3.
51. Albert H. Leake, *The Means and Methods of Agricultural Education* (Boston: Houghton Mifflin, 1915), 201–2.
52. Fippin, *Rural New York,* 40.
53. "A Growing Question: How Can You Keep Women on Farms?" *Wall Street Journal,* Aug. 30, 1984, 1.
54. "Daughter Chooses the Farm," *Farmer's Wife,* June, 1917, 8.
55. *Farm Journal,* Sept., 1944, 37.
56. Ward, *Farm Woman's Problems,* 8.
57. Newell Leroy Sims, *Elements of Rural Sociology* (New York: Thomas Y. Corwell, 1928), 274–75.
58. Ward, *Farm Woman's Problems,* 11.
59. Fred A. Shannon, *The Farmer's Last Frontier: Agriculture, 1860–1897* (New York: Holt, Rinehart and Winston, 1945), 368–69.

60. Mary E. Wilkins Freeman, *The Revolt of Mother and Other Stories* (Old Westbury, N.Y.: Feminist Press, 1974).
61. Mary E. Wilkins Freeman, "Who's Who and Why," *Saturday Evening Post,* Dec. 8, 1917, 25, 75.
62. *Farm Journal,* Jan., 1948, 92–93.
63. "Running Water Runs Up Profits," 125.
64. Sims, *Elements of Rural Sociology,* 264.
65. U.S. Department of Agriculture, *Economic Needs of Farm Women,* 64.
66. "Giving the Farm Girl Her Chance," *Banker-Farmer,* Apr., 1914, 7.
67. *Farm Journal,* Jan., 1944, 44.
68. *Farm Journal,* May, 1947, 117.
69. *Farmer's Wife,* May, 1938, 30.
70. "I Resolve to Grow," *Farmer's Wife,* Jan., 1917, 173.
71. "Electric Cooking Saves *Me!*" *Farm Journal,* Oct., 1948, 93.
72. "600 Ways to Get That Running Water," *Farm Journal,* Apr., 1948, 138, 140–41. Other articles include "How Some Women Got the Water Piped In," *Farmer's Wife,* July, 1930; and "Running Water: Victory Tool—and Here's How Some Families Got It Piped In," *Farm Journal,* Nov., 1942.
73. *Farm Journal,* Feb., 1942, 45.
74. "600 Ways to Get That Running Water," 141.
75. *Rural New Yorker,* Jan. 20, 1900.

Technology and the Redesign of Work in the Insurance Industry

Eileen Appelbaum

Financial corporations in the United States are undergoing a rapid transformation as a result of the convergence of three powerful forces for change: high and volatile interest rates, rapid deregulation, and the diffusion and systematic application of computer and information technologies. The interaction of these forces is presenting financial corporations with the impetus to create new products and to alter the production process. While the consequences of these changes are just emerging, it is already apparent that major adjustments in the work force of the financial sector will be required.

The insurance industry is a case in point. Automation began in this industry around 1960 with the introduction of mainframe computers to handle customer billing and to provide management with detailed and timely accounting data. The carriers established data processing centers physically separated from other insurance operations. Employment of professional and clerical workers increased as these centers were staffed, while jobs elsewhere in the firms were largely unaffected. The automation of routine underwriting and rating procedures, which began in the 1970s, at first also involved the computerization of discrete tasks. Some underwriting and rating functions were transformed, but initially automation meant the transfer of codified knowledge from a set of manuals to a computer program. The work process was largely unaffected and, despite the capabilities of the technology, an insurance application continued to pass routinely through five or more hands before a policy was issued. Not until the financial environment was radically altered by the doubling of the inflation rate and the associated increase in interest rates in the 1970s did the industry begin to exploit the capabilities of computer and information technologies to develop new products and to experiment with the redesign of jobs and the reorganization of work. Driven by market forces and the capabilities of new technologies, changes in the work process began in earnest in 1979.

This study investigates the nature of these changes and their implications for the insurance industry work force. The findings are likely to have application far beyond the insurance industry. Nearly half the U.S.

labor force works in an office. "Information workers"—managers, technical/professional, clerical, and sales personnel—currently comprise 53 percent of the labor force. Clerical workers alone represent nearly one-fifth of all workers. Office automation and other information technologies are permanently altering the nature of white-collar and pink-collar work. The insurance industry is on the cutting edge of these developments. The effects of technology on the nature of work in the insurance industry may very well signal the future direction of change in office work acrosss the U.S. economy.

Study Approach

This investigation of adjustments in the insurance industry work force focuses on several important dimensions of change: the effect on the number of jobs, the distribution of occupations, the level of skills, the nature of clerical work, and the opportunities for upward mobility. Two major issues considered in this paper are the implications of these changes for women workers and for education.

The salient features of both the economic environment and the automation technologies are described in the next two sections. While this is a necessary beginning point for evaluating and forecasting the effects of automation on the work force, it is not sufficient; for the impact of new technology depends fundamentally on the way in which it is implemented.

For this reason, aggregate data available from the U.S. Department of Labor and a careful study of the specialized literatures on the various segments of the insurance industry as well as on office automation were supplemented with on-site visits and interviews at a small number of insurance carriers and agencies. Executives responsible for the implementation of new technology and for the design (or redesign) of jobs were interviewed. The vice-president for human resource development was interviewed at every carrier and, where appropriate, the vice-president for technical systems was interviewed as well. At one carrier, in which automation of the sales force was the major technological priority, the assistant vice-president for personal lines marketing, who had been charged with developing the software and training the agents, was also interviewed. Interviews at agencies were conducted with the president of the agency as well as with agents and clerical staff.

In all, interviews were conducted at six carriers and two independent agencies. Two of the carriers are in the life/health segment of the industry, three are in the property/casualty segment, and one sells personal lines (life, health, auto, homeowner's, accident) as well as group health. Four of the companies sell their products through independent agents, one has a captive agency sales force, and one is a direct writer using mail, television, and other forms of direct solicitation to sell its products without a sales force. Assets at the carriers varied from $60 billion down to $0.2 billion. The sample, while small, is representative of the range of firms in the industry. These interviews, together with aggregate employment data and published descriptions of the technologies provide the basis for the remaining sections of the article.

Economic Environment

Interest rates doubled in the course of the 1960s and nearly doubled again in the 1970s, reaching double-digit levels by the end of the decade. Financial markets encountered difficulty performing well in these circumstances. Rising and increasingly volatile interest rates fueled a wave of financial innovation and deregulation as financial institutions sought to develop strategies for coping with the economic environment. "Financial institutions pushed out in all directions, and financial practices became highly flexible as financial deregulation proliferated both in fact and in formal law" (Sametz 1984, 8). Competition developed among large financial institutions whose functions and operations had been segregated by law since the 1930s.

Rising interest rates had a marked effect on the insurance industry, which depends primarily upon investment returns, not underwriting, for its overall profit. Traditionally, insurance carriers were major participants in the capital markets as they matched the maturities of their portfolios to expected claims. Inflation in the late 1970s resulted in negative yields on long-term assets, however, and encouraged insurance companies to find ways around regulatory standards on investment. Turbulence in financial markets increased the risks involved but also raised the possibility of large payoffs for carriers whose investment managers outperformed the market. The large cash flow characteristic of the industry, and the possibility of high returns, attracted new entrants. Increased competition in all segments of the industry drove down the price of insurance. Average premiums per $1,000 of coverage dropped sharply.

For property/casualty firms the late 1970s were a period of high profits; following the initial adjustment to an inflationary regime, however, competition dangerously narrowed the margin between premium income and the cost of writing policies on commercial risks and also eroded the market share of some established carriers. Carriers turned to technology to reduce costs and to improve margins and regain market position.

For carriers in the life/health segment of the industry adjustment to inflation was more difficult. Whole life, the industry's predominant product, combines insurance with a savings plan yielding a 4 to 6 percent return. With interest rates on competing savings instruments rising, the ability of life insurance products to attract savings declined. Sales of term insurance increased, but since term is much cheaper than whole life, premiums stagnated. Life insurance companies were under pressure to develop new products.

Variable annuities were developed during the 1960s. Variable life was proposed in 1972 and approved by the Securities and Exchange Commission in 1976. Both are based on a portfolio of common stock and pay benefits that are not guaranteed but are contingent on the actual performance of the portfolio. Universal life, introduced in 1979, splits the premium and allows the consumer to decide how much goes to the death benefit and how much to savings. As with variable life, the premiums are placed in separate accounts and invested in securities whose returns are more sensitive to market rates of interest. Not until 1983, when carriers began providing their sales forces with computers and software capable of calculating death benefits and cash value under a variety of interest rate projections and with the premium split in different ways, did these so-called new wave policies become significant. Universal life accounted for 18 percent of new premium income in 1983 ("Upheaval in life insurance" 1984, 61). Life insurance companies have had to upgrade their computer systems and retrain their sales forces in order to sell these products. Moreover, competition from financial supermarkets not dependent on agents who collect commissions has created pressure on life insurance companies to use technology to upgrade the productivity of their traditional distribution system.

Office and Information Technologies

The production process in the insurance industry was rationalized decades before the introduction of office automation. Jobs were fragmented and functionally specialized, and paper wended its way around the office floor as surely as if it were on an assembly line. Introduction of the mainframe computer into the industry in the 1960s left this process largely untouched.

Computers at first were used to process routine or repetitive transactions. Mainly, they were used to keep track of and process all premium transactions. Claims disbursements were also automated early.

In addition, the computer was used from the beginning to generate the numerous reports needed by the accounting department. Separate electronic data processing departments were established. The resulting growth of computer specialists and operations research personnel contributed to the increase in professional employees during the 1960s, while keypunch operators and computer operators increased the number of clerical workers.

In the 1970s the capabilities of the central computer were used to support the underwriting aspects of the insurance business. The technology allowed underwriters at field or central offices to accept applications. If accepted, the application would undergo overnight processing by the computer, which would also calculate the premium. The output would then be mailed from central processing to the field office or printed via remote printer. In addition to processing applications, the computer could generate activity reports for field offices.

To implement the technology, programmers translated the manual processing procedures into programs. Decision algorithms were incorporated into the programs, systematizing the decision-making process for underwriters. In the early period, underwriters still had to make judgments. Now, however, personal lines underwriting rarely requires decisions that are not machine generated, and the computerization of underwriting for small or routine commercial risks is proceeding. At some carriers, low-level underwriting functions have been assigned to newly created clerical positions. Moreover, as underwriting jobs have been systematized, women have been hired into them.

Access to computer programs for underwriters is provided through telephone lines and cathode-ray tubes (CRTs). Initially, use of this technology required substantial clerical staff to code information and type attachments as well as to assemble and mail the policy packages. Currently, policies are entered on-line as they are issued, and word processing handles the attachments. Routine keyboarding is declining.

Electronic typewriters and word processing equipment spread rapidly in insurance offices in the 1970s. Electronic sorting of incoming mail, document control, electronic filing, and electronic mail are other important technologies in use in insurance. On-line processing of policies and optical character recognition (OCR) techniques adopted over the last decade have reduced the need to code information on worksheets and to keypunch it into the computer. Substantial savings in labor time in routine clerical work have already been achieved.

The next stage of office automation is integrated information processing, in which components that do word and data processing are linked through high-speed communications networks. These systems are used to support both clerical and decision-making functions. Important problems have slowed the adoption of this technology in insurance offices. These include high cost, the expectation of future improvements, and unresolved questions of access to and responsibility for central files.

Software is currently being developed to provide the on-line data and information services essential for middle and senior management and for professional staff. There are two aspects to the required technology: an appropriate data base and data base technology, and terminals or small computers capable of transparent interface with the central computer, other terminals, and a variety of peripherals. Data base management systems are now being developed and implemented. Since the batch-oriented accounting support systems already in place do not lend themselves readily to the demands of the decision support system, firms face difficult and expensive choices. The technology is expected to improve the performance of managers, but it has run into difficulty being accepted. The issue is not reluctance to use a keyboard per se, but more general complaints about access methodology. Managers complain that with existing menu-based keyboard systems, the personal time and effort required to get into the system are too great in terms of what can be gotten out of it. For the present, professional support staff are increasing as some companies establish separate programming staff responsive to the needs of managers.

Cost-effective software services are being made available to property claim departments. These include computerization of automobile and property claim estimates as well as damageability and management report information. Computerization does not yet extend much beyond auto, though other personal lines and worker's compensation claims are being automated. Computerization automatically captures all estimate information without duplicate keypunching. Data can then be summarized into management reports and used to improve the efficiency of the claims management operation. Linking the claims data base to other data bases will also allow insurers to predict claim frequency and to estimate loss ratios.

Carriers are actively engaged in automating the sales force. Although some agencies have used microcomputers for several years, the cost proved difficult for most to justify. Originally it was believed that the expense of computerizing agencies would not be warranted without interface between agents and carriers. In the last year, however, the carriers have recognized the importance of computerization in improving agents' productivity. Moreover, new wave life policies cannot be marketed without the high-speed calculating capability of the computer. As a result, some carriers are currently helping their high-volume agents obtain sophisticated equipment and specialized software, either providing them outright or subsidizing their purchase. The computer is used mainly to prepare sales proposals or to expand and focus marketing efforts. A few carriers have established interface with a small number of high-volume agents, enabling them to underwrite, rate, and issue policies directly. Independent agencies that do not produce a volume of business high enough to warrant computerization by the carrier have established a common network to interface with agencies that have this capability.

Technologically advanced firms have targeted the distribution system and the management function for cost cutting via technology during the remainder of the 1980s. Interest in networks that allow otherwise noncompatible machines to interact is high, but implementation of the paperless electronic office is a low priority for most carriers.

The Redesign of Jobs

An important insight that has emerged after several years of experience with office technologies is that the technologies used to automate clerical, underwriting, and processing functions differ fundamentally from older industrial technologies. The management of office automation must likewise differ. The logic of scientific management in a factory setting meant that work was rationalized and fragmented as it was automated. Productivity increased, but in the process worker skills were devalued, tasks became repetitive, and a sense of responsibility for the company's product was diminished. When automation was first introduced into an office environment, the same logic prevailed. In the insurance industry, where work had long since been fragmented, computerization was applied to discrete tasks. Skill levels tended to decline and the automated tasks were routine and repetitive.

As experience with office automation increases, however, it appears that in contrast to earlier factory automation, computer and communication technologies are often most effective in reducing costs when control, communication, and decision making are decentralized and when hierarchic organization and the functional specialization of tasks are reduced. Recent applications of these technologies have involved the elimination of both low-skill clerical and routine technical and professional jobs, and the creation of new, multiactivity, skilled clerical positions to handle these functions. A less common alternative is to broaden the agent's job by folding routine underwriting and rating functions into it and providing for the printing and issuing of policies at the point of sale. The result has been a significant reduction in unit labor requirements and an increase in the average skill levels of the remaining clerical, sales, and professional work force. The following examples illustrate the point.

In the property/casualty segment of the industry, competition has driven down premiums on small or unexceptional commercial risks—condominiums, stores, commercial auto, worker's compensation—despite rising costs, thereby substantially reducing the profitability of these lines. One major insurer has developed a strategy that reduces the costs of processing an application and improves the efficiency of its distribution network. The carrier is developing computer programs that assist in underwriting and rating these commercial lines, and agents are being trained to use the programs. The carrier is providing its highest volume, most professional agents (about 10 percent of its sales force) with intelligent terminals linked to its central computer. The terminals are also linked to printers capable of issuing a policy at the point of sale.

When the procedures are fully implemented, all clerical processing will be eliminated for sales generated by these agents. Policy typist, rater, and underwriter's assistant—jobs that provided career paths from clerical to lower-level professional jobs as underwriters—are disappearing. In fact, the lower-level jobs as insurance professionals are rapidly declining as well. Jobs for the most skilled underwriters remain, but the jobs have changed. Skilled underwriters no longer manage risk, they manage agents. They oversee the agent's "book of business," assessing the agent's success at underwriting, offering advice, developing customer profiles, focusing marketing efforts, ensuring the professionalism of the agency—and encouraging the agent to do a volume of business that warrants the carrier's investment. A few of the displaced clerical workers are being retrained and given basic programming and troubleshooting skills in order to provide technical support to agents using computer terminals. But most of the traditional clerical and professional functions previously involved in accepting or rejecting an application and in issuing a policy will be performed by the agent.

A very different example is provided by the carrier that sells personal lines insurance. These products are standardized and can be mass marketed without agents through direct mail and television solicitation. Direct writers, as they are called, are the most profitable and most rapidly growing carriers. New companies have entered this market, undercutting existing firms and causing wide swings in market share. One established company, which experienced a sudden drop in market share in 1980, had previously automated mail handling and filing, thus eliminating nearly all unskilled clerical jobs. Policies were entered online, and the system could handle inquiries for current information about coverage immediately. The work process was extremely fragmented, however, to the extent that customer inquiries were answered by different people with different job titles depending on whether they came by mail or telephone.

The first step taken when business declined was to integrate some of the tasks to facilitate reductions in staff. This first round of integration made no use of computer technology. But by 1983, information technologies had been used to create highly integrated multiactivity jobs in the operations area. Since the company's products were standardized, underwriting and rating functions could be entirely computerized and those jobs eliminated. Instead of these positions, a new highly skilled clerical position has been designed. Customer service representatives handle sales, access the computer program that assesses risk, access the rating program, explain rating procedures to customers, answer customer questions, and respond to complaints by telephone or mail.

Thus the company responded to the loss of business and the need to "skinny down" by a change in job design. Success is apparent in the fact that by 1983 the company was again doing its 1979 volume of business, but with half the number of employees.

Skill Levels and Upward Mobility

Job redesign has included both the integration of tasks into multidimensional jobs and the elimination of the lowest-level clerical and less skilled professional jobs. The resulting configuration of jobs varies from firm to firm, but in every case job categories have become more abruptly segmented while the avenues of mobility between them have been sharply reduced. Many of the newly created jobs are characterized by few opportunities for the exercise of judgment and increased managerial control over the pace and content of work as compared with the professional jobs they replace. Yet these very jobs are less fragmented, less centralized, involve considerable training, and often require significant knowledge of the product.

The effects of automation on skills in the insurance industry vary from carrier to carrier. It can be said, however, that the new techniques neither eliminate skilled workers nor reduce required skills to the barest minimum. The clerical jobs that remain fall into two categories: routine keyboarding (text or data entry, accessing of underwriting and rating programs) and skilled positions (customer service representative, claims representative, secretary). Routine keyboarding is decreasing in importance as office technology continues to advance and as work is reorganized so that sales are entered on-line. Skilled clerical work continues to increase, however, as the more routine aspects of professional work are automated and become part of the clerical function. The requirements for skilled clerical work are high general literacy, good verbal communication, and an aptitude for arithmetic, but not specific business or insurance skills.

The remaining professional jobs—exceptions or special risks underwriters, lawyers, electronic data processing professionals, actuaries, financial managers—require years of formal training in insurance or other disciplines. As a result of the automation of underwriting and claims estimating for standardized insurance products, career ladders from skilled clerical to insurance professional positions have been eliminated. The gap between the skills of clerical workers and those of professionals has widened despite the elimination of unskilled clerical work such as sorting mail and much filing, and the reduction of routine keyboarding. Skill requirements for clerical workers have increased at the same time that the jobs have become overwhelmingly dead-end.

The effect has been to eliminate a range of middle-level jobs within this industry and to close off avenues of upward mobility for those in clerical occupations. Male clerical workers always had opportunities for advancement to insurance professional and managerial positions. But until the 1970s women were prevented from advancing by the sex segregation of occupations; underwriters, managers, and even clerical supervisors and office managers were usually men. Today, partly as the result of successful affirmative action suits against several carriers, sex is a much less effective barrier to mobility. Now it appears that newly opened avenues of advancement from clerical work to professional jobs are being blocked by new structural barriers—the elimination of less skilled professional positions. While the more routine kinds of underwriting are being computerized, credentials necessary for entry into commercial lines and special risk underwriting are increasing. They often include a college degree plus the requirement that the employee obtain professional certification. The gap between the skills required in skilled clerical work and those required in the remaining insurance professional and professional staff positions appears to be unbridgeable in the context of how work is currently being organized. Avenues of mobility that have only recently opened up for women clerical workers are already disappearing.

Thus the introduction of microprocessor-based technologies and the dramatic redesign of jobs is altering the distribution of occupations in insurance. Office automation has wiped out thousands of jobs for low-skilled clerical workers, created new jobs for skilled clerical workers, and eliminated many professional jobs that comprised the middle of the occupational distribution—and that used to constitute the rungs of a career ladder by which clerical workers could climb up into more highly

TABLE 1.   Insurance Industry Employment, Selected Years

Year (annual average)	Property/ Casualty	Life/ Health	Agencies/ Brokers	Total Insurance
1960	288,700	502,600	207,200	1,008,600
1970	365,800	619,500	288,000	1,273,300
1978	460,600	661,400	392,800	1,514,800
1980	490,500	680,500	454,100	1,625,100
1981	484,400	679,600	457,500	1,621,500
1982	472,100	680,900	475,500	1,628,500
Period	Percent Change in Employment (annual average)			
1960–70	2.7	2.3	3.9	2.6
1970–78	3.2	0.9	4.6	2.4
1978–81	1.7	0.9	5.5	2.5
1980–82	−1.9	0.0	2.9	0.1

Sources: U.S. Department of Labor, *Employment and Earnings, United States, 1909–1978* (Washington, D.C.: GPO); U.S. Department of Labor, *Employment and Earnings,* table B-2, Mar. issue, various years.

Note: Figures do not include insurance industry labor force employed in real estate offices, stock brokerage houses, etc. (approximately 6 percent of the industry labor force, but increasing).

skilled professional jobs. Declines in unskilled clerical jobs have limited the entry-level job opportunities for minority and working-class women. What is more, the opportunities for advancement by even the more highly skilled clerical workers are being closed. The bottom and the middle of the occupational distribution are both shrinking in the insurance industry.

Changes in Employment and Occupations

The introduction of automation in the 1960s, characterized by the use of mainframe computers, did not discourage employment growth at carriers. Property/casualty firms experienced average annual employment growth of 2.7 percent through the decade (table 1). Job growth was paced by rapid increases in the numbers of professional/technical and clerical workers (table 2).

Not until the 1970s—when the costs of mail sorting and word processing equipment dropped, OCR technology became available, and software to automate most personal lines rating and underwriting was developed—did automation slow the growth of employment. The slowdown was most apparent in the life/health segment of the industry, which

TABLE 2. Insurance Industry Employment by Selected Occupations, 1960, 1970, 1978, and Projected 1990

Occupation	1960		1970		1978		1990	
	Number	Percentage	Number	Percentage	Number	Percentage	Number	Percentage
Managers/Officers	144,000	13.3	160,011	11.8	194,200	12.1	289,663	14.8
Professional/Technical Workers	34,700	3.2	77,773	5.8	96,468	6.0	108,487	5.5
Accountant			24,188	1.8	28,805	1.8	39,762	2.0
Systems analyst			3,833	0.3	5,514	0.3	5,514	0.3
Programmer			11,078	0.8	12,388	0.8	11,580	0.6
Clerical Workers	512,000	47.4	675,427	50.0	730,242	45.4	869,847	44.3
Computer operator			9,751	0.7	21,374	1.3	20,640	1.1
Keypunch operator			24,026	1.8	18,763	1.2	12,278	0.6
Statistical clerk			37,799	2.8	40,214	2.5	40,153	2.1
Bookkeeper			48,099	3.6	44,549	2.8	36,611	1.9
Adjustor, examiner			99,082	7.3	157,354	9.8	227,506	11.6
File clerk			34,185	2.5	27,440	1.7	31,021	1.6
Mail handler			9,334	0.7	8,332	0.5	5,947	0.3
Secretary			178,161	13.2	192,853	12.0	275,433	14.0
Typist			92,472	6.9	81,661	5.1	95,306	4.9
Clerical supervisor			15,134	1.1	16,739	1.0	16,702	0.9
Sales	363,000	33.6	404,846	30.0	555,408	34.5	663,667	33.8
Agents, brokers			403,700	29.9	554,083	34.4	662,828	33.8
Other	29,650	2.7	32,844	2.5	31,488	1.9	30,682	1.6

Sources: U.S. Department of Labor, Bureau of Labor Statistics, *Tomorrow's Manpower Needs,* vol. 2, *National Trends and Outlook: Industry Employment and Occupational Structure,* Bulletin no. 1606 (Washington, D.C.: GPO, 1969); U.S. Department of Labor, *The National Industry-Occupation Employment Matrix, 1970, 1978, and Projected 1990,* vol. 1, Bulletin no. 2086 (Washington, D.C.: GPO, 1981).

deals entirely in personal lines. Employment growth in this segment averaged 0.9 percent per year. In contrast, employment growth at property/casualty carriers, whose business is dominated by commercial risks that are only now being automated, averaged 3.2 percent per year between 1970 and 1978. It slowed to 1.7 percent in the last years of the decade as automation of office clerical and professional work accelerated.

While employment of raters and underwriters is not reported in the National Industry-Occupation Matrix, their numbers appear to have declined. This may have been offset to some extent between 1970 and 1978 by the 120 percent increase in computer operators, a category that includes operators of peripheral equipment such as CRTs (table 2). The spread of word processing equipment and electronic dictating machines is reflected in declines in the absolute numbers of typists and stenographers. The effects of increased on-line processing can be seen in decreases in the numbers of keypunch operators and file clerks. Data for the 1978–81 period are available, though they are not strictly comparable with figures cited in table 2 (U.S. Department of Labor, n.d.). The trends reported in these data are consistent with those reported for the earlier period. Most clerical categories show a relative decline (i.e., in employment share), while some occupations registered absolute declines. These include manual bookkeeping clerks, correspondence clerks, file clerks, and raters as well as typists and stenographers.

Two recent studies look ahead to the years 1990 and 2000 and examine the effect of office automation on employment (Roessner 1984; Leontief and Duchin 1984). Roessner is concerned with the effects of automation on clerical employment in insurance and banking. His study identifies several "breakthrough" technologies with the potential to reshape clerical work, examines their impact on a matrix of clerical tasks and functions, and concludes that the most likely path for clerical employment in insurance is "flat clerical employment through about 1990, then a decline in employment by 2000 to 61 percent of the 1980 level, or from 924,000 to 568,000 employees. . . . At minimum, we foresee *absolute* reductions in clerical employment of 22 percent in insurance . . . by 2000" (Roessner 1984, 26–27).

Leontief and Duchin examine the automation of office operations in business enterprises generally. They consider two scenarios, the more modest of which assumes slower adoption of computer-based workstations and integrated electronic systems. Since integrated electronic systems ("paperless offices") are expected to be slow in penetrating the insurance industry in this decade, the more modest scenario is of greater interest. In the scenario Leontief and Duchin conclude that the number of stenographers, typists, and secretaries required to produce the output of 1977 with the technology of 1990 will be 85 percent of the 1977 number. For office machine operators it will be 45 percent and for other clerical workers it will be 88 percent. By 2000 the proportions will fall to 76, 15, and 74 percent respectively. While labor requirements per unit of output are falling, the labor force and demand for output are both growing over time. Weighing reductions in unit labor requirements against growth in production, Leontief and Duchin conclude that office employment in the U.S. economy will continue to grow, though they do not report predictions for particular industries such as insurance.

The interviews I conducted with insurance executives suggest that Roesner's conclusion that there will be substantial drops in insurance industry employment is correct. His findings may, however, exaggerate the decline in clerical employment. Cost-cutting strategies at insurance carriers rely heavily on eliminating professional jobs by standardizing more routine professional functions and turning them into skilled clerical work. Thus, some part of the decline in traditional clerical jobs that he identifies may be offset by the creation of new clerical functions. In addition, many carriers expect a shakeout in insurance agencies in which only the larger, more professional ones survive. They anticipate a leaner sales force with fewer agents writing a larger volume of business as automation proceeds.

Finally, the carriers anticipate slow growth or a decline in management ranks. Excessive growth in management and supervisory personnel characterized both the life/health and property/casualty segments of the industry between 1970 and 1978. Reasons for this vary. Some firms, locked into compensation schemes geared to low inflation rates, promoted employees to raise salaries when inflation exploded. Others quietly used "title inflation" to achieve affirmative action promotion goals. Some firms rewarded their professional staff with managerial designations. By 1982 many carriers had succeeded in breaking this promotion cycle. In addition, most carriers set increases in white-collar productivity and the elimination of redundant management ranks as high priorities. The Leontief and Duchin study estimates that increases in productivity of managers as a result of automation, even in the more modest scenario, will allow the 1977 volume of work to be done with 99 percent of the 1977 managers in 1990 and 88 percent by 2000.

Changing Opportunities for Women: Race, Class, and Gender Issues

Shifts in the occupational distribution in the insurance industry have important implications for employment opportunities for women. Women comprise virtually 100 percent of the employees in clerical occupations in which employment has declined. Because of the high turnover rates in clerical jobs in insurance, reductions in staff were accomplished largely through attrition. Nevertheless, traditional clerical jobs for which noncollege-bound women frequently train while in high school declined by a total of 28,556 positions between 1970 and 1978. At the same time, skilled clerical positions are being penetrated by women and new skilled clerical jobs are being created. Thus, women insurance adjustors, examiners, and investigators (occupations classified as clerical) were 9 percent of total employees in those occupations in 1962, 26 percent of the total in 1971, and 58 percent of the total in 1981 (U.S. Department of Labor 1982). Employment in these occupations increased more than 58,000 between 1970 and 1978, while the percentage of female employees nearly doubled. As a result, the number of women holding such jobs increased by approximately 56,000. Thus the feminization of insurance adjustor, examiner, and investigator occupations more than offset the declines in traditionally female clerical jobs before 1978. These jobs will be affected, however, as the automation of claims procedures progresses.

As a result of both the technological dynamic and the penetration by women of male occupations, the level of skill required of women clerical workers is rising. Insurance companies have adopted several strategies for hiring women with the appropriate skills. These include moving the work from central cities to small towns, suburbs, and rural areas where the work force is mostly white and pay for women is lower. A second strategy firms have followed is to hire college graduates for career clerical positions. Clerical work does not require any specific skills learned in college, not even computer literacy, since computer tasks required in clerical jobs are easily mastered. However, college graduates are hired to ensure that general literacy and the problem-solving requirements of the jobs will be met.

Minority women have only recently penetrated clerical work and are still found mainly in the less skilled clerical jobs. Thus automation is eliminating precisely those jobs in which black women are present in significant numbers. The movement of clerical work to small towns and suburbs and the increased hiring of college-educated women for these jobs also limits opportunities for black women. These developments have a similar negative impact on employment possibilities for less educated urban white working-class women, as well.

The issue of upward mobility is also an important consideration. As argued above, job categories have become more segmented. The gap between skilled clerical and professional employees has grown larger, and jobs that constituted the career path from clerical to professional work have largely been eliminated. This does not mean that professional, technical, sales, and lower level management jobs are likely to become entirely male again. On the contrary, jobs for college-educated women professionals, and to a lesser extent managers, continue to open up. Women increased from 10 percent of insurance agents, brokers, and underwriters in 1962 to 12 percent in 1971 and 24 percent in 1981 (U.S. Department of Labor 1982). This is reflected in the employment growth of women in the agencies/brokers segment of the industry (table 3), though most of these jobs of course are clerical. In nonclerical jobs, it appears, desegregation will continue. The ongoing recruitment of women as computer programmers, marketing managers, and underwriters is seen by the carriers as obviating the need for promotion of women from clerical to professional or managerial ranks.

Men continue to dominate those departments from which the carriers choose their top managers and executives, namely, finance, marketing, investment, and actuary. But women have been entering professional and lower managerial ranks and can be expected to continue doing so. Some of the specialized occupations within these categories may become majority female, since educated women can be hired more cheaply than similarly qualified men. The result could be lower pay and lower status in those jobs, with the work devalued because it is done by women.

The occupational structure for women in the insurance industry is becoming increasingly two-tiered. It has been observed that the occupational hierarchy is not as gender-segregated as in the past, but occupational stratification occurs increasingly along class and race lines (Baran and Teegarden 1983). Educated white women with the appropriate credentials and class background enter the upper tier as jobs there continue to be desegregated. The vast majority of women in insurance, however, are relegated to totally segregated clerical jobs. Technology is eliminating the least skilled of these, but literate clerical workers, especially if they are white, will find their situation essentially unchanged.

Implications for Education

The combined effects of technology and changes in the economy are placing new demands on the U.S. instructional system. As exemplified by the insurance industry, office automation has raised skill requirements for clerical workers. Employers have made it clear that they want high schools to provide a strong foundation in reading, math, written and verbal communication, and problem-solving skills. Computer literacy is viewed as a less pressing requirement, since the computer skills

TABLE 3. Employment of Women in the Insurance Industry, Selected Years, in Thousands

Year (annual average)	Property/Casualty		Life/Health		Agencies/Brokers		Total	
	Number	Percentage	Number	Percentage	Number	Percentage	Number	Percentage
1960	165.8	57.4	252.7	50.3	112.2	54.1	530.7	52.6
1970	207.8	56.8	314.7	50.8	158.8	55.1	681.3	53.5
1978	283.4	61.5	371.6	56.2	239.1	60.9	894.1	59.0
1980	308.8	63.0	396.9	58.3	282.1	62.1	987.8	60.8
1982	294.0	62.1	401.3	58.9	301.4	63.4	996.7	61.2

Sources: U.S. Department of Labor, *Employment and Earnings, United States, 1909–1978* (Washington, D.C.: GPO); U.S. Department of Labor, *Employment and Earnings,* tables B-2 and B-3, Mar. issue, various years.

required by nonspecialists can be acquired through company training by workers who have reading and problem-solving capabilities.

Thus automation is blurring the distinction between vocational or commercial education and academic education in secondary schools, as new technology increases the importance of reading and analytical skills for clerical workers. With job content changing as automation progresses, employers want—and workers require—broad occupational preparation as well as specific technology-related vocational skills. A broad education is essential because it increases individual career choices, provides a foundation for learning new skills, and allows an individual to adjust effectively to a job change or a change in the work environment. These are qualities workers need in order to deal with likely future changes in skill requirements in office industries.

Specific vocational skills related to current office technologies which are useful for business students are word processing, data processing, electronic mail handling, and electronic records management. It should be noted, however, that the insurance industry has a long history of providing company- and industry-sponsored training programs to teach specific vocational skills (including word processing, telephone speaking skills, even use of BASIC), as well as insurance concepts and procedures, to workers who require them. As unskilled clerical and routine keyboarding jobs decline, the proportion of workers requiring such training is increasing. Carriers are stepping up their training and retraining programs, and industry-wide educational organizations are responding by developing new courses. Employers' primary concern, therefore, is to hire workers who will be successful in these training and educational programs and for whom training costs can be kept to a minimum.

Women need college degrees to enter professional jobs now that the jobs that once constituted internal career ladders are declining. Opportunities for college education need to be made more generally available. Inner-city high schools need the resources to prepare students for entrance into degree programs. Otherwise the desegregation of occupations by gender will mask an equally invidious exclusion of inner-city women, especially black women, from these jobs.

The need for increased emphasis on training in mathematics for women is also apparent. Arithmetic as well as problem-solving and analytical skills are necessary in both clerical and professional jobs. Moreover, women need advanced training in mathematics in order to enter top professions (for example, actuary, operations researcher, or financial manager in insurance), from which the upper ranks of corporate management are often filled.

By shifting the occupational distribution toward skilled clerical and highly trained professional jobs, office automation is challenging the educational system to design instructional programs that provide a sound foundation in basic skills for all students and that prepare high school graduates for a lifetime of continuing education, either in college, other postsecondary schools, or industry-based instructional programs. The educational establishment is also being asked to develop programs to meet the newly emerging lifelong need for education for those in the labor force.

The capacity of the educational system to meet these requirements is in doubt. Funding of public secondary and higher education is inadequate to enable educators to design and deliver instructional programs that will significantly broaden and improve basic education, especially when the needs of workers in other industries that require scientific education and technical training or proficiency in a foreign language and a knowledge of history and culture are also taken into consideration. Educational goals continually run into resource constraints, a situation that can only be reversed by a change in national priorities.

Conclusion

Automation is changing the job opportunities for clerical workers. In the insurance industry it has eliminated thousands of traditional clerical jobs for file clerks, data entry clerks, typists, bookkeepers, stenographers, and mail handlers. At the same time, women have penetrated previously male clerical jobs such as insurance examiner, adjustor, and investigator while automation has created new skilled clerical jobs such as underwriter's assistant and customer service representative, which are filled mainly by women. The result is an increase in the skill levels of clerical workers.

Automation has also reduced the upward mobility of clerical workers who want to move from skilled clerical to professional positions. This has happened because the routine aspects of professional work have been automated and folded into clerical jobs, and lower-level professional jobs have been eliminated. These jobs used to serve as a career ladder for clerical workers. Declines in unskilled clerical jobs have limited the entry-level job opportunities for minority and working-class women while opportunities for advancement even by skilled clerical workers are also being closed.

Women constitute 61 percent of the insurance industry's current labor force and nearly 100 percent of the workers in traditional clerical jobs. Educational systems have a key role to play in preparing those women workers who are most affected by automation for remaining employment opportunities. Women must be college educated in order to compete for the remaining professional jobs. They must be literate, with good communication and problem-solving skills, to compete for skilled clerical jobs. Failure to improve the quality of inner-city schools will close off clerical employment for minority and white working-class women.

REFERENCES

Baran, Barbara, and Suzanne Teegarden. 1983. Women's labor in the insurance office. Department of City and Regional Planning, University of California, Berkeley. Mimeo.

Leontief, Wassily, and Faye Duchin. 1984. *The impact of automation on employment, 1963–2000*. Final Report to the National Science Foundation. New York: Institute for Economic Analysis, New York University.

Roessner, J. David. 1984. *Impact of office automation on office workers*. Final Report to the Employment and Training Administration, U.S. Department of Labor. Atlanta: Georgia Institute of Technology.

Sametz, Arnold W. 1984. *The emerging financial industry*. Lexington, Mass.: Lexington Books.

Upheaval in life insurance. 1984. *Business Week,* June 25.

U.S. Department of Labor. n.d. *Occupational employment survey, insurance 1978, 1981*. Unpublished report, Bureau of Labor Statistics, Washington D.C.

———. 1982. News release, Bureau of Labor Statistics, Middle Atlantic Region, Nov. 2.

Office Technology and Relations of Control in Clerical Work Organization

Valerie J. Carter

Among critical analysts of the labor process, in the established tradition of Harry Braverman's *Labor and Monopoly Capital* (1974), it has become almost a truism to say that new technology is utilized by capitalists to deskill and otherwise weaken the working class. It is seen as in the interests of capitalists and managers to use technology to routinize and degrade labor with the intention of obtaining greater productivity or efficiency, and hence greater profits. In addition to cutting labor costs, both through deskilling and actual job loss, new technology may increase managerial control over workers. Worker autonomy becomes reduced as workers perform more narrowly defined, repetitive work and become more easily replaceable. Furthermore, as Richard Edwards suggested in *Contested Terrain* (1979), managerial control over workers has become increasingly structural in nature; that is, it has become embedded in the actual technology used in the workplace (such as in the assembly line) or in the bureaucratic structure of the complex organizations within which most people work.

Within the past ten years or so, many analysts working within this critical labor process tradition have turned their attention to clerical workers as a crucial segment of the working class. The theoretical framework of deskilling and work degradation has often been extended to the office workplace to describe the consequences of new microelectronics-based technology for clerical work (e.g., Machung 1983; West 1982; Murphree 1982). This literature suggests that clericals working with video display terminals (VDTs) will tend to become increasingly deskilled—that is, they will perform more narrowly circumscribed, repetitive tasks and will be deprived of an overall knowledge of the productive process of which they are a part. Presumably they will also be subjected to greater managerial control through such means as work quotas, computer surveillance or monitoring of one's work, a greater subdivision of labor, truncated mobility ladders, and so on. All this suggests that clericals will find themselves increasingly unhappy with their work, simultaneously more bored and under greater stress.

The main alternative to Braverman's approach in analyzing the

202

impact of office automation upon office work has until recently been in the business-oriented literature, which usually emphasizes the positive consequences of automation in terms of enhanced skills for workers, as well as increased productivity generally, without explicit references to the issue of control in the workplace (e.g., Meyer 1983; Teger 1983; Hubbartt 1983). Much of this literature has also suggested, in direct contradiction to the critical labor process literature, that the new "information age" office will result in job enlargement or enrichment, more interesting work, and increased job opportunities for more highly skilled workers (Zisman 1978; Hubbartt 1983; Giuliano 1982; Matteis 1979).

Now some researchers within the critical labor process tradition, without accepting the enthusiastic proautomation attitudes of management-oriented analyses, have begun to question whether this deskilling model is always appropriate for analyzing the current work situations of clerical workers. My own research on the impact of office automation on control and autonomy within clerical work also indicates that there is a need to modify and extend Braverman's model of deskilling when analyzing clerical work. Much of the testimony I have heard thus far from clerical workers themselves suggests that the situation is more complex than that portrayed in most of the critical office automation literature.

In assessing how the deskilling model might be revised or modified to take into account the complex and diverse situations of clerical workers, it is first necessary to discuss some of the problems in formulating adequate concepts of control and autonomy in the clerical workplace. Next, I will suggest some possible explanations for the apparent contradiction I have found between the deskilling hypothesis and my own fieldwork, and describe my own research on office workers in a large public university. Finally, I consider some of the implications of the research findings for theories about how women office workers are affected by computerization, and more generally for theories about women and technology.

Control in the Office

Among clerical workers, and especially among secretarial workers, the issues of control and autonomy in the workplace are complicated, both conceptually and in terms of finding concrete ways of studying them. A conceptual understanding of control in the office must begin with the fact that clerical work is predominantly done by women, as it has become transformed into a female sex-typed occupation (Davies 1982). This apparently simple fact helps to explain why clerical workers tend to be subjected to specifically sex-linked forms of control, which have been termed "patriarchal" or "patrimonial." Many of the recent analyses of control among clerical workers have focused on the complex relationships among patriarchal control and the other forms of workplace control outlined by Richard Edwards (1979): simple, technical, and bureaucratic control.

According to Edwards, three major forms of workplace control developed historically in the United States. Simple control, which characterized most firms through the late 1800s, is still most characteristic today of small, competitive firms. This term refers to direct, personal, and relatively arbitrary forms of control by entrepreneurs or supervisors over workers. The other two types of control, technical and bureaucratic, are both more structural and more formal in nature; they developed along with the transition to monopoly capitalism (from 1890 to 1920). Technical control refers to control that is embedded in the physical structure of the labor process, for example, in the machinery used to manufacture commodities or in the continuous assembly line. Bureaucratic control, on the other hand, is embedded within the social structure of an organization in the form of bureaucratic procedures, company policy, and impersonal rules. Although bureaucratic control did not completely replace simple and technical control (in fact, Edwards emphasizes that in reality workplaces tend to utilize some combination of all three types), it developed as the major control system in large corporations, as they became increasingly centralized and concentrated.

Patriarchal control can be seen as a form of simple control, in that it tends to be manifested through personal, direct forms of supervision by superordinates over subordinates. In addition to being based on differences in hierarchy or authority per se, however, patriarchal control carries the additional dimension of traditional male dominance over women. Insofar as female clerical workers are viewed as conforming to the traditional stereotype of women as passive, obedient, emotional rather than analytical, and in a service role to men as helpmates, the role expectations for clerical workers will be based both on differences in hierarchy and on perceived sex differences. Davies (1982) and Glenn and Feldberg (1977), for example, have described how being "nice," pleasant, loyal, courteous, and well-groomed (if not "attractive") has become a built-in and often explicit role demand for clericals (and for secretaries in particular). The frequent role expectation for clericals to help maintain a pleasant and cheerful environment can be seen as a form of invisible labor, that is, it only becomes noticeable when it is not being done, or is not done well. And as with housework, another form of invisible labor, it is performed predominantly by women.

While almost everyone would agree that clerical workers, like other workers, are usually subjected to more than one form of control, there is some disagreement over how the mosaic of control in the office is changing. Several analysts have described how technical and bureaucratic forms of control in the office are increasing, while patriarchal control becomes eroded; they suggest that this process is being heightened by office automation. These changes can have mixed consequences, however, and their implications for office workers are not clear.

These coexisting forms of control are not only different in kind but may be actually contradictory, as Roberta Goldberg (1983) argues. Under patriarchal control, for example, women clerical workers have often been expected to accept, or at least to put up with, various forms of explicit and implicit sexual harassment. In a bureaucratically controlled system, however, sexual harassment may be expressly prohibited. Clerical workers can utilize bureaucratic rules and regulations to resist such harassment. Having clear-cut job descriptions under a bureaucratic system can also undercut traditional expectations for secretaries to perform sex-based tasks such as making coffee, watering the plants, buying a gift for the boss's wife, and so on. Hence increased bureaucratic control, while it tends to increase stratification in the office, can actually be "more liberalizing," she says. Goldberg suggests that it is in the interests of employers to maintain patriarchal control, although this form of control is no longer sufficient by itself.

In a similar vein, Machung (1983) also sees some potentially positive consequences for women workers coming out of the transition from predominantly patriarchal to predominantly technical forms of control. This transition may ultimately result in greater class consciousness and greater receptivity to union organizing among secretaries and word processor operators, as the supposedly special privileges of office work become eroded.

On the other hand, both Barker and Downing (1980) and Machung (1983) see the structural forms of control—technical and bureaucratic—as undermining the traditional "social office," in which clerical workers have developed their own modes of resistance to patriarchal systems of control. For example, clericals have developed their own "culture of the office" in which personal and family matters become shared topics of conversation; clericals thereby maintain a separateness or distance from managerial authority and may be excused for their "idle chatter" because they are women. These analysts argue further that conventional notions of deskilling do not apply to clerical work, which is a predominantly female labor process, since many of the necessary office skills are in fact unrecognized and devalued—albeit important—social and diplomatic skills.

As Machung puts it, clerical work was not historically deskilled in the same sense that craft workers were; instead, clerical work was "feminized." Along with the rise of monopoly capitalism from roughly 1890 to 1920, the demand for clerical workers increased dramatically as the need for corporate record keeping grew. As the size of the clerical labor force expanded, clerical work also changed from a predominantly male occupation to an increasingly female one. It became sex-typed as appropriate for women, due to their supposedly greater manual dexterity, patience for repetitive work, and attention to detail. The fact that women could be paid less than men was also an obvious advantage.

As part of the growing sex-typing of clerical work as naturally "women's work," the occupation was transformed into a "feminine" craft in which social and emotional traits or skills in dealing with people became centrally important. Machung has characterized this type of occupational role demand for clericals as "emotional labor," in which clerical workers are expected to maintain a cheerful, friendly demeanor as well as help to keep the office atmosphere itself pleasant and nonthreatening through a variety of social skills and personality traits. Although this type of skill is not recognized or valued highly as a form of work, it takes its toll nonetheless by adding to the stress of clerical workers who must often swallow their own anger in order to keep office interactions meshing smoothly, seemingly without effort.

Since coexisting and contradictory forms of control characterize the clerical workplace, the existence of one form of control can actually provide the basis for resistance to another; there may also be a contradictory potential for clerical resistance within the *same* mode of control. Within patriarchal control, for example, women who encounter sexually suggestive remarks from their bosses may utilize traditional gender expectations by feigning ignorance, or they may refer casually to their large, jealous male partners (whether or not such partners exist).

Analyzing the relationship of new office technologies to workplace control is further complicated by the great diversity among clerical workers. Clerical jobs vary by level of hierarchy and type of work, by the type of organization, by location in the public versus the private sector, and so on. The situation of private secretaries differs greatly from that of file clerks, clerk-typists in the typing pool, or word processors. This diversity often serves as a "divide and conquer" mechanism, since it obscures both the differences between management and workers and the underlying similarities in clerical work. Glenn and Feldberg (1979) and Goldberg (1983) have also described the increased segmentation and diversity among clericals as a barrier to class consciousness.

To summarize, the early consensus among researchers who have studied the effects of office automation—especially word processing—on control has been that a transition to an automated office results in greater technical and bureaucratic control, as well as in general deskilling. Usually this is described as being manifested in decreased discretion on the job, narrowed skills, increased surveillance and machine monitoring, increased use of quotas, less control over personal space and movement, greater standardization in work, and a heightened division of labor. Some very recent work suggests greater complexity regarding this issue, but this complexity has yet to be fully explored.

Studying Office Workers

Although I fully expected to find these predictions confirmed in my own research, my preconceptions were greatly shaken during my initial fieldwork with office workers from two organizations and with clericals attending a union-sponsored conference on health and safety. As I had expected, many clericals were concerned about real and potential health and safety problems associated with VDT use, especially eyestrain, headaches, and the possibility of pregnancy-related problems such as miscarriages and birth defects. But, Harry Braverman notwithstanding, my conversations with clericals at various levels and my survey pretest results did not substantiate my other predictions.

Many of the clericals who worked with VDTs gave them lavish praise and said that thanks to them, they had been relieved of much of the drudgery of typing repeated drafts. Clericals who were not working with VDTs often lamented that fact, and many looked forward to getting them. My pretest survey results did not suggest any relationship between whether an individual worked on a VDT and whether she found her work repetitive, stressful, boring, or difficult. Clericals working with VDTs who were asked to compare their pre-VDT and post-VDT work were just as likely to say their work was easier and more interesting after they began using VDTs, as not.

I also found evidence that some clericals were seizing the opportunity to get VDT training and skills as a means of obtaining promotions into the lower professional job categories, for example, from administrative secretary to administrative assistant. One source familiar with this area said explicitly that during the past few years several clericals had made the transition into the professional ranks. She thought this transition was often related to these persons having acquired computer skills. While this transition may not have made a substantive difference in the nature of the work they did, they were nonetheless able to obtain both higher status and higher pay.

Why was I not hearing stories from my clerical contacts about deskilling and greater managerial control, especially greater technical control, in offices that were automated? One possible reason for the discrepancy between my investigations and the findings of other researchers may be the great diversity among clericals and among work situations. In fact, most of the critical clerical research I have come across so far has dealt with clericals in large, centralized settings, usually in the private sector. Word processor operators in banks and in insurance companies seem to represent the typical clerical worker under scrutiny, and such workers are rarely unionized. Not all clericals work in such large settings, however, and clericals in the government sector have become heavily unionized over the past decade or so. More specifically, the discrepancy may be explained by more systematic differences in the structural or organizational setting, such as the size of the office, centralization, and the division of labor.

Most of the research thus far has failed to look at the *conditions* under which new office technology is introduced. This issue is, I believe, a crucially important one, and one that bears directly on the notion of technological determinism, which often characterizes many of these analyses at least implicitly. Are deskilling and greater workplace control over employees necessary consequences of the introduction of new office technology? Are they a more or less universal consequence under capitalism, as many people would suggest? Or does the impact of office technology depend greatly on the structural conditions of the workplace—such as characteristics of the organization itself in its larger historical context, as well as characteristics of the particular office setting? This is the main focus of my research in this area.

To be fair, most of the researchers are careful to point out that diversity does exist among clerical workers, and that office automation need not *necessarily* lead to greater managerial control, less worker autonomy, deskilling, or proletarianization. However, the conditions under which it might not produce such effects are left unspecified.

In my own research on the problem of how office automation affects control and autonomy in clerical work, I studied clerical workers at a large public university. I used survey questionnaires as well as conducting fieldwork. The survey questionnaire allowed information to be gathered from a large number of people, while the field research permitted greater depth and breadth in the kind of information I could obtain.

At this large university, which employs literally hundreds of clerical workers, I compared a large sample of office workers across two dimensions. One is the size of the office or unit, and the other is the intensity or degree of automation. This ranges from offices entirely without automation to those with partial and/or recent automation to those in which automation (such as word processing or automated student records) is well established and affects most or all of the workers in the office.

The types of offices sampled were quite diverse, ranging from small academic offices with one or two clerical workers, with no VDTs or one VDT used occasionally by the clericals for word processing exams, to large academic offices with six or seven clerical staff. In some of these large offices there were no VDTs at all, in others, recently-installed VDTs that the staff were only beginning to use, and in others, there were VDTs that had been in use for quite some time by some or all of the clerical staff. There were also many nonacademic offices: financial offices dealing with accounts, student services–oriented offices where there was a great deal of ongoing contact with students, administrative offices such as a dean's or vice-president's office, which might have a combination of clerical and professional staff. Some small units had only one or two professional staff, who might or might not use VDTs on the job, while other large offices had twenty or more clerical and/or professional workers—some computerized, some not. In other words, there was a diversity of office configurations in terms of type of service, size, presence and use of VDTs, and presence of clerical and/or professional staff.

The major hypothesis in my research is that the consequences of office automation for the type and degree of control over clerical workers will vary according to structural differences in office settings, even within the same organization. Structural features of the office setting—in particular, the size, centralization, division of labor, and type of supervision—may be important in determining what effects automation has on workplace control and worker autonomy. I hypothesized that clericals working in relatively small, decentralized office settings will not be adversely affected by office automation in terms of control over their own work, while workers in large, centralized automated settings will be subjected to greater control and will hence have less autonomy. Thus the question is this: Will working on a VDT, in and of itself, produce more repetitive work, with greater control by management and less discretion on the job? I expected that the answer would be dependent on the kind of immediate office setting within which it is implemented (everything else being equal).

Explaining Autonomy and Routinization

To test this hypothesis, I began by examining the relationships between two sets of independent variables (individual, i.e., relating to the worker; and structural, i.e., relating to the office setting); and two sets of dependent variables, used respectively as indicators of job autonomy and of work routinization. The sample used in this analysis is actually a segment ($N = 78$) of the larger sample of clerical and lower-level professional ("nonclerical") workers surveyed at the large university (total sample $N = 296$). The sampling design was a stratified random sample, with respondents chosen randomly but by different proportions within the office type categories (large computerized, large noncomputerized, small computerized, small noncomputerized).

The individual-level independent variables include number of hours worked on a VDT per day, whether the respondent is a clerical worker or in a nonclerical job category (coded as a dummy variable), months of experience using a VDT, and the age of the respondent. The structural level independent variables are office size (coded as a dummy variable, where small equals five or less office staff, and large equals six or more office workers); and whether the office is computerized (Office Computerized), i.e., whether the office has VDTs actually in use by the office staff (also coded as a dummy variable). The exact office size in terms of numbers of staff was not yet available for this analysis (but see Carter 1986).

The two indicators of routinization were "learning new things," the extent to which respondents' jobs require them to keep learning new things, and "repetitive," the extent to which their jobs require that they do things that are very repetitious (table 1). The two dependent variables used as indicators of job autonomy were "decide tasks," which measured the extent to which the respondent determines the order or priority of tasks in his or her job, and "freedom," or the extent to which the respondent has the freedom to decide how to do his or her own work (table 2). See appendix A for the exact wordings of the dependent variables.

For each of the four dependent variables, a multiple regression was run for the full subsample ($N = 78$), as well as separately by categories of office size. I also repeated the analysis for clericals only and for nonclericals only, to determine whether the results for these groups were different from those of the sample taken as a whole. The regression model used in these analyses looks at the effect of each variable as a predictor of the dependent variable, after the effects of all the other independent variables are taken into account. In other words, the regression coefficient for each variable shows what additional effect that variable had as a predictor, treating it as the last variable entered into the regression equation.

TABLE 1. **Standardized Regression Coefficients of Routinization**

Independent Variables	Whole Sample ($N = 72$)	Clericals Only ($N = 49$)	Large Offices ($N = 46$)	Small Offices ($N = 26$)
	Dependent Variable: Job Requires Learning New Things			
VDT hours	.27*	.41*	.22	.41
Clerical	−.23*	—	−.25	−.09
Office size	.12	.12	—	—
Office computerized	−.005	.03	.13	−.18
Experience	−.13	−.37*	−.17	−.15
Age	.26*	.38*	.28	.26
R^2	.21*	.17	.23*	.12
	Dependent Variable: Job Is Repetitious			
VDT hours	−.12	−.26	−.04	−.35
Clerical	.15	—	.14	.17
Office size	.34*	.38*	—	—
Office computerized	.005	−.02	−.11	.47
Experience	−.02	.11	.00	−.46
Age	−.18	−.17	−.14	−.31
R^2	.14	.14	.06	.31

*Significant at .05 level, 2-tailed test

Effects of Computerization

The results for "learning new things" on the job for the entire subsample showed that as the number of hours worked on a VDT increased, respondents were more likely to be in jobs requiring them to learn new things on the job, and hence less likely to be in routinized jobs. The relationship between individual VDT hours and learning new things remains statistically significant even after the effects of the other independent variables are controlled. Clerical workers were also less likely than nonclerical workers to be required to learn new things, and older workers were more likely than younger workers to be required to learn new things. In other words, clerical workers found their work more routinized than nonclericals, and older workers tended to find their jobs less routinized than younger workers. (See Carter 1986 for detailed regression results.)

In the separate analyses of "learning new things" for large versus small offices, and for clericals versus nonclerical workers, only one re-

TABLE 2. Standardized Regression Coefficients of Autonomy

Independent Variables	Whole Sample ($N = 73$)	Clericals Only ($N = 50$)	Large Offices ($N = 46$)	Small Offices ($N = 27$)
	Dependent Variable: Able to Decide Order or Priority of Tasks			
VDT hours	−.23	−.10	−.29*	.64*
Clerical	.09	—	.11	−.08
Office size	−.11	−.10	—	—
Office computerized	−.05	.02	−.07	−.67*
Experience	−.20	−.40*	−.25	.06
Age	.07	.13	.15	.07
R^2	.21*	.28*	.19	.27
	Dependent Variable: Freedom to Decide How to Do Work			
VDT hours	−.10	.06	−.20	0.35
Clerical	.11	—	.15	−0.004
Office size	−.09	−.08	—	—
Office computerized	−.21	−.18	.08	−1.00*
Experience	−.04	−.35*	−.08	0.57*
Age	.03	.10	.05	0.07
R^2	.15	.21	.07	0.51*

*Significant at .05 level, 2-tailed test

gression, that of the clerical workers, showed any statistically significant relationships. The strongest variable was age, with a positive slope indicating that, as for the sample as a whole, older workers were more likely to learn new things on the job, or less likely to be in routinized jobs. Individual VDT hours was again a significant positive predictor of learning new things, while those workers with greater computer experience were somewhat less likely to be in jobs where they were expected to learn new things—in other words, amount of computer experience was a negative predictor.

While these findings may appear contradictory, they might be explained by three sometimes conflicting tendencies: (1) older workers are more likely to be in jobs with greater responsibility and diversity; (2) people with more hours on the VDT may often be learning VDT skills for the first time; and (3) those workers with the most computer-related experience are sometimes those who have done data-entry for many years.

To summarize the results for the "learning new things" dimension of routinization, individual characteristics seemed to be more important predictors than structural characteristics such as office size, and hence these results do not support my research hypothesis.

For the other routinization variable, "repetitive," a similar set of multiple regressions was performed. First, for the sample as a whole, although the model itself was not significant, there was one significant predictor variable. The coefficient for office size indicated that workers in larger offices found their work more repetitive than workers in smaller offices. Taking the results of regressions separately by office size and for clerical versus nonclerical workers, again only the clerical group showed any significant predictors. Among clerical workers, as with the total sample, people working in large offices found their work more repetitive and more routine.

To summarize the results for doing repetitive work, then, the importance of office size as a predictor indicates that this structural characteristic matters more than individual characteristics, which supports my research hypothesis. In this case, the number of hours worked on a VDT was not at all important. Repetitive work is probably more a function of the extent to which labor can be divided, and office size seems to reflect this.

Going on to look at the multiple regression results for the two autonomy variables, "decide tasks" and "freedom," we find for the sample as a whole that the regression model for deciding on the order or priority of tasks was strongly significant, taking all the variables together, but there were no statistically significant predictor variables taken individually.

The subgroup analyses for this autonomy variable are much more revealing. Looking at clericals alone, the most important predictor or independent variable in the model was amount of computer experience. The results indicated that as clerical workers accumulated more experience, they actually had less autonomy on the job, as measured by the degree to which they could decide on the order or priority of their tasks, rather than having this decision determined by others. This finding may possibly be explained by the fact that clericals with the most experience may be most likely to be doing tasks such as data entry or similar tasks in which there is little latitude for variation in decision making. Alternatively, there may be differences in subjective perceptions of how much autonomy one's job offers among workers with varying levels of experience. These are questions that cannot be answered in this analysis, however.

For persons working in large versus small offices, the most interesting finding was that the effect of number of hours on a VDT was different for each of the groups, with the regression coefficient positive for small offices and negative for large offices.

For people working in small offices, both VDT Hours and Office Computerized were statistically significant predictors of decision-making latitude. The regression coefficient of $b = .64$ shows that as number of hours using a VDT increased in small offices, actual autonomy on the job increased as well. People working in computerized offices, however, had less autonomy on the job than people in noncomputerized offices. In large offices, on the other hand, individual VDT hours had a regression coefficient of $-.29$, meaning that in these offices people were likely to have *less* autonomy in terms of deciding on the order of tasks, as the extent of time they spent on the computer increased.

A summary of the results for "decide tasks" as a measure of autonomy, then, shows that the structural characteristic of office size is an important variable in determining the importance of individual VDT hours. In this case, office size is a mediating variable: in small offices, working on a VDT is positively associated with being able to decide on the order or priority of job tasks, while in large offices, working on a VDT is negatively associated with deciding tasks. This finding supports the research hypothesis that structural characteristics help to determine the relationship between office automation and autonomy.

The other variable used as an indicator of autonomy, freedom to decide how to do one's work, was not significantly related to any of the independent variables for the sample taken as a whole. However, among clericals, amount of experience on a VDT was the only significant predictor of freedom. The regression coefficient indicates that among clericals, as months of experience on a VDT increased, the actual level of freedom decreased, similar to the pattern shown for the "decide tasks" dependent variable.

While the analysis for large offices showed no significant results, in small offices the model as a whole explained a large degree of the total variable in freedom to decide how to do the work. Two individual variables, amount of computer experience and whether the office was computerized, were strong predictors of freedom on the job. These results indicate that for people in smaller offices, those working in computerized offices had less freedom, but that people with more VDT experience tended to have greater freedom. While this may seem somewhat contradictory, this suggests the interesting possibility that while office automation may produce an initial drop in freedom to do the work as one pleases, workers may subsequently be able to increase their freedom or autonomy as they gain more experience with and knowledge about the computer.

Overall, the results for freedom to decide how to do the work also support the idea that office characteristics may play an important role in determining the consequences of working on a VDT for office workers, although job characteristics of individuals, such as clerical versus non-clerical status, obviously continue to be important as well.

In summary, then, these analyses showed that both structural and individual-level independent variables were in some cases important predictors of routinization and autonomy on the job. The results for "learning new things" on the job, the first routinization measure, showed that individual predictors were most important: number of hours worked on a VDT, age, and clerical status. The results were quite different for doing repetitive work, however; with this variable, the only important predictor was the structural characteristic of office size. This discrepancy suggests that perhaps "learning new things" and repetitive work cannot both be subsumed under the conceptual rubric of routinization, or else that they are simply measuring quite different aspects of work routinization.

The results for the autonomy variables, "decide tasks" and "freedom," show that the analyses are more revealing when done within subgroupings of the sample rather than for the sample as a whole. The importance of computer experience among clerical workers and in small offices, combined with the negative effects of the Office Computerized dummy variable among small offices, suggests that automation of work can have negative consequences for autonomy under some circumstances, but that as workers gain greater experience over time it is possible for autonomy to increase, at least in small office settings. In addition, the effect of working more hours on a VDT on "deciding tasks" was totally opposite for workers in small versus large offices. In small offices, more VDT hours meant greater autonomy in deciding the order or priority of tasks, while in large offices, more hours worked on VDTs meant less autonomy. These results strongly support the idea that office size helps to determine how autonomy is affected by working on a VDT.

More detailed analyses of the entire sample are currently in progress, and it will be interesting to see how such variables as supervisory relations may influence the relationship between these independent variables and the measures of autonomy and routinization utilized here.

Theoretical Implications

Why should the consequences of office automation be different depending on the size of the office setting? First, size is strongly related to how centralized an office or organization is; the larger the office, the more centralized it usually is in terms of authority and assignment of tasks. Second, there tends to be a more extensive division of labor in a large setting, such that people become more specialized in performing more narrowly defined sets of tasks.

Third, in smaller offices, clerical workers are more likely to have a monopoly on knowledge, in particular their knowledge of the information systems with which they work. In a large setting, managerial, supervisory, or management information systems (MIS) personnel may control the overall technical knowledge of how information is stored and processed, as well as knowledge of the information itself. In a smaller office, on the other hand, a clerical worker can often retain a great deal of control in this area by developing and maintaining her technical expertise in a position of scarcity. For example, one university clerical worker said to me, "I've set up three data bases, and I'm the only one who knows how to use them." If, for example, a clerical worker is the only one who understands the accounts receivable information system, she (and usually it is a she) can wield a great deal of leverage.

It is clear that retaining or developing one's own autonomy depends on the resources available to do so. Such resources include not only formal, legitimate power (authority), but also informal, sometimes unrecognized forms of resistance. Since clerical workers have been largely unable to depend on official organizational channels of power to maintain their autonomy (even high-level executive or other private secretaries who can often exercise considerable informal power), they have had to depend on other resources.

Such resources can be collective—for example, the backing of a union in an organized workplace, or direct actions by workers such as organized forms of sabotage or work stoppages—or individual. Individual resources include such things as the possession of valuable skills, maintaining a position of scarcity in the market, and the possession of valuable organizational and/or technical knowledge that may not be directly accessible to others. This may be especially true in an office that is only beginning to be computerized, since those who deal most directly with the computer system may have privileged access to it and hence maintain a position of influence.

In sum, two related issues must inform our analyses of how automation affects the labor process in the office workplace: first, office workers are active subjects as well as passive objects of technological change in the workplace; and second, office workers who attempt to utilize such technological change for their own purposes may have more success in some settings than in others.

I suggest that the discrepancy between the predictions of critical labor process theorists and the initial testimony I have gathered may be due to a lack of recognition of the dialectical nature of the relationship between new technology on the one hand and workplace control and worker autonomy on the other. As some critics of Braverman have pointed out (e.g., Stark 1982; Wright 1978), it is necessary to look not only at the attempts of managers and capitalists to reorganize the workplace and/or control workers, but also at the responses of workers and the strategies they develop. Stark (1982) argues further that the reorganization of work can produce new problems of control for managers or capitalists, while Wright (1978) suggests that changing technology can create new job categories in which workers have greater immediate control over the labor process.

It is only too easy to forget that clericals, whether they work in automated offices or not, do have some resources available to them. People can and do actively work to maintain or develop those resources in order to further their own interests (individual or collective) and in particular to retain their autonomy in the face of attempts to limit it. It seems clear that we need to be sensitive to both sides of the control-versus-autonomy and technology question. On the one hand, there is much evidence that under certain conditions office automation can be used to enhance managerial control over workers as well as to deskill their jobs. In many large, centralized settings such as insurance companies, banks, telephone companies, or the postal service, there has been eloquent and compelling testimony that new office technology can indeed be used to make work life more authoritarian and stressful for hundreds of thousands of office workers. In this study also, clerical workers in larger offices experienced more negative effects of office automation and fewer benefits.

On the other hand, we must be open to the possibility that the implementation of new office technology, under certain structural and historical conditions, may actually enhance the skills, leverage, and autonomy of workers. Further, there may actually be ways in which clerical workers can utilize new technology for their own advantage, whether or not managers intended it that way. In explicitly recognizing the likelihood of continuing change and ongoing struggles in the workplace, and in acknowledging the possibility of contradictory tendencies brought about by such changes in office technology, we must keep in mind the time-bound nature of this study. In those situations in which office workers have managed to work for and develop some degree of leverage and autonomy in automated offices, for example, in some of the small offices studied here, it seems likely that their control over their own labor will continue to be challenged. Thus the question of whether and how workers in the automated office can maintain their autonomy over time remains to be answered by future research.

REFERENCES

Barker, Jane, and Hazel Downing. 1980. Word processing and the transformation of the patriarchal relations of control in the office. *Capital and Class* 10 (Spring): 64–99.

Braverman, Harry. 1974. *Labor and monopoly capital.* New York: Monthly Review Press.

Carter, Valerie J. 1986. New technology and the clerical labor process: The impact of office automation on relations of control. Ph.D. diss., University of Connecticut.

Davies, Margery W. 1982. *Woman's place is at the typewriter.* Philadelphia: Temple University Press.

Edwards, Richard. 1979. *Contested terrain.* New York: Basic Books.

Giddens, Anthony, and David Held, eds. 1982. *Classes, power and conflict.* Berkeley and Los Angeles: University of California Press.

Glenn, Evelyn Nakano, and Roslyn L. Feldberg. 1977. Degraded and deskilled: The proletarianization of clerical work. *Social Problems* 25 (Oct.): 52–64.

————. 1979. Women as mediators in the labor process: Explorations in class and consciousness. Paper presented at the American Sociology Association meetings, Boston.

Goldberg, Roberta. 1983. *Organizing women office workers.* New York: Praeger Publishers.

Giuliano, Vincent E. 1982. The mechanization of office work. *Scientific American* 247, no. 3 (Sept.): 149–64.

Hubbartt, William S. 1983. A personnel policies primer. *Office Administration and Automation,* Jan., 40–42, 72–73.

Kanter, Rosabeth Moss. 1977. *Men and women of the corporation.* New York: Basic Books.

Kim, Jae-On. 1975. Multi-variate analysis of ordinal variables. *American Journal of Sociology* 81, no. 2:261–98.

Machung, Anne. 1983. *From psyche to technic: The politics of office work.* Ph.D. diss., University of Wisconsin.

Matteis, Richard J. 1979. The new back office focuses on customer service. *Harvard Business Review* 57, no. 2 (Mar.–Apr.): 146–59.

Meyer, N. Dean. 1983. The office automation cookbook: Management strategies for getting office automation moving. *Sloan Management Review* 24, no. 2 (Winter): 51–60.

Murphree, Mary C. 1981. Rationalization and satisfaction in clerical work: A case study of Wall Street legal secretaries. Ph.D. diss., Columbia University.

————. 1982. The secretary: A review of selected research. Paper presented at the Business and Professional Women's Foundation conference, Research to Make a Better Living for Working Women, Washington, D.C., Jan.

Quinn, R. P., and L. J. Shepard. 1974. *The 1972–73 Quality of Employment Survey.* Ann Arbor, Mich.: Survey Research Center.

Stark, David. 1982. Class struggle and the transformation of the labour process: A relational approach. In *Classes, power and conflict. See* Giddens and Held 1982.

Teger, Sandra L. 1983. Factors impacting the evolution of office automation. *Proceedings of the IEEE* 71, no. 4 (Apr.): 503–11.

West, Jackie. 1982. New technology and women's office work. In *Work, women and the labour market,* ed. Jackie West, 61–79. London: Routledge and Kegan Paul.

Wright, Erik Olin. 1978. *Class, crisis, and the state.* London: New Left Books.

Zisman, Michael D. 1978. Office automation: Revolution or evolution?" *Sloan Management Review* 19, no. 3 (Spring): 1–16.

APPENDIX A: QUESTION WORDINGS FOR DEPENDENT VARIABLES ("DECIDE TASKS," "LEARNING NEW THINGS," "REPETITIVE," AND "FREEDOM")

---

1. Are you usually able to decide for yourself the priority or order in which you do various tasks on the job, or is this decision typically determined by others—such as requests by students, the public, or your supervisor?
   _____ usually decide for myself
   _____ often decide for myself but sometimes determined by others
   _____ sometimes decide for myself but more often determined by others
   _____ usually or almost always determined by others

The following questions refer to various aspects of people's jobs. For each question, please indicate how true that aspect is *of your job.* [Respondents were then asked to check under the appropriate column, rating the statements as "Very True," "Somewhat True," "A Little True," or "Not at All True."]

2. My job requires that I have to keep learning new things.
3. My job requires that I do things that are very repetitive.
4. I am given a lot of freedom to decide how I do my own work.

Technological Advances and Increasing Militance: Flight Attendant Unions in the Jet Age

Frieda S. Rozen

Technology is only one variable in a complex framework at the workplace, so when technology changes, the change may set off elaborate interactions (Grzyb 1981; Cotgrove and Vamplew 1972; Dunlop 1958; Baker 1964; Kennedy, Craypo, and Lehman 1982). American flight attendants and their unions have experienced important changes in recent years, changes that must be attributed to the complex interactions stemming from the introduction of technological innovations in aircraft design. In contrast to other workers' experiences, these technological changes have had little impact on flight attendants' actual tasks. There has not been a shift from mechanical to clerical or professional work, nor have skilled jobs using tools been transformed into unskilled jobs paced by machines or computers (Dunlop 1958). The major change that attendants have experienced as a result of advances in aircraft technology has been in the size of their work groups. A single stewardess worked alone on the 21-passenger DC-3 in 1945, whereas a dozen attendants work together on a flight of the 450-passenger jumbo jet today. This increase in work group size has interacted with other factors in the industrial relations system to change flight attendants' relative bargaining power within the industry.

In the days of smaller planes and fewer passengers, when flight attendants were still called stewardesses, theirs was the lowest-paid occupation in the airline industry. Their unions were under the domination of larger unions committed to other more powerful occupations or work groups, and their leaders did not challenge the restrictive company rules that cut stewardesses' work lives short. The airlines' adoption of wide-bodied jets in the early seventies, however, caused the number of flight attendants to increase at a faster rate than that of pilots or other airline occupations. The result was a radical change in the relationship between flight attendants, their own unions, and the larger unions to which their unions belonged. Other articles in this volume examine the kinds of technological change that make skills obsolescent, alter job content, shift the workplace from home to factory, or, like the new information systems, bring waged labor back to the home. But the transformations that the newer, faster, more powerful, and immensely *larger* aircraft have wrought in the lives of flight attendants are just as much a result of technology as are the changes that emerge for other workers from the introduction of assembly lines, automation, or microelectronics.

Theoretical Framework

Sociologists, organizational theorists, and administrative scientists spent a generation focusing on the internal characteristics of organizations; then they "rediscovered" the importance of an organization's environment, and, as part of that environment, they discovered technology (Zey-Ferrell and Aiken 1981; Woodward 1965; Perrow 1967). Yet some social scientists who studied work settings and industrial relations had never lost sight of the importance of the environment—or of technology—even during the years when their colleagues overlooked everything external to the organizations being studied (Levinson 1971; Blauner 1964; Baker 1964).

Dunlop's theory of industrial relations systems (Dunlop 1958) is a multivariable approach that includes technology as an important variable. Although it antedates much of the sociological work on organizational environments, it provides an appropriate theoretical framework for examining the effects of technological change because it makes it clear that technology interacts with a different constellation of variables in each setting. Dunlop has recognized that managers, workers and their unions, and government are all actors in relationships that affect work; he also includes economic factors and the political power of the actors in the larger society, along with technology, as the contexts that are critically important for analysis.

His work has served as a useful framework for research and theoretical discussion (Blain 1972; Wood et al. 1975), and anyone studying airline occupations or airline unions finds his systems approach essential. If we are going to understand the growth, the problems, and the changing status of flight attendants, it is impossible to ignore the airline industry's history and its relations with government. In addition, the technology available, the market in which the industry has operated, and changes in the political power of the airlines, of pilots, and of women in the larger society—all have been important in the transformation of the flight attendant occupation and its unions.

Regulation and Industry Growth

The United States government played a critical role in shaping the airline industry. It encouraged the growth of the industry and regulated it. It also insisted on competition between airlines at the same time it discouraged competition. This seeming conflict in public policy toward the industry, which lasted nearly five decades, is important in understanding why the stewardess occupation developed as it did.

The earliest U.S. government interest in aircraft stemmed from their potential military and postal uses, but from the beginning, visionaries in the government also dreamed of encouraging the growth of passenger lines. After passage of the Kelly Act of 1926, the government was able to use airmail contracts to foster the growth of companies that might begin to develop passenger routes. By awarding or withholding airmail route contracts, the Post Office Department actually determined which companies would survive and grow and which would fail.

Under early government policy, contracts were awarded to potentially strong companies rather than to the lowest bidder, because airline enthusiasts in the government feared that the infant industry's small companies would eliminate each other through unbridled competition (Baitsell 1966).[1] By the early 1930s, however, when suspicion of big business was at its height, the fear of excessive competition between airlines was tempered by a strong public and congressional distaste for apparent Post Office Department encouragement of monopoly. This ambivalence was reflected in legislation that was enacted to regulate the industry and that, with only minor changes, governed the industry from 1938 to 1978.

The regulatory legislation called for "limited competition" while specifically restricting *price* competition, which would have been one of the most natural ways to compete.[2] Airlines were not permitted to alter prices, add routes, or abandon unprofitable routes served by a single airline without going through elaborate and lengthy procedures before the regulatory authority. At the same time, the government insisted on "limited competition" by assigning two to five carriers to profitable routes like those between New York and Los Angeles or New York and Miami. Curiously, the airlines perceived the industry as extremely competitive because of this "regulated competition."

But there was another reason why competing airlines eschewed price competition. The government policies that encouraged the growth of more stable companies also discouraged the entry of new companies, made mergers almost inevitable, eliminated weak companies, and had the long-run effect of creating an oligopolistic structure in the industry.

And oligopoly discouraged price competition while it encouraged other forms of competition.

An oligopolistic industry is one in which a few large firms divide the bulk of the market between them and yet succeed in differentiating themselves through advertising or product changes. Each firm fights to maintain or increase its share of the market, but each firm also believes that price cutting is more dangerous than it would be in a truly competitive market or industry. Each firm is so visible that if one firm cut prices, competitors could immediately retaliate, and the result would be a price war that would benefit no one and hurt everyone, in the view of oligopolistic firms (Heilbroner and Thurow 1984). Competition within an oligopolistic industry therefore centers on the adoption of new technology and on elaboration and differentiation. In the auto industry, it has meant new models, often incorporating minor technological innovations, and lots of elaboration and differentiation, e.g., style and color changes, that cause consumers to choose one brand over another.

In the airline industry, oligopolistic structure further strengthened the trend toward nonprice competition that regulation had fostered (Caves 1962; Douglas and Miller 1974). Competition within the industry centered increasingly on the adoption of new technology and on differentiation and elaboration of services. Periods of major innovation in aircraft design, when the airlines have competed to adopt the new technology, have alternated with periods of relative stability in aircraft design, when airlines have emphasized services and other forms of nonprice competition. Bigger and better planes and busier and more beautiful stewardesses were the two most visible results of this industry structure, especially from the 1950s to the early 1970s.

The New Planes

Airline executives believe that offering the fastest, safest, smoothest, and most comfortable trip is critical to winning passenger loyalty, and most airline analysts agree with them. Airlines have given highest priority on competitive routes to the adoption of the most advanced aircraft design available, although they have retained older styles of aircraft on noncompetitive routes (Kahn 1971, 1976).

Government policies facilitated this rapid adoption of improved technology in several ways. Early on, subsidylike payments—rewards, really—were made for investment in larger, safer aircraft; and under the Civil Aeronautics Act of 1938 the government guaranteed loans for certain kinds of equipment purchases. The regulatory agency also adjusted rates and subsidies if airlines suffered a temporary loss of profits as a result of their fleet improvements (Richmond 1961). Airline management knew that the government would not let them suffer even if they purchased or leased equipment beyond the judicious dictates of the market. This safety net, combined with competitive zeal, promoted unusually rapid adoption of new technology,[3] especially when breakthroughs in aircraft design seemed to lead to greater public acceptance of flying.

Each new model of aircraft increased the overall number of airline employees,[4] as airline travel became more popular; but in particular each new design increased the ratio of flight attendants to other airline employees. How could this be? One pilot, one copilot, and one stewardess had served on the 21-passenger DC-3 that dominated the airlanes from 1936 to the later 1940s. One pilot, one copilot, and two stewardesses served on the 58-passenger DC-6 that became the industry mainstay from 1948 to about 1958. In the late 1950s and early 1960s, while some airlines were converting to turbojets, others skipped that stage and bought true jets, the Boeing 707 and the DC-8. These planes carried 100 or more passengers. They were still flown by one pilot and one copilot, but now there were several stewardesses on each flight.[5] In the early 1970s, conversion to wide-bodied jets on major routes increased the number of passengers threefold, to 345 or even 450 (Kahn 1980). About a dozen stewardesses served a wide-bodied jet. In short, the number of pilots and copilots per plane did not increase, but the number of stewardesses did increase steadily in proportion to the number of passengers on board.

Flight attendants comprised only 5.4 percent of the total domestic airlines' labor force in 1950 and 6.7 percent in 1960; by 1970 their numbers had risen to 11.8 percent, and by 1975 to 13.1 percent. This rapidly increasing ratio of flight attendants to other airline personnel, in the industry labor force as a whole but even more markedly on each jet flight, brought about important changes in the working relationship between flight attendants and pilots and between the flight attendants' union and the pilots' union. These changes will be discussed after the following short history of the stewardess occupation.

The Stewardess Occupation: From Nurse to Advertising Copy

Flight attendants today have basically the same duties that the first stewardesses had in 1930: they are prepared to help passengers to safety in an emergency and they provide the services that make a passenger's flight pleasant. The same airline industry structure that led to competition in adopting advanced technology also led to competition in offering services and differentiating the product through advertising and image. This competition focused increased public attention on the services that stewardesses performed and on the stewardesses themselves. This competition is the key to understanding how the image of the stewardess was transformed during the 1950s and 1960s.

The first stewardesses were hired in 1930, and by the mid-1930s most airlines were hiring women—registered nurses until World War II—for the job of cabin attendant or stewardess. A recent airline commercial included photographs of those early stewardesses; it showed charming, smiling but serious young women in professional-looking uniforms helping passengers. In the early 1950s, however, the airlines began to change the stewardess image so that it lost its professional aspect and gained a sexual overtone with which the occupation was identified until the early 1970s.

The 1950s were a period of increasing competition in the industry. With adoption of the DC-6, airline travel was finally moving toward accelerated growth and broad public acceptance; yet it is clear, when one studies the industry journals of the period and reads their editorials and news stories, that airline executives feared the end of an *expanding* market and hence gave increasing attention to winning a larger share of the *existing* market. As the industry approached maturity, individual firms were growing larger and fewer, and the forms of competition characteristic of an oligopolistic market were becoming more evident.

Because their fleets had already been almost totally converted in the early 1950s to the best new plane available, the airlines turned their competitive zeal to services, as they have done whenever they found themselves between waves of technological advance in aircraft design. In the 1930s and 1940s service had consisted of the distribution of chewing gum to prevent ear popping at takeoff and landing, the serving of simple meals, the passing out of magazines, and little else. In the 1950s, the competition began in earnest, with free alcohol in first class, photogenic gourmet meals, "club lounges," first-run movies, and other luxuries, some of which have survived while others are long forgotten. Each of these services resulted in increasing the visibility and therefore the importance of stewardesses.

But the stewardess role changed in other ways as well. Airlines became aware—or decided—that it was stewardesses themselves, and not just their meal trays, free chewing gum, and magazines, who were attracting passenger loyalty.[6] The typical passengers of that period, to a larger extent than today, were male business travelers. To attract them, airlines began to change the stewardess image in a sexually explicit direction.

From the beginning, most airlines had hired friendly, attractive, unmarried women within a narrow age, height, and weight range. By the mid-1950s, all of this was codified in a rigid set of rules. Stewardesses were forced to resign when they married and to "retire" at twenty-eight or thirty-two. They signed prehiring agreements in which they agreed to resign or be fired if it was discovered, for instance, that they were secretly married. Stewardesses were dismissed if they could not maintain the prescribed weight. According to one apocryphal story, which did achieve a certain respectability through publication in the *New York Times,* a major airline even sent a special plane to London to pick up a stewardess who had her critical birthday while in London between flights. She had been on duty on the way over, but the airline considered it unseemly for her to serve on the way back, since she was now overage.

Public relations experts made increasing use of stewardesses in advertising and publicity during the 1950s. They called press conferences, with stewardesses there to be photographed, on every imaginable anniversary or whenever they had concocted another statistic about the number of miles stewardesses walked on a plane, the number of bottles they had heated for infant passengers, or the number who had retired because of marriage. The publicists succeeded in giving the occupation a reputation for glamour and for leading to upwardly mobile marriage. More and more women aspired to stewardess jobs and the airlines made a science of selecting only the most beautiful applicants, who then stayed an average of only eighteen months as a result of the rigid rules on age, marriage, and weight.

This image manipulation was heightened in the 1960s and into the 1970s. During that period, flight attendant uniforms became the focus of competition. Some airlines hired top designers; others were more direct, simply making uniforms tighter and skirts shorter, or even putting stewardesses into hot pants.

The final chapter was the "battle of inuendo." Airlines outdid one another in appealing to the prurient interests of passengers through double entendre. The stewardess stereotype was already loaded in the public consciousness when in the early 1970s "Fly Me—I'm Karen" or "We Work Our Tails Off For You" and other, only slightly more subtle advertising campaigns were launched. Hiring and personnel policies made the stewardess job glamorous and sought-after, but the same policies had also transformed it from the professional status of the original nurses to the questionable status of women as sex objects, women who would be dismissed when they lost their youthful appeal.

Stewardess Unions: Organizations without Power

Government regulation and industry structure had led the airlines to place great emphasis on stewardesses' youth and good looks, and the result was stewardesses who seldom stayed on the job more than eighteen months. Unions with a membership that turned over every year and a half remained relatively ineffectual. There had been stewardess union groups since shortly after World War II, when some stewardesses at United Airlines organized and successfully negotiated contracts for themselves and for stewardesses at several other airlines. Even though they began to organize before many other women's occupations were unionized, and despite the fact that stewardesses on most airlines were covered by union contracts within a few years, stewardess unions did not get stronger or more independent during the 1950s and 1960s. Instead, their power seemed to diminish, and other unions dominated them and subordinated their interests to those of other airline occupations.

When the stewardesses initiated their organizing campaign in 1945, the Airline Pilots Association (ALPA), the pilots' union, refused to assist them because it had a strong commitment to a craft rather than an industrial model of unionism. In addition, ALPA's president Dave Benecke believed that the Railway Labor Act, which governed collective bargaining relations on the railroads and airlines, prohibited unions made up of more than one craft.[7] Soon after the first stewardess contracts were signed, however, the pilots started a rival steward and stewardess union. ALPA agreed to merge this union with the stewardesses' own union, keeping the merged union under the wing of ALPA.

Why did ALPA suddenly change course? It had just refused to help the stewardesses to avoid compromising its position as a union representing only one craft, and now it was actively soliciting membership of another craft. The change was motivated by ALPA's desire to keep other unions over which it had no control from organizing airline employees, especially those who worked on the aircraft itself (i.e., flight engineers or stewardesses, in contrast to ground crews or ticket agents). In 1945 it seemed unlikely that other crafts would succeed in organizing, and pilots had enough bargaining power on their own so that they had no motivation to help the other crafts organize. Within a year or two, however, it became obvious that other airline crafts *were* about to organize, either in independent unions or with the help of unions other than ALPA. If they did organize without ALPA, the collective bargaining goals or strategies of nonpilot unions might conflict with those of pilots. If another union decided to call a strike against an airline, the planes and the pilots would be grounded whether the pilots liked it or not. But if unions of stewardesses, flight engineers, or other crafts were subdivisions of ALPA itself, their decision making could be controlled.[8]

Once it became clear that the other crafts would organize, with or without ALPA, the pilots changed their policy and authorized several groups for other crafts to form under the ALPA umbrella. The new union that resulted from the merger agreement between the stewardess union and ALPA was named the Airline Steward and Stewardess Association (ALSSA). It operated under a charter reserving all real power to ALPA and allowing ALPA to expel the new body at ALPA's discretion, without consultation.

Although most stewardesses spent only a year or two on the airlines and in the union, the male stewards and a minority of stewardesses stayed on,[9] and several ALSSA officers were reelected through most of the 1950s. After a few years in office, they chafed under the charter's restrictions. One incident in particular exacerbated the deteriorating relations between them and ALPA's officers. In preparation for a strike (which did not, in fact, materialize), ALSSA made a mutual assistance pact with the machinists' union of the airline they expected to strike. This was an example of exactly the kind of independent decision that ALPA wanted to avoid in union groups subordinated to it. In 1960, ALPA decided that ALSSA's officers had gone too far in asserting their independence and in flouting the charter, and expelled ALSSA.

Within a few months it became clear to ALSSA that it could not survive as an independent union,[10] and so it joined the Transport Workers Union (TWU), which already represented most crafts on Pan American Airlines as well as some workers on other airlines. TWU let ALSSA come in as a large "local" union so it could retain its identity as a stewardess union. TWU made some other concessions in its agreement with ALSSA, and at first the group enjoyed more autonomy than it had in ALPA.

Over the next two years, however, almost half of ALSSA's membership defected (or returned) to a new stewardess structure that ALPA initiated, the Steward and Stewardess Division (SSD-ALPA). The largest stewardess group, those at United Airlines, and the stewardess groups from most of the small airlines were among the defectors. Stewardesses from the small airlines had close relationships with pilots and wanted to stay in ALPA. This time ALPA made sure that the group was unequivocally defined as a subdivision, completely subordinate to the parent union. Once again, ALPA's right to expel the stewardess group without consultation was clearly stated.

When half its membership returned to ALPA, ALSSA's bargaining power within TWU was sharply reduced. As a result, TWU unilaterally altered the terms of its original understanding with ALSSA, and the stewards and stewardesses suffered a major loss of autonomy, ending up with little more control than ALSSA had had in ALPA, or SSD-ALPA now had.

From the early 1960s on, then, both stewardess union groups—ALSSA in TWU, and SSD-ALPA—were completely subordinate to their international or parent unions. TWU or ALPA officials, rather than ALSSA or SSD-ALPA officers, did most of the negotiating, grievance handling, and other work for the stewardesses and the few stewards. When attendants did sit on negotiating committees, it seemed to be only for show. The internationals had the power to make final agreements with the airlines, and they often ignored priorities that attendants considered important. For instance, single rooms for layovers became a symbolic issue for stewardesses, but it was some time before their unions negotiated hard on the issue. The airlines paid for single rooms for pilots on layover, but they paid only for double rooms for stewardesses, even if a stewardess had to share her room with a stewardess whose hours were completely different from her own. Stewardesses complained that either they were asleep—and woke with a jolt—when a strange roommate came stumbling in; or they had just gotten to sleep—and were awakened—when a roommate got a wakeup call for her own very different schedule. The issue of single or double rooms may seem minor; however, it came to symbolize not only discrimination against females (there were so few male attendants at the time that they had single rooms like pilots), but also the right of union members to choose the issues they considered important.

If stewardesses stayed on the job long enough to get active in the union, TWU and ALPA officials dismissed them as self-seeking and unrepresentative of the "real" stewardess. In the unions' view, a real stewardess was young and did not stay long enough to care whether the union got anything for her in negotiations or protected her from arbitrary employer rules.[11] The unions seldom if ever challenged company rules about marriage, age, or weight during the 1950s and well into the 1960s.

External Influences on the Status of Stewardesses: The Civil Rights Act and the Women's Movement

Passage of the Civil Rights Act in 1964 and the resurgence of the women's movement in the late 1960s offered the potential for great change in women's occupations. In some occupations, little of this potential was realized, but for stewardesses both the Civil Rights Act and the women's movement led to important changes.

The Civil Rights Act forbade discrimination on the basis of race, religion, or national origin, *or* on the basis of sex.[12] If the courts redefined discrimination and the redefinition applied to restrictions practiced in a workplace or occupation, important changes could result. The more pervasive the restrictions and the more definitively the courts judged them discriminatory, the greater the change in the occupation.

The chief effect of the act in other occupations was to give a small proportion of the workers upward mobility, or to give new categories of workers access to the occupation. Some blacks and women got promotions previously denied them, some men became telephone operators and some women climbed telephone poles, and some of the largest airlines started to hire male flight attendants after four decades of hiring only females. However, these were relatively minor changes.

It is reasonable to argue that the act caused more change for flight attendants than for any other occupation. Restrictions on them were more pervasive than those in other occupations, and the court decisions that defined discrimination clearly applied to those airline rules. For example, the marriage and age restrictions affected every stewardess (on most airlines). One of the earliest, most decisive court rulings under the act suggested that an employer's refusal to employ a married woman or a mother, though married men, fathers, or unmarried and childless women were hired, was discrimination. The courts' reasoning in this and similar cases had obvious implications for the airlines.

The reason that stewardesses experienced greater change than any other occupational group was that *all* female workers in the occupation were affected. The majority of women *already* on the job, as well as women who had been *terminated* long before but who sued for reinstatement, and even women who *would* enter the occupation in the future— all were free, after the implications of the law became clear, to go on working, even when they married, got older, or had children. The rules that had forced premature termination were overturned on one airline after another, either through court decisions or as the unions took courage from those decisions and began to press the companies in negotiations. The marriage restrictions were eliminated first; next, the unions took up age restrictions. (In the days of the marriage restrictions, most stewardesses had been terminated long before they reached twenty-eight or thirty-two, so only a minority cared that the age limit existed.) The most dramatic proof of the transformation caused by the Civil Rights Act was the steep rise in average seniority, which went from eighteen months in the late 1960s to over six years in 1975.

The women's movement also affected the occupation. Steward-esses, or rather the popular image of the stewardess, epitomized all the female stereotypes derided by the movement, and stewardesses some-times felt personally belittled by movement leaders.[13] However, a sig-nificant number of stewardesses heard the message of the movement and responded positively. A women's movement organization, Steward-esses for Women's Rights (SFWR), was formed in 1972. Although it did not grow very large or achieve all its goals, it made stewardesses aware of the women's movement and it challenged the image—or stereotype—of the stewardess promoted in airline advertising. In fact, one of its first projects was to combat the "Fly Me—I'm Karen" campaign and others like it. SFWR's newsletter also dealt with health issues, for example, calling for research into the causes of persistent health problems that some stewardesses began to experience after the introduction of jet planes. In this way, SFWR raised the job consciousness of many steward-esses. The newsletter also challenged the unions' commitment to stew-ardesses. Not surprisingly, TWU officials grew hostile to SFWR.

A number of the women who were active in SFWR decided after a couple of years that they could be more effective on work-related issues if they became active in the unions. Some agreed with SFWR that the unions were not committed to their occupation, but they decided to change the unions from inside. Others became convinced that SFWR might be effective in consciousness-raising and might succeed in talking to the companies about stewardess complaints, but that only the unions could negotiate and win signed agreements that had legal force. The stewardess unions, especially groups that were represented by TWU, gained a significant group of activists from the women who cut their leadership teeth in SFWR and then moved on.

In SFWR one can see that stewardesses were learning to use their natural advantages. Airline publicists had always known they could get newspaper coverage by offering interviews with stewardesses; now the stewardesses themselves became adept at using their reputation for glam-our to get press coverage. They had always valued their airline passes for personal travel; now they realized they could use those passes to attend SFWR conferences or to carry their message to unconverted steward-esses. They even found that the leadership of the women's movement was more eager to address their conferences than those of women in shoe or garment factories, and Gloria Steinem and other media person-alities came to their national meetings.

Why did a significant number of stewardesses respond to the mes-sage of the women's movement despite the conflict between the move-ment's ideas and the female stereotypes linked to the occupation? Because their response to that message was not inhibited by a network of traditional relationships or institutions that would counteract the message of the women's movement. Unlike most women's jobs, stewardessing involved irregular hours and constant travel. Stewardesses' work schedules and their physical mobility (Coser 1975; Dunlop 1958) limited their participation in their communities of origin as well as in the communities where they resided. For the few years that they were flight attendants, their community was their occupational work group, consisting of other stewardesses and pilots (Salaman 1974; Lipset, Trow, and Coleman 1956). So they may have come into the occupation accepting the stereotypes, proud to be pretty enough to be hired as stewardesses; but their working conditions left them free to consider new ideas, especially if those new ideas were relevant to their fellow stewardesses, the people with whom they also had most of their social relations.

The Civil Rights Act was important in bringing an end to restrictive employment rules for stewardesses, and as a result, a stable work force began to emerge. At the same time, the women's movement raised the consciousness of those women about the sexual image of the occupation that had been fostered by the airlines, about health issues on the job, about the unions, and about their own ability to achieve results. Stewardesses began to recognize their own potential power.

When Technology, Law, and a Social Movement Interact

When the changes that resulted from new aircraft technology were joined with those from the Civil Rights Act and the women's movement, stewardesses found that they could alter both their name and image from "stewardess" to "flight attendant," and they realized that they had the power to take their unions into their own hands. Adoption of jets had led to a greater increase in flight attendant employment than in other airline occupations and to a larger cabin crew on each flight; union agreements and court cases following passage of the Civil Rights Act had led to increasing seniority; and the women's movement had developed flight attendants' consciousness of their rights and, perhaps, their sense of sisterhood.

The increased ratio of flight attendants to other airline occupations meant, for one thing, that SSD-ALPA had a growing block of votes inside ALPA; pilots feared that at some future date flight attendants might "take over the union." The pilots voiced their fears even before most SSD leaders had recognized the potential increase in their power. Once the pilots did articulate these thoughts, SSD officers began to study the implications.[14]

The greater number of flight attendants working on each flight had other important consequences. Flight attendants now had more of a work relationship with fellow attendants than in the days of one- or two-stewardess flights. Therefore, they were less dependent on the advice, support, or even company of the pilot and copilot. This naturally loosened their dependence on the pilot union and on pilot advice regarding union matters.

Another effect of the larger crew of coworkers was that attendants widened their network within the occupation. Flight crews did not necessarily work together for more than a single flight: a different set of fellow attendants might be scheduled for each flight. With these large and varied crews, effective communication networks were easily developed among flight attendants, and news, new ideas, or even revolts could spread among them quickly.[15]

Though they were slow to realize that their political power within the union had increased, the officers of SSD-ALPA and of ALSSA did recognize the effect of rising seniority. They realized that flight attendants' interest in their jobs was growing now that they could expect to go on working. ALPA and TWU officers, the people who did most of the negotiating with airline managements, were not as quick to recognize the changing expectations as were SSD-ALPA and ALSSA officers, who dealt with members daily.

The first flight attendant group to seize the opportunities made possible by the juxtaposition of technology, the Civil Rights Act, and the women's movement was SSD-ALPA. When delegates at the 1970 ALPA convention voiced their fear over the increase in stewardess votes in their union, the officers set up a joint study group with SSD-ALPA. Although the study group could not resolve the issues, SSD-ALPA leaders continued to study alternatives to subdivision status. They recognized the positive implications of the pilots' fear: their own potential bargaining power had increased. They continued to study and negotiate, and after three years, they and ALPA agreed to a change in the terms of the relationship. In 1974, SSD-ALPA became an affiliate rather than a subdivision. It was now the Association of Flight Attendants (AFA). In 1984, the AFL-CIO granted AFA an independent charter, and AFA is now totally independent of ALPA.[16] Kelly Rueck, who was president of SSD-ALPA in the first half of the 1970s, developed the union's potential further by instituting programs to train officers for more effective leadership.

The coming together of technology, the Civil Rights Act, and the women's movement also caused major changes in the ALSSA groups. They, too, gained autonomy, but in a less amiable or evolutionary fashion than SSD-ALPA. ALSSA's constituent groups disaffiliated from TWU and from each other. In 1977 the flight attendant groups from TWA and from American Airlines voted to leave TWU, and in 1978 flight attendants from Pan American followed suit. These groups formed their own separate, independent flight attendant unions, totally autonomous groups that are not affiliated with other unions, with the AFL-CIO, or with each other. Each of the disaffiliations can be traced to the recognition by flight attendant officers that the membership wanted a larger role in determining collective bargaining priorities than the TWU negotiators were willing to give them.

Additional groups originally in SSD-ALPA or ALSSA have also changed their affiliation: one joined the Teamsters Union (Northwest Airlines); another formed a small independent union that has since been swallowed up as a result of bankruptcy followed by merger (Continental Airlines); and another moved from AFA to TWU (National Airlines).

In summary, every flight attendant group experienced some kind of reaffiliation, challenge to its leadership, or other internal restructuring during the period from 1974 to 1978. Turmoil so widespread within the unions of one occupation is probably unique; what is most surprising is that we find this turmoil in an almost totally female occupation, one in which women initially accepted greater job restrictions and greater sexual stereotyping than those in other occupations. Today flight attendants lead their own unions, set their own priorities, and do not depend on male leaders from another occupation to decide what their unions will do. They have moved from dependency to autonomy in a short time. If autonomy means power, flight attendant unions have been strengthened, not weakened, by interactions that developed from technological change in the airline industry.

NOTES

1. The current price wars among the airlines lend credence to those fears. Even industry members who benefit from the competition voice fear of the long-run effects on the industry.
2. The Airline Deregulation Act was passed in October, 1978, ending the regulation that had been in effect since the 1934 and 1938 acts. The Civil Aeronautics Board's power to regulate entry, routes, and rates is ended, and the agency is now disbanded.
3. The current technological race among the computer giants is similar in its intensity, if not in governmental encouragement. In many industries, especially those that were more monopolies than oligopolies, the dominant giants managed to discourage competition leading to technological progress.

The Singer Sewing Machine Company in the first half of the century is a good example. It fought off the introduction of major changes until the late 1940s. One might also say that Henry Ford tried, with temporary success, to stay with a tried-and-true model, his black Model T.

4. Some advances in design did make certain skills obsolescent. Aircraft mechanics and flight engineers no longer have the role in the control cabin that they once did. The story of their occupation and their unions makes a fascinating counterpoint to that of the flight attendants, but the details belong in a separate treatment of the subject. See Baitsell 1966 for their history; the implications for flight attendant unions are discussed elsewhere in my own writings.

5. In some cases, there *was* a third pilot on the plane, but his presence was due to a compromise with the flight engineers who were no longer needed in the air thanks to increasingly sophisticated flight panels. Some airlines allowed redundant flight engineers to qualify as third pilots (Baitsell 1966).

6. Georgia Panter Nielson suggests that one airline hired its first stewardesses in the thirties because an investigation of a crash indicated that more of its passengers would have been saved if there had been a stewardess there to assist them (Nielson 1982). However, safety considerations do not explain the increasing popularity of stewardesses in the fifties, when one airline that had been hiring male attendants only for two decades began to hire females only.

7. It is clear that at that time the National Mediation Board, which administers the Railway Labor Act, did favor separate representation for each craft. Correspondence between the stewardesses who were organizing and the president of ALPA is on file with the Association of Flight Attendants, the flight attendants' union that is now a member of the AFL-CIO. The ALPA president's general union philosophy is clear in discussions of the relations between ALPA and the flight engineers union as well as from his actions as union president (Baitsell 1966; Hopkins 1971).

8. ALPA's reluctance to compromise pilots' priorities in support of other airline crafts has been a continuing problem. During the recent United Airlines strike, ALPA leaders referred to their own long history of unbrotherly acts as they called for the support of other unions, and they promised to mend their own ways. It is not hard to understand why pilots do not want the planes grounded unless they themselves are calling the strike. Their incomes are five to eight times higher than those of many other union workers. They think of themselves as having more to lose (measured in dollars) than other workers. They have not had to develop strong feelings about unity or class consciousness, because until recently, their bargaining power was so great that they were able to achieve their goals without the support of other workers. As a result, they did not worry about *giving* support to other workers, either.

9. The age restrictions were not instituted by some of the companies until the

early 1950s. Up to that time, even senior stewardesses were still relatively young, since real growth of air travel started after World War II, and few stewardesses had been hired earlier.

10. ALSSA's officers had petitioned the AFL-CIO for an independent charter as a steward and stewardess union, but the AFL-CIO did not grant the request, operating on the assumption that ALPA and the Transport Workers Union had prior claim to jurisdiction over airline employees, since both already had AFL-CIO charters to organize workers in the airline industry. Under the circumstances, ALSSA had no alternative but to join another union.

11. These attitudes are apparent in statements made by ALPA officers, recorded in the proceedings of ALPA conventions; from my interviews with TWU officials in charge of the Air Transport Division, the division ALSSA belonged to; and from my interviews with flight attendants who had been officers in the ALSSA-TWU and SSD-ALPA years.

12. The Equal Pay Act of 1963 was actually the first prohibition of sex discrimination, but it applied only to pay, and it had limited relevance to flight attendants.

13. In interviews with the author, flight attendants referred to their own feelings when they read disparaging remarks about stewardesses in *Ms.* magazine articles by women's movement leaders.

14. Proceedings of ALPA and of SSD-ALPA, and of SSD special study committees for 1970 through 1974.

15. In the mid-1970s, flight attendants at National Airlines and those at TWA refused to ratify contracts that had been negotiated for them by their unions. The decertification campaigns I discuss next succeeded in part because flight attendants had more effective communication networks than in the days of the DC-6.

16. It is clear that there is much more mutual respect between ALPA and flight attendants than in the days of the subdivision. ALPA announced on July 2, 1985, that pilots would increase their dues so they could give strike assistance to flight attendants as well as to pilots, especially those in AFA who honored the 1985 pilot strike againt United. In the past, the pilots would have taken flight attendant support for granted, or, more likely, they would have assumed that it was unimportant.

REFERENCES

Baitsell, John M. 1966. *Airline industrial relations.* Cambridge, Mass.: Harvard University Press.

Baker, Elizabeth Faulkner. 1964. *Technology and women's work.* New York: Columbia University Press.

Blain, A. N. J. 1972. *Pilots and management: Industrial relations in the U.K. airlines.* London: George Allen and Unwin.

Blauner, Robert. 1964. *Alienation and freedom.* Chicago: University of Chicago Press.

Caves, Richard. 1962. *Air transport and its regulators.* Cambridge, Mass.: Harvard University Press.

Coser, Rose Laub. 1975. Stay home, little Sheba: On placement, displacement, and social change. *Social Problems* 22, no. 4:470–80.

Cotgrove, Stephen, and Clive Vamplew. 1972. Technology, class and politics: The case of the process workers. *Sociology* 6, no. 2:169–85.

Douglas, George W., and James C. Miller, III. 1974. *Economic regulation of domestic air transport: Theory and policy.* Washington, D.C.: Brookings Institution.

Dunlop, John T. 1958. *Industrial relations systems.* New York: Henry Holt and Co.

Grzyb, Gerard J. 1981. Decollectivization and recollectivization in the workplace: The impact of technology on informal work groups and work culture. *Economic and Industrial Democracy* (Beverly Hills) 2, no. 4:455–82.

Heilbroner, Robert L., and Lester C. Thurow. 1984. *The economic problem.* 7th ed. Englewood Cliffs, N.J.: Prentice-Hall.

Hopkins, George E. 1971. *The airline pilots: A study in elite unionization.* Cambridge, Mass.: Harvard University Press.

Kahn, Mark L. 1971. Collective bargaining on the airline flight deck. Part 4 of *Collective bargaining and technological change. See* Levinson 1971.

———. 1976. Labor-management relations in the airline industry. Chapter 4 in *The Railway Labor Act at fifty,* ed. Charles M. Rehmus. Washington, D.C.: National Mediation Board.

———. 1980. Airlines. Chapter 7 in *Collective bargaining: Contemporary American experience,* ed. Gerald G. Somers. Madison, Wisc.: Industrial Relations Research Association.

Kennedy, Donald, Charles Craypo, and Mary Lehman, eds. 1982. *Labor and technology: Union response to changing environments.* University Park, Pa.: Department of Labor Studies, Pennsylvania State University.

Levinson, Harold M. 1971. *Collective bargaining and technological change.* Evanston: Transportation Center, Northwestern University.

Lipset, Seymour Martin, Martin A. Trow, and James S. Coleman. 1956. *Union democracy.* Garden City, N.Y.: Doubleday and Co., Anchor Books.

Nielson, Georgia Panter. 1982. *From sky girl to flight attendant: Women and the making of a union.* Ithaca: ILR Press, New York State School of Industrial and Labor Relations, Cornell University.

Perrow, Charles. 1967. A framework for the comparative analysis of organizations. *American Sociological Review* 32:194–208. Reprinted 1980 in *Organizations, structure and behavior,* 3d ed., ed. Joseph Litterer. New York: John Wiley and Sons.

Richmond, Samuel B. 1961. *Regulation and competition in air transportation.* New York: Columbia University Press.

Salaman, Graeme. 1974. *Community and occupation: An exploration of work/ leisure relationships*. Cambridge: Cambridge University Press.

Walker, Kenneth F. 1977. Toward useful theorising about industrial relations. *British Journal of Industrial Relations* 15, no. 3:307–16.

Wood, S. J., A. Wagner, E. G. A. Armstrong, J. F. B. Goodman, and J. E. Davies. 1975. The "industrial relations system" concept as a basis for theory in industrial relations. *British Journal of Industrial Relations* 13, no. 3:291– 308.

Woodward, Joan. 1965. *Industrial organization: Theory and practice*. Oxford: Oxford University Press.

Zey-Ferrell, Mary, and Michael Aiken. 1981. *Complex organizations: Critical perspectives*. Glen View, Ill.: Scott, Foresman and Co.

**Part 3
Access and Action**

Introduction

Gail O. Mellow

If the movie *The Graduate* were made today, Dustin Hoffman would be advised to choose a career in computers instead of plastics. He would be just one of many who are being encouraged to ally themselves with the new technologies. But we might ask whether a woman would be given the same advice, and whether the rewards for her would be as great. When, for example, the chair of the Hartford High Technology Council defines high technology as "any business which is going to create jobs in the 1980s and 1990s," it becomes apparent that the introduction of technology is associated with increased employment opportunities. But are these promises of employment real, and how likely are women to reap the benefit? What *is* the potential of paid employment in high technology fields to improve women's economic status? And how can that potential be realized?

The articles in this section attempt to answer these questions. First, they examine whether women do have equal access to jobs in high technology fields and to the economic prosperity that such employment is supposed to offer; and second, they consider what actions can be taken to rectify inequity, where it exists, for all workers, but especially for women and minorities. As we measure access, we must be clear that women are not newcomers to technology; they have always played a role in its creation, implementation, and utilization. The problem is that women have been underrepresented, underpaid, and unrecognized in a labor market that, for the most part, has been conceptualized and structured as part of the male domain.

This section opens with a look at the past and closes with speculations about our economic future. Most of the contributions to this section focus on today's high-profile computer industry. "High technology" is a term applied to a vast range of technology made possible by the microprocessor, including robotics, automation, fiber optics, and telecommunications; but it is the computer that is the quintessential representative of the new technologies. In assessing women's access to employment in the computer field, the contributions to this section examine such issues as wage discrimination, training, segregation and stratification, and unionization. These articles describe the underlying dynamics of the sexual division of high-tech labor, whereby a largely female labor force operates machines while a largely male labor force controls what happens inside those machines; and the authors outline new opportunities for changing those dynamics, so that women will not become the "techno-peasants" of the twenty-first century.

The thread that ties these seemingly disparate contributions together is education. Education may serve to help workers get jobs; but beyond that, if we choose, education may be used to transform the workplace. Education, like technology itself, cannot be viewed in a vacuum, removed from social, political, or economic values. It exists and functions in a context where it can be used to promote a variety of goals and to advance the interests of various groups or classes. Taken together, these papers demonstrate that our use of education must have wide-ranging and complex interplay with the existing employment structure and with personal life-styles if education and work are to be appropriately transformed.

This dual transformation of both technology *and* education is precisely what Helen Marot was after. Janet Polansky's essay opens the section by reclaiming this visionary management theorist whose work challenges the traditional climate of thought about the implications of technology for workers. Marot's analysis of technology in industry emerged from a strongly feminist and holistic perspective. Combining the need for human education with technological innovation, she produced a new paradigm for organizational management theory and a radical new way to implement technological change. For Marot, education was an essential and integral aspect of work, and she posited a curriculum within industry that would not only train workers for their specialized jobs, but prepare them for organizational responsibility and full participation in a democratically transformed workplace. Her vision, forged from her union activism at the turn of the century, provides an exciting antidote to the deskilling and routinization typically associated with the introduction of technology both then and now.

Marot looked at workers holistically: she refused to slice them into "eyes, arms, fingers and legs," instead insisting that all humans possess an intrinsic capacity for creativity and intellectual growth. Marot criticized both labor and industrial organizations for failing to provide the educational means to enhance these human assets. Aiming at a new synthesis of manual and managerial skills, Marot set education at the center of a form of production controlled not by machines but by human cognition, of which machines were only an extension. Industry's ability to use technology for human advancement would rest on its willingness to fully educate its work force; that, in turn, meant educating workers not merely to produce quality products but to control their industry and their lives.

Just as Marot rejected a narrow and fragmented view of workers, so, too, she rejected linear and compartmentalized views of education. Then as now, traditional education was conceptualized as a linear process, with the student expected to progress steadily and incrementally toward a single credential and career objective. There are a number of problems with this model. One of them is its masculine bias: many women enter education, especially higher education, later in life; or they enter, leave to bear and care for children, and then reenter. Neither is this model adequate for, say, a twenty-two-year-old black man who began to work in the automobile manufacturing industry when he was nineteen, is now laid off because of the introduction of robotics, and needs education and retraining. Nor is this model adequate in the face of rapid and continuous technological change, which demands that education and training become lifelong processes. Moreover, the content of that education must become broadly transferable to avoid technological obsolescence.

These trends call for an educational system that educates intermittently with increasing levels of sophistication as people move through their lives, and that incorporates the whole person into the learning process. Similarly, a feminist perspective leads to a view of education as an ongoing, multifaceted, and cyclical process in which work and family are interwoven as parts of a blended life plan. This is not just a way to accommodate women; it is a more accurate way to conceptualize the relationship between work and education for everyone. Marot's theory offers a foundation for just such a reconceptualization of education; at the same time, precisely because Marot's vision of education is so startlingly different from what we are accustomed to, she helps us to see the values that characterize much of traditional education and to which we are otherwise blind: materialism, managerial authority, and technological determinism.

The importance of using education for humanistic as well as technical ends is echoed in the next article. Linda Lewis investigates the relationship between access and education by examining sex-based disparities in the acquisition of computer literacy. Focusing on the classroom, Lewis documents differences between girls and boys in enrollment patterns and rates of computer usage. Although equal interest in the computer is demonstrated by girls and boys in first grade, by sixth grade boys outnumber girls in computer classes by two to one; the ratio increases to three to one in high school, with even greater disparities in advanced classes. Educators are often oblivious to this situation. For example, at a recent national three-day conference on education and computers, only one session was devoted to encouraging women to enter the field.

Lewis illuminates the attitudes, policies, and practices that discourage young women's participation in computer-related education. She then presents new ways to capitalize on young women's different styles of reasoning and expression, so that these can serve as the basis for girls' inclusion in computer education rather than as barriers. Lewis challenges educators to rethink their computer pedagogy, to change the ways in which computers are introduced into the classroom, and to make the education of girls and minority males a priority. Through the alternatives she offers, Lewis, too, forces us to become aware of specific values embedded in computer-education-as-usual, e.g., gamesmanship, competitiveness, and violence, as well as biases favoring mathematical rather than verbal facility and field-independent rather than field-dependent learning styles. She also suggests that the incorporation of "feminine" values into the computer curriculum will help to integrate humanistic concerns with technical means.

Sandy Weinberg's contribution stands as a counterpoint to Lewis's article. Lewis outlines the barriers women face in obtaining educational credentials, whereas Weinberg challenges the appropriateness of the credentials themselves. The standards are derived, he maintains, from the engineers and mathematicians who pioneered in the computer field. These pioneers, primarily white men, embraced a particular "macho-aggressive" culture that is reproduced in the work and educational environments where computers are present. Weinberg argues that the macho-aggressive ethos rewards the values of competition, domination, and isolation from the users of the hardware, and thus it perpetuates myths that render computer experts dysfunctional in real-world computer applications. In this type of cultural milieu, formal bans on female participation are not necessary, since the artificial standards function to exclude those persons (typically women) who do not exhibit macho-aggressive characteristics. Moreover, Weinberg argues that these attributes are not necessary for understanding, using, or creating the third generation of computers. Thus he disputes the need to find mechanisms for drawing women into traditional math and science courses; instead, he advocates a radical change in education and in the credentials required of all computer specialists.

What is the myth and what is the reality when we turn to those women who have cleared the educational hurdles and are entering the high technology work force? The economic promise of high-tech employment for women emerges from characteristics of both the work and the labor force. The work appeals to women because it seems clean and classy—not demanding the physical strength said to limit women's employment in smokestack industries. We imagine a well-dressed employee sitting in a quiet office, performing interesting, challenging, and creative work with a high-powered computer. The gender-neutrality of the machines themselves seems to bode well for women—the machines are oblivious to whether a woman or a man pushes their keys. In addition, high technology fields are unencumbered by an entrenched group of workers who have performed this work since its inception and passed jobs on to their sons. Moreover, statistics suggest an expanding job market, which promises not only easy access to entry-level positions but also job security and advancement. The U.S. Department of Labor predicts that by 1995 over 2 million people will be employed in occupations directly related to computers (e.g., computer programmers, manufacturers, or repair technicians), and millions more will be indirectly employed (in areas such as advertising, clerical work, or retailing). Thus the prospect of interesting and appealing jobs for women, together with easy entrance into the field, creates a rosy picture.

The research of Katharine Donato and Patricia Roos shows that some of the promise of high-tech employment for women can indeed be realized. Their article documents that women *are* better paid in the computer industry relative to other fields; more importantly, wage disparities between women and men are smaller in the computer industry than the national average, although this is most true at the lowest levels of the industry's wage/classification scale.

Industry and labor analysts, including the International Labor Organization (ILO), have maintained that women's lower wages are not a function of gender-based discrimination but occur because women are clustered in companies that provide poor salaries generally. Donato and Roos's analysis decisively challenges that thesis, demonstrating that women's lower wages are *not* explained by employment in lower-paying industries. Interestingly, they also find that self-employed women in the computer field average two thousand dollars more per year than women working with computers for the government or for private industry. Perhaps women are more equitably paid when they desert the hierarchy of an established firm and found their own businesses.

Donato and Roos's study reveals that an analysis of sex differences in the levels of education obtained by those in the computer industry provides a critical vantage point from which to view the status of women. They find that gender differences in job classification and in salary are partially explained by women's lower level of education. But women also receive a lower return on their investment in education than men do; men's salaries, in other words, reflect increases proportionate to the years they spent in education to a greater extent than do women's salaries. Donato and Roos's findings suggest that simply ensuring that women obtain educational credentials equal to men's will not alone create employment equity in the high-tech labor market.

How the introduction of new technologies within an industry will affect women's employment prospects depends, as the next contribution to this section shows, on the racial, ethnic, and gender stratification of the work force. Since most women, particularly most black women, are found within specific job classifications or industries, the implementation of technological change will differentially affect job opportunities for those groups. Some trends in employment initially augured well for women, especially women of color, because of their representation in the service sector. It was thought that manufacturing jobs lost to "offshoring" would be replaced by an increase in service sector jobs. But newer technologies, specifically developments in satellites and telecommunications technology, now allow corporations to send clerical and data processing jobs "offshore" to other countries, just as manufacturing jobs were. Underpaid and unorganized women in Jamaica, Korea, Singapore, Barbados, Mexico, and Haiti now perform much of the clerical work for New York City corporations.

These newer technologies also allow companies to relocate businesses from inner cities, where the pool of female minority employees is greatest, to the suburbs, where clerical workers are predominantly white and married. Because they are subsidized by their husbands, these women are more likely to settle for lower pay and fewer benefits. Detroit stands as an example of the differential effect on various labor pools: clerical jobs in the city have decreased by 40 percent since 1980, while the suburbs have maintained their 1980 levels of employment despite economic contraction. With about 35 percent of all women in the paid labor force working at clerical jobs, the loss of clerical jobs due to automation seriously threatens the well-being of all women workers, but the threat is particularly acute for women of color who have only recently entered white-collar employment.

The volatility of employment in high-tech fields may also have a particularly adverse effect on women and minority men. San Jose, in California's "Silicon Valley," can serve as an example. In 1985, unemployment claims were up 50 percent over 1984, while the proportion of Hispanic workers employed by the industry dropped by 36 percent. Minority women, brought into the lowest skill levels of high-tech employment, are now being squeezed out as better and more highly skilled jobs emerge through continued technological innovation. Problems of access are compounded by the fact that women, especially minority women, have been steered away from the science and mathematics courses that could lay a foundation for more highly skilled computer-related occupations. It is essential, therefore, that evaluations of women's access not lump all women together; instead, researchers need to make careful distinctions between specific groups of women and their relative ease of access, and they need to chart access across time, so that volatility may also be gauged.

The next contribution to this section, by Evelyn Glenn and Charles Tolbert, draws precisely those kinds of distinctions. Analyzing employment in the computer industry by job classification, race, and gender, the authors argue persuasively that not all women will benefit from the relatively good wages in the computer industry. Documenting a desegregation/resegregation cycle, they find that racial ethnic women have entered the white-collar computer occupations only to be resegregated at the lowest levels of the industry. Although Anglo women do not fare much better, Glenn and Tolbert reveal an earning disparity that derives from salary discrimination based on a racially stratified labor market and on differential job classifications. Once again, the importance of an adequate education is stressed, particularly the need to train women of color to fill positions as programmers, computer scientists, and computer analysts—the higher-status jobs within the industry.

Just as it is important to look at all workers in a highly differentiated way, so, too, we must look carefully at the work itself. All high-tech work is not alike, and differences in autonomy, transferability of skill, and salary require close examination. While new jobs have been (and will continue to be) developed as a result of high technology, any evaluation of new job opportunities must include a consideration of layoffs, plant closings, and job redesign that may result. We know that the introduction of new technologies is most likely to create new jobs in those occupations such as data processing and clerical work in which the current labor force is predominantly female. Will the overall effect be to employ more women, or to create a net loss in traditional women's jobs?

Whether and how workers are trained to perform redesigned or newly created jobs becomes a crucial issue. Management can offer workers job training that provides increased (and transferable) skills, or minimal training that emphasizes only basic tasks, thereby deskilling a woman's job and providing no real facility with the new technology. Or management can offer no training at all, so that workers quit, thus terminating a company's financial obligation to them. Drawing upon models developed by European unions, Maria-Luz Samper argues that when workers educate themselves about new technologies, they can develop truly creative strategies to humanize the introduction of technology into the workplace.

Of the 44 million women in the American work force today, fewer than 7 million belong to unions or employee associations. But unionized women workers earn approximately thirty percent more than nonunionized women. For a variety of reasons, unions have historically been reluctant to organize women workers. At present, none of the major computer industries in the United States, and very few of the predominantly female service industries, are unionized. Samper's paper shows how collective action on the part of workers can help to ensure that technological innovation will be used to enhance the status of all workers, and to meet human as well as corporate needs. In an interesting variation on the theme of education, Samper exhorts the academic community to make its findings about the implications and hazards of technology accessible to workers; at the same time, she invites workers themselves to pursue this information so that they can come to the bargaining table with a knowledge base equal to that of management. Within this context, unions can see themselves as educators and actively promote women's acquisition of technical knowledge.

Samper envisions a potentially positive role for higher education and research in workers' high-tech future; the closing article suggests, however, that the research university, wittingly or unwittingly, may be entering into a close alliance with corporate interests. In a coda on the theme of education, Barbara Wright examines the university-affiliated technology park, its close relationship to academic research in high-tech fields, and its implications for women and work. This final article shifts the focus from workers and jobs per se to the larger economic structure in which those workers and jobs are embedded, and it suggests changes in economic structure that loom as collaboration between the academic research community and industry grows. By outlining the benefits of this partnership for universities (primarily financial gain and enhanced prestige) as well as for business (increased profits through access to cheap, highly skilled labor pools and to university researchers' discoveries), Wright shows us the magnitude of the stakes for both business and research universities. She argues that the new economic structures emerging out of university/industrial collaboration will not necessarily be any more hospitable toward women or minority men than the traditional ones have been; in a worst-case scenario, these workers may even find themselves more severely disadvantaged than before. She delineates the risks to the university associated with this involvement, including the privatizing and commodifying of knowledge, limitations on free scholarly exchange, compromise of the university's "objectivity," and exploitation of the university community's labor pool (especially students and faculty spouses); and she wonders whether participation in private, profit-making ventures is compatible with the university's traditional mission to serve the common good.

In her analysis, Wright uses insights and ideas presented in this volume to sketch how a feminist perspective might be effectively brought to bear upon planning and policy development of university-affiliated technology parks. She notes that women and minority men remain under-represented among the high-level university and corporate leaders who will plan these parks; consequently, a strong voice from within the university must demand equity as a fundamental principle of technology park policy. Wright notes that this is also a good time for academic feminists to reach out to their sisters in the local community: hiring plans, pay scales, education and training policies, child care provisions, and zoning laws will all affect the community, and academic and community women can take action together to ensure access with equity for those who have traditionally been excluded from high technology's promises.

Together, the articles in this section lay the foundation for a comprehensive analysis of women's access to paid employment in the computer field, and by extension to other high technology fields. Education emerges as critical, both heralded as the key to women's success and denounced as a formidable obstacle. As with any polarity, the trick is not to force the issue into one dimension or the other, but to expand the analysis so that the social and situational variables that allow education to be both villain and savior are more fully understood. A serious reconsideration of what education means in the field of high technology and what role educational institutions are to play is essential if equitable access to this field is to be obtained.

Economic and social justice alone would certainly be reason enough to work for women's full access to employment in this arena. As Eleanor Roosevelt said to the General Assembly of the United Nations in 1952, "too often the great decisions are originated and given form in bodies made up wholly of men, or so completely dominated by them that whatever special value women have to offer is shunted aside without expression." But there is more at stake here than justice. Beyond the need to respond to women, the very quality of life and work is at issue. Whether the focus is on the failure of women to gain adequate entry into all levels of employment, or the creation of routinized and numbing work, or the increasing diversion of new technology to create armaments capable of destroying all human life, the authors of these articles document the failure of the new technologies to produce a better life for all humanity. No longer is it a question of responding to women; rather, it becomes clear that high technology is in critical need of an influx of the kinds of ideas and perspectives that could come with responsiveness to and inclusion of women.

Helen Marot: The Mother of Democratic Technics

Janet Polansky

During the first half of the 1980s, lowered productivity, lags in plant retooling, and media attention to the alternative, people-centered management styles credited for Japanese corporate success have challenged traditional authoritarian, hierarchical modes of management. Mainstream management theorists have begun to show interest in decentralization, quality orientation, and worker participation, as articulated in such best-sellers as Kanter's *The Changemasters* (1983) and Peters and Waterman's *In Search of Excellence* (1982). While this trend in management theory might appear new, in fact it is part of a larger and older search for an inclusive, holistic understanding of the means and activities by which our environment is transformed. This search for holism and inclusiveness has long been central to the progressive critique of technics.[1]

Mainstream historians of technology and management theorists have tended to ignore holistic approaches to technics, concentrating chiefly on the development of tools but not on the history of dwellings, or advocating management by "experts" rather than worker participation. It is important for us now to trace alternative traditions in technological history as they were shaped and used not only by social scientists and historians but also by management theorists and feminist and trade union activists. During the early part of this century, these theorists and activists challenged fragmented, hierarchical technological ideologies, seeking a view of technics, industry, and culture that balanced the authoritarian with the democratic and studied the machine in the context of the human actors who created it and upon which it impinged. In this alternative tradition, technology was not only machines but also—and perhaps more importantly for contemporary organizations—systems, languages, process, and education.

The Underpinnings of a Critique of Technological Ideologies

In the beginning of this century, as industry increasingly relied on mass production and scientific management, intellectuals from many disciplines began to refashion their understanding of technological culture to reflect the changing environment and to generate an expanded, more inclusive concept of technology. Central to this new paradigm for technics was the concept of balance between male and female cultural and productive roles. Progressive intellectuals such as Otis T. Mason, curator of the Department of Ethnology at the U.S. National Museum, studied "primitive" and non-industrial technologies, challenging orthodox notions of women's role in culture, noting women's crucial contributions to technological development, and bringing attention to neglected aspects of women's role in production as, for example, dyers, basket makers, potters, boot makers, and weavers (Mason 1910; Mumford 1934; recent feminist anthropology has expanded this critique, as in Reiter 1975). This shift in understanding brought into focus not only women's role in production, but also the question of how technologies extend themselves through generations to meet changing needs. Thorstein Veblen, for example, in his *Instinct of Workmanship and the State of the Industrial Arts* (1914), saw technology as fundamental to the "scope and method of civilization" (vii).

We can see a related shift in perspective among Progressive Era management theorists, who responded to the authoritarian implications of scientific management by fashioning a critique of the American workplace based upon democratic, participatory ideals. James Hartness criticized scientific management as overly mechanistic and ignorant of human nature in *The Human Factor in Works Management* (1912), while Horace Drury, in *Scientific Management* (1915) attempted to restore workers' participation to a central place in contemporary theory. R. F. Hoxie, in *Scientific Management and Labor* (1915) and *Trade Unionism in the United States* (1917) examined the relationship between workers' organizations and progressive management theory, while Ordway Tead explored industrial democracy from a psychological perspective in *New Adventures in Democracy* (1939) and *Instincts in Industry* (1918). Much current theory since then, particularly in motivation and organizational development (MacGregor 1960; George 1968), builds upon these early critiques.

Perhaps no figure from mainstream management theory in this period illustrates the revisionist contribution better than Lillian Moller Gilbreth, whose work affected both corporate vision and the working lives of many people, particularly women. In *The Psychology of Management* (1914), Gilbreth incorporated psychological considerations into suggested reforms of industrial engineering curricula and into contemporary time-and-motion analysis. Her influence became even more widespread through her work as a consultant to such companies as Burroughs, Macy's, and Sealy.

Helen Marot: Beyond Theory, Beyond Reform

However neglected many of these pioneering contributions to a more holistic management theory may be today, they at least enjoy the advantage of association with a history of mainstream enlightened corporate practice. The same is not true of critiques of industrial organization that issued from feminist and trade union circles. One such contribution is the little-known management theory of Helen Marot (1865–1940). Since the discipline of management theory tends to be generated either from corporate management itself or from academe, it is hardly surprising that Marot rarely appears in histories of management theory. As an activist woman of socialist bent, she was excluded from such circles in a way Lillian Gilbreth, for instance, was not.

Marot argues for the reshaping of American industry not by manipulating the worker with wage incentives but by appealing to the innate creative capacity and hunger for responsibility in each of us. Her theory was given shape in her organizational writings for the National Women's Trade Union League (NWTUL), in the liberal and trade press (she worked as an editor of both the *Dial* and the *Masses*), and especially in a thin volume called *The Creative Impulse in Industry: A Proposition for Educators* (1918).

The Creative Impulse in Industry

Drawing upon her activist background and organizational expertise, Marot wrote *The Creative Impulse* at the request of the Federal Bureau of Educational Experiments in order to suggest reforms in vocational and technical education. Her work, however, goes far beyond the schoolroom to propose a plan for regenerating American industry. It draws on John Dewey's educational philosophy (especially *Democracy and Education* [1916]), on Veblen's social psychology (Veblen 1914), and on the ideals of participatory democracy as they were developed by theorists and activists in the Progressive Era.

Although nominally a plan for curricular reform of industrial education in the schools of Gary, Indiana, *The Creative Impulse* is principally a critique of the industrial organization, management theory, and trade union philosophy of her day. Consonant with the spirit of the times, Marot's volume is sometimes overreaching and abstract, but her critique offers a revolutionary view of education within industry and proposes the creation of a democratic workplace. The goal of Marot's transformation of both the curriculum and the workplace is to enable people to work with what she called "conscious creative intention . . .

[which] requires the ability to associate with others in the administration of industry as well as to take the place of an individual in the routine of factory work" (1918, 114). Participating in all aspects of workplace tasks, workers would direct production, organizational development, and industrial planning, using their creative powers to free American industry from a system that values business goals (i.e., exploitive profit making) over the industrial goals of productivity and quality. One result of this transformation would be that work and workplace become, paradoxically, more communal as a result of unleashing each individual's creative potential. The environment of transformed industry would lead not only to satisfaction but in fact to "joy," a central concept for Marot: "It may be possible for each worker to experience the joy of creative work as he takes part with others in the planning of the work along with the labor of fabrication" (137), thus ending the isolation and alienation characteristic of the Industrial Revolution and its aftermath.

When Marot was writing *The Creative Impulse,* American industry was enraptured with German industrial and educational methods because they seemed to result in increased production and to serve as an antidote to labor's expanding influence. Marot provided a progressive critique of the German model, arguing that the price of efficiency was militarism, authoritarianism, and paternalism—in short, the enslavement of the people. Marot maintained that Americans were deluded who thought that they could have German-style production without the concomitant authoritarian institutions, which functioned at "the sacrifice of individual life and development" (91). Marot envisioned instead a "democracy of industry."

The Creative Impulse is also antithetical to most versions of contemporary scientific management, which, she said, reduces the human to "eyes, arms, fingers, legs" (5). Scientific management, she charged, functions by "plucking out some of [the worker's] faculties and discarding the rest of the man as valueless" (5). To counter this mutilation, she posited, against the prevailing notion of business, the "creative impulse, . . . a strong emotional impulse, a real intellectual interest in the adventure of productive enterprise" (24). Marot maintained that modern industrial organization, although relying on "the common people's productive energy, has discounted their *creative potential*" (7).

Marot criticized not only conservative scientific management but also contemporary liberal industrial psychology, which she did not cite directly but which we can find in writers such as Lillian Gilbreth and Ordway Tead. Marot thought it inappropriate to emphasize workers' "instincts" (or lowest-level needs), or to see humans as collections of passive, static buttons to be pushed. By contrast, her notion of "creative impulse" suggests a more comprehensive and intrinsically self-motivating dimension of human character, and presupposes a dynamic need to create, achieve, and define the self through *techne,* creation in work.

Focusing always upon what Maslow would later call "self-actualization" and what she called "satisfaction in the process of completion [of a task]" (136), Marot did not see work as a simple mechanical process, in which workers were composites of behavioral "instincts." Rather, she viewed both work and worker as complex and creative interactions of the cognitive with the material, moving in a dialectical pattern that is, like Veblen's "instinct of workmanship," teleological in nature (Veblen 1914, vii), transforming technics as well as human civilization. Marot wrote, "The creative impulse is concerned with the transforming of a concept or some material into an expanded concept or a new object" (1918, 135). This definition posits no dichotomy between conceptualization and production. Product and producer alike are dynamic and fluid, growing and developing in a dialectic that moves both industry and the individual forward.

Reflecting not only her Quaker but also her feminist ties, Marot advanced "the highest coordinating factor in life—the principle of giving," in direct contrast to the "egoism of modern enterprise," with its emphasis upon "individual desires as the reason for existence" (1919b, 133). She believed this egoism caused a displacement that underlay industry's failure to utilize its human resources and its creative potential. "Industry under the influence of business prostitutes effort" (1918, xiv), which she thought would render the American plant unable to meet the challenge of Europe's retooling once the war ended.

Marot thought that scientific management, for all its advances, had been unable to support "initiative" (what we would probably call "motivation"), because rather than fostering authentic involvement in the productive process, it relied on such "short lived reaction to stimulus" as bonus pay and similar incentives unconnected with the work itself. In fact, Marot was suspicious of all "humanitarian schemes" and "welfare work," from profit sharing to company baseball teams, which served ultimately to maximize not workers' participation and fulfillment but company profits. She found in liberal (what she called "diplomatist") management theory such as Tead's and in "benevolently imposed" bureaucratic reform measures (1914, 9) no means of promoting production or quality, her key criteria for industry. Protective legislation, for instance, makes workers more productive for the owners' benefit rather than for their own. Perhaps because she was a worker and an organizer herself, Marot distrusted the outside expert, no matter how well intended: "Experts can successfully handle inanimate things, but the fundamental interests of men are neither successfully nor finally directed from above" (9). For this reason, her plan in *The Creative Impulse* was for change to come from workers' initiative through organization and well-placed confrontation.

According to Marot, trade unionists and other workers must learn organizational as well as mechanical skills in order to maintain their status in industry and to participate fully in a democratically transformed workplace. Mechanical skills, no matter how varied and complex, were quickly becoming fragmented and downgraded, alienated from the workers themselves; meanwhile, workers' mental skills, e.g., conceptualizing, planning, and organizing, were being reassigned to managerial employees through the predations of scientific management. Marot argued that by learning organizational skills, workers would and should assume responsibility for the industrial enterprise as a whole, "nothing more or less than sharing in the decisions, the determination of procedure, as well as suffering from the failure of those decisions and participating in their successful eventuation" (1918, 58).

For all her class consciousness, Marot's writings show a distrust of class conflict that reflects her Fabian background. She saw "class isolation" as an inevitable but regrettable result of industrialization (54). Class isolation was antagonistic to the goal of "association" or cooperation. She argued that "the need the workers have had for the cultivation of class isolation will disappear . . . as the workers become in the estimation of a community and in their own estimation, responsible members of a society" (60). In an essay on revitalizing the rail industries, she spoke of a "distinctly American method which would not be concerned with rights but with opportunity for increased accomplishment" (1919b, 131). This attitude, somewhat curious for one who practiced confrontation on a daily basis, distinguishes conflict that is neither productive nor participative from conflict that advances or clarifies an essentially cooperative relationship. She opposed "class isolation," or manifestations of conflict that occur when parties lack the rationality and empathy needed to protect the interest of industrial civilization as a whole. This interest lay for Marot not in capital, ownership, or even in the advance of workers, but rather in *techne:* human creativity used to advance civilization.

Although a lifelong socialist, Marot saw both capital and labor as essentially "exploitive" rather than creative users of technology and resources, both demonstrating "the universal attitude towards wealth production, which is to take as much and give as little as one can get off with" (1918, 23), and to seek short-term gain rather than long-term goals. A socialist state, she believed, "would lean exclusively on the consumption desire for production results, just as the present system of business now does" (24). While the socialist and the trade union movements mouthed the goal of increased worker participation, Marot believed that neither saw in industry a source of adventure or fulfillment, concentrating instead on bread-and-butter issues, trading participation for wages, and reproducing capitalist attitudes through false consciousness. As a result, the labor movement, like management, pursued consumptionism.

Marot's vision depended upon the cooperation of labor and managerial workers—technical and organizational "experts," not agents of capital. Common ownership, although not the root of creative industry, could help promote cooperative relationships. In Marot's transformed socialism, a type of participatory democracy buttressed by high productivity and living standards was necessary to fulfill both the "lower" needs, i.e., security and society, which must be satisfied before the creative impulse can be given full reign. Further, the new synthesis required not only altered standards of production but also a transformation of human consciousness through education.

More than a conventional syndicalist paean to workers' self-management, Marot's theory recognized that owing to the false consciousness (1918, 22–23) created by an unabashed profit motive, few American workers could be induced to trade wage increases for "responsibility." In the *Dial,* Marot and Veblen (both editors) had followed the contemporary debate on workers' supposed biological "limitation"—in which it was argued, for example, that only 1 to 5 percent of workers were capable of "initiative." In *The Creative Impulse* Marot assigned creative potential, the "skill and intellectual power which is latent in the working class," to everyone as part of being human (49). But she conceded the limiting effects of negative socialization, which blunted people's capacity for self-direction and creativity; these limits could be overcome only through training in positive skills.

Marot's vision of the transformed workplace offers a holistic view of the human being and provides a model for technological practice that incorporates a fluid, modern mode of production, controlled not by machines but by extensions of human cognition. Thus, she gives human thought a primary role, whether in education, in human relations, or in work itself. Her detailed plan for workshops in the Gary school system was not only to be applied to other lines of industry by enlightened managers (117), but also would be reproduced in successive generations through education. Marot's curriculum balanced the study of technical skills with the humanities and social sciences. For instance, in running a toy shop, which would serve both educational and productive purposes, students would not only deal with the technical problems of manufacture, with keeping financial accounts and estimating costs, and with maintaining the workplace and the health of the work force; they also would study economics, aesthetics, literature, and history. The humanistic content was to be integrated into the industrial process, transforming both the mechanical and the human, rather than remaining a frill upon a workplace essentially barren of human values, fit only to "embroider the system with the history and aesthetics of textiles . . . or introduce the story of past processes" (technological history) into an otherwise "impoverished" industrial mode (93). While this insistence on the importance of liberal studies may seem a well-worn concept today, Marot's proposal that the humanities and social sciences be fully integrated into technical study was noteworthy, and her main point revolutionary: the key objective of industrial education was to give all future workers "the ability to control industry" (92), without which any other reform would be pointless. *The Creative Impulse* is a model for democratic industry based upon true workers' participation, a model that begins with educaton in conceptualization, planning, and problem solving for all students—a full education that she saw as "incident to the development of the creative impulse in the individual, and . . . incident to the development of industry as a socially productive enterprise" (126).

Compared to the work of her contemporaries, Marot's treatise is at once more inclusive than Lillian Gilbreth's reports on, say, a department at Macy's, and also more practical than the work of academic management theorists such as Ordway Tead, who applied generalizations from psychological models to hypothetical workers. Marot shared with Lewis Mumford the generalist's outlook which enabled her to observe the individual worker in a job "Taylorized" for a particular segment of industry and then to propose an organizational theory that critiques industrial civilization at its roots and formulates an overarching plan for change. Marot, in fact, was an important influence in the intellectual development of Lewis Mumford, whose work was to become much better known than hers and to reach a much wider audience. Marot herself was keenly aware of her audience. Whereas the diction and tone of *American Labor Unions* (1914)—her earlier study of organizational patterns in contemporary trade unions—was fashioned for activist workers, the understated, practical, authoritative tone of *The Creative Impulse* was crafted for professional managers and educators. Absent is the overblown rhetoric characteristic at the time of the usual syndicalist tract on workers' self-management; missing is the pompous socio-psychological jargon of contemporary industrial psychology.

The Personal and the Political

Helen Marot's analysis of industrial society arose directly from her experience in contemporary trade union and feminist movements, where she gained first-hand exposure to industrial organization and to the forms of networking and bonding among activists that served as a model for humanizing industry. The self-sufficient, independent spirit present in all Marot's writing is evident in her life as well. Although enjoying a childhood rich in intellectual and social advantages (Cohen 1971; O'Sullivan and Gallick 1975), Marot, always intellectually adventurous, chose to become not an orthodox academic but a self-supporting, independent researcher and organizer. Her position at the margin, so familiar to activist women, detached Marot from both academic and corporate culture, but her involvement with feminist, trade union, and reform networks provided a model for her vision.

Marot's early projects, the *Handbook of Labor Literature* (1899) and *The Makers of Men's Clothing* (1903), a comprehensive study of the Philadelphia textile trades published by the Free Library of Economic and Political Science, a Philadelphia-based progressive think tank that she helped organize, provided the conceptual background and observational technique necessary for sustained work on organizational theory. At the turn of the century, Marot moved to New York, where she was invited to be an organizer and researcher for the Child Labor Committee, working with her associate and lifelong friend, Caroline Pratt, the well-known educator and founder of the City and Country School in New York City. Marot dedicated *The Creative Impulse* to Pratt because Pratt "intensified for the author the significance of the growth processes in industrial and adult life." As the two women assumed an active role in Greenwich Village life, Marot found intellectual stimulation and a network supportive of her creative work in a pioneering area.

Both Marot and Pratt were "allies," feminist activists associated with the National Women's Trade Union League, which had been chartered by the American Federation of Labor (AFL) to educate and organize women workers. Allies acted as links between trade unions, working women, and progressive, socialist, and feminist activists. Marot served as staff secretary during NWTUL's most productive period (1906–13). Appealing to "women of all groups who endorse the principles of democracy and wish to see them applied in industry" (Boone 1942, 233), the NWTUL, often in conjunction with settlement houses and other reform efforts (Costin 1983; Fishel 1967; Flexner 1973; Foner 1979; Kessler-Harris 1982), spanned both class and ideological barriers. Working alongside Margaret and Mary Dreier, Rose Schneiderman,

Leonora O'Reilly, and Melinda Scott, Marot helped steer NWTUL through the most volatile period of its long and sometimes stormy history (Boone 1942; Cantor and Laurie 1977; Dye 1980; Davis 1964; Eisenstein 1983; O'Neill 1969).

Always, Marot's organizational and theoretical strategy was to incorporate experience and observation into a comprehensive matrix. Marot coordinated NWTUL's administrative work, writing most of its reports and correspondence and speaking frequently at union meetings. Her involvement peaked with the 1909–10 shirtwaist makers' strike, the "Uprising of the 20,000," which transformed New York's largely female garment industry workers from diffident immigrant girls to union activists and made the ILGWU a major trade union force (Buhle 1981; Woloch 1984; Cook 1979; Kessler-Harris 1982). The NWTUL, rather than the male-dominated, conservative craft unions, emerged as a link between trade unionists, working women, and the so-called mink brigades of upper-class reformers who supported them in picketing, speaking, raising bail, and marshaling public opinion.

Unlike most of the other allies and despite her privileged background, Marot was a charter member of her local chapter of the Bookkeepers, Stenographers, and Accountants (AFL Local 12646); she identified herself as a wage-earning woman who saw her interests lying with other workers. Marot struggled against channeling NWTUL energies into efforts that seemed to detract from organizing or to emphasize gender over class (for example, campaigns for some forms of protective legislation). Although called the most class-conscious of the NWTUL allies (Dye 1980, 58), Marot continued to look to the conservative AFL for organizational, if not ideological, support. On the other hand, her regard for effective organization and administration sometimes led her to criticize the frequently incompetent leadership of mainstream trade unions, whether the conservative AFL or the radical socialists of United Garment Workers of America Local 25.

Although Cohen (1971) says that the reason Marot resigned in 1913 was to protest NWTUL's footdragging in efforts toward its stated goal of placing working-class women in leadership positions, that goal was to a large extent realized by 1914, when every officer was a working woman (Dye 1980, 116). Marot herself was not forthright about her reasons for resigning, but it seems that she reacted to a deepening division between cultural and socialist feminist sentiments in the group and to the growing split between NWTUL and the AFL, a split fueled by traditional labor organizations' failure to develop strategies appropriate for women.

Marot's writings in the political press at the end of World War I tell us much about her appraisal of industry and labor relations then, for she speaks of the failure of trade unionism and reform alike to guarantee lasting security for workers, especially women workers: "Now, dumb as usual, we are watching with the helplessness of little children," as a labor movement that had relied more on "state machinery" than its own initiative was stripped of its wartime prerogatives. With a "disquieting sense of the futility of government protection in labor affairs" (1919a, 165), workers watched business interests reassert themselves against a largely legislative reform movement whose "roots . . . are too tender to penetrate beyond the surface of our political and industrial institutions" (1919c, 294). Moreover, she saw in the wartime advances no increased opportunity for workers to participate in the creative, satisfying aspects of production. It was in this sober climate that Marot turned from trade union and reform activism to organizational management for a vision of a "new industrial economy" as well as a new psychology that she saw developing in the wake of wartime industrial strategy.

Women, Work, and Technology

Marot devoted surprisingly little direct attention to women workers in *The Creative Impulse,* having addressed them specifically in a chapter of *American Labor Unions* and of course exhaustively in the NWTUL analyses. Perhaps because the particular industries she addressed tended to be those traditionally employing men, her work appears, on the surface at least, neutral in the matter of gender. Marot's organizational experience acquainted her most deeply with textile trades long staffed by women, and with largely unskilled work. Her personal work was professional, however, and she considered skilled workers more receptive to organization and more effective in negotiation, a position that sometimes aligned her with Melinda Scott's "pro-American" wing rather than with the radical socialists more favored among immigrant workers (Dye 1980, 116). Her class analysis, however, always kept her from the bias against non-Anglo-Saxons that sometimes appeared among the other allies.

Her feminism, too, is not as self-consciously cultivated as that of others in her group, perhaps because she identified more with the socialist than with what we would call the "cultural" wing of the feminist movement. But whereas Marot rarely spoke of "sisterhood," her regard for the supportive network the NWTUL had established was apparent in the efforts she made, often at the expense of her own preferences, to keep alive the tenuous alliance among such different groups. Cooperation, even at the sacrifice of one's own immediate wishes, was central to her vision of industrial culture. In her view, conflict based upon either class or gender hurt women workers while leaving caste divisions intact, forcing women to rely on protections essentially patriarchal in character. This view may have been rooted in the conflict she witnessed not only between female and male trade unionists, but also between working- and middle-class women in the NWTUL, and even between young female textile workers socialized to traditional family values and prostitutes who heckled them during the strike.

Marot was exquisitely sensitive to context and present reality. Her understanding of the way false consciousness worked was fostered, no doubt, by her observation of women workers' conditioned lack of self-assertion in the workplace and in their private lives. Indeed, the belief that women were too disadvantaged in this way even to organize themselves was one of the chief rationalizations for protective legislation, and one which Marot opposed as paternalistic and degrading. Working-class men, too, had been deprived of opportunities to develop their leadership capacities: "He has not the habit of formulation [planning]. He is not practiced in directing others [managing]" (1914, 6). Thus, educating both men and women workers to responsibility, self-reliance, and initiative became a chief element of Marot's plan. These practical remedies for the predations of contemporary capitalism challenged the more sanguine, abstract view taken by many other progressive and syndicalist writers.

Marot always saw women workers as especially disadvantaged, owing to their status as reproducers as well as producers. Her chapter in *American Labor Unions* entitled "Organization of Women" commented both upon women's "double day" and upon their exclusion from decision-making roles in the trade union movement, showing how these had led women to undermine their own efforts. She saw trade union women being subjected like all women to sex-role socialization: "labor union women are like other women; they lack the courage and determination to overcome the prevailing attitude that women are unfit to assume executive responsibility" (1914, 68), a harsh indictment, which, in Marot's terse way, points out the negative effects of a false consciousness about one's own potential. Nevertheless, Marot saw the NWTUL, for all its faults, as "persistent, strenuous, militant" (75–76)—perhaps the only means at present for working women to deal on a somewhat equal basis with men who had "no confidence" in women's ability to manage their own affairs.

On the other hand, Marot does not discount the importance of women's work in the home: "They are expected to settle home problems and make home adjustments as they did before industry was transferred from homes to factories" (1914, 71). Unlike some other feminists and reformers, Marot never used women's nurturing role as a means of differentiating them from men, nor did she mystify their biological status.

In addition to being disadvantaged in the workplace by their roles as mothers and housewives, women workers were also, in Marot's view, disadvantaged by their lack of job skills, which made craft unionism untenable for them. Since women organized by the NWTUL were sometimes placed in unions indifferent or even hostile to their concerns, independent women's networks were essential to self-assertion and self-determination. It is perhaps because of Marot's unique sensitivity to women's presence in industry that she was among the very earliest and strongest advocates of industrial as opposed to craft organization, since women workers tended to be widely distributed in unskilled positions ("Industrial and Trade Organizations," chap. 6 in Marot 1914).

Perhaps nowhere is the difference between Marot's feminist perspective and that of the progressive management theorists more apparent than in the latter's apprehension of women's status in the workplace as marginal. The industrial psychology of a prominent liberal manager like Tead, for instance, lists women's presence in the workplace as a sexual fringe benefit for male managers and workers, placing "sex" along with "security" and "recognition" as incentives for male workers (Tead 1918). In reality, the sexual harassment of women workers by male supervisors had been a key issue in the Kalamazoo garment workers' strike and was frequently commented upon by NWTUL organizers (Dye 1980, 12; Foner 1979, 357).

Marot's critique, although curiously gender-neutral on its face, nonetheless attacks patriarchalism in several of its guises, including Prussian industrial paternalism or romantic schemes to return to premodern industrial forms. "Interdependence" among workers was possible only in a modernized, industrialized economy; that is, only upon the demise of home production, which could never lead to "democracy of industry" because it was based upon the patriarchal (i.e., hierarchical) family rather than upon the society as a whole.

Marot's vision is, in fact, not in any sense a nostalgic evocation of a bygone era of home production or guilds. Scientific management, although sometimes unwisely applied, marked an advance over previous arbitrary, haphazard systems in that it injected standards, guidelines, and rationality into industry. Marot distrusted absolutes and idealism; she placed her faith in technology, science, and education. From her experience in the textile industry, Marot knew that machines had long made women's participation possible and that technological progress was sorely needed: owners' historic reliance on cheap labor rather than on upgraded industrial plants had resulted in routine, inefficiency, and danger (Baker 1964; Levine 1924). Marot's experience in industry kept her so far from what Autumn Stanley has called "neo-Luddism," in fact, that she said quite explicitly in *The Creative Impulse,* "The proposition to revert to an earlier period suggests nothing more than the repetition of an experience out of which the present state of affairs has evolved" (1918, 21).

Marot maintained that no one had yet been able to make an accurate assessment of the value of either technology or the division of labor in industrial organization: are they inherently "antagonistic to individual growth and to the interests of workers in productive effort" (135) or have they only been *used* that way? Marot argued that our understanding of technology and its proper uses is limited by our assumption that creative effort is the same thing as individual expression. What technology in modern industry offers is the opportunity for growth in *associated* effort, which she thought would prove to be even more rewarding than individual expression. Associated effort, in fact, not only enables us, in Marot's view, to work together fully and creatively in particular factories; it also can lead us to sympathy or understanding on a global scale.

Marot saw the modern world, especially business, as being inescapably interdependent. Because this interdependence had resulted from the "industrial motive of exploitation of people and of wealth" and not from "mutuality of interest," it had led to rivalry and misunderstanding of disastrous proportions:

> While our institutional life is an acknowledgment that interdependence is a necessary factor in modern wealth production, we still measure the strength of a man, or a society, or a nation, and say of all that they are strong or weak as they are able apparently to stand alone. We have not yet discovered that a desire to stand alone in an enterprise where people are of necessity dependent, is a weakness and that our ability to cooperate with others in such an enterprise is a measure of our strength. . . . [Dewey says that] "From a social standpoint dependence denotes a power rather than a weakness; it involves interdependence. . . . [The attempt to become self-sufficient] often makes an individual so insensitive in his relation to others as to develop an illusion of being really able to stand alone, an unnamed form of insanity which is responsible for a large part of the remediable suffering of the world." (140–41)

What Marot's vision of transformed industry ultimately leads to, then, is a sane world based on international mutuality of interest and understanding. Marot argued that industry could become the locus for recovery from the limitations of personal interest and the addiction to self-expression as an end in itself:

As industry through the ages has changed from the isolated business of provisioning a family to the associated work of provisioning the world, it has blazed a pathway for relationships which are socially creative. But art in social relationships will not be realized until a passionate desire for the unlimited expression of creative effort overcomes inordinate desires of individuals for self-expression. Art in living together is possible where the intensive interest of individuals in their personal affairs and attainments, in their social group, in their vocation, in their political state, is deeply tempered by a wide interest and sympathetic regard for the life of other groups and people. (144)

Marot saw world peace becoming possible only within the context of a fully operative, participatory technology in which cooperation ends the fight for resources, and exercise of the creative impulse by all workers eliminates the need for their exploitation and coercion (144). Instead of Mary Cunningham's *Powerplay* (1984), corporate messiahs, or a Japanese model based upon the feudal warlord, we have in the work of Helen Marot a theory and a practice for industrial democracy that synthesize technological history and feminist values.

NOTES

I would like to thank Robert Asher, Barbara Wright, and the members of the editorial collective for their helpful criticisms and suggestions. In particular, I am grateful to Patricia Miller for her valuable editorial assistance.
  1. "Technics" is a term used by Lewis Mumford in *Technics and Civilization* (1934) more or less interchangeably with "technology," although for the most part he uses the term to refer to the practical application of theory rather than knowledge about, for example, history of theory or application. His definition reads: the "translation into appropriate, practical forms of the theoretic truths, implicit or formulated, anticipated or discovered, of science" (52).

REFERENCES

Abbott, Edith. 1910. *Women in industry: A study in American economic history.* New York: D. Appleton and Co.
Baker, Elizabeth. 1964. *Technology and women's work.* New York: Columbia University Press.
Bendix, Reinhard. 1984. *Work and authority in industry: Ideologies of management in the course of industrialization.* Berkeley: University of California Press.

Boone, Gladys. 1942. *The women's trade union leagues in Great Britain and the United States of America.* New York. Columbia University Press.

Buhle, Mari Jo. 1981. *Women and American socialism: 1870–1920.* Chicago: University of Illinois Press.

Cantor, Milton, and Bruce Laurie, eds. 1977. *Class, sex, and the woman worker.* Westport, Conn.: Greenwood.

Cohen, Sol. 1971. Marot, Helen. In *Notable American women, 1607–1950,* ed. E. T. James and J. W. James, 2:499–501. Cambridge, Mass.: Harvard University Press.

Cook, Blanche Wiesen. 1979. Female support networks and political activism. In *A heritage of her own: Toward a new social history of American women,* ed. Nancy F. Cott and Elizabeth H. Pleck. New York: Simon and Schuster.

Costin, Lela B. 1983. *Two sisters for social justice: A biography of Grace and Edith Abbott.* Chicago: University of Illinois Press.

Cunningham, Mary. 1984. *Powerplay: What really happened at Bendix.* New York: Simon and Schuster.

Davis, Allen F. 1964. The Women's Trade Union League: Origins and organization. *Labor History* 5:3–17.

Dewey, John. 1916. *Democracy and education.* New York: Macmillan.

Drury, Horace B. 1915. *Scientific management: A history and criticism.* New York: Columbia University Press.

Dye, Nancy Schrom. 1980. *As equals and as sisters: Feminism, the labor movement, and the Women's Trade Union League of New York.* Columbia, Mo.: University of Missouri Press.

Eisenstein, Sarah. 1983. *Give us bread but give us roses: Working women's consciousness in the United States.* New York: Routledge and Kegan Paul.

Fishel, Leslie H., Jr. 1967. The problem of social control. In *Technology in western civilization,* ed. Melvin Kranzberg and Carroll Pursell, 2:499–515. New York: Oxford University Press.

Flexner, Eleanor. 1973. *A century of struggle: The women's rights movement in the United States.* New York: Atheneum.

Foner, Philip S. 1979. *Women and the American labor movement.* New York: Free Press.

George, Claude S. 1968. *The history of management thought.* New York: Prentice-Hall.

Gibson, Jane, and Rensis Likert. 1976. *New ways of managing conflict.* New York: McGraw-Hill.

Gilbreth, Lillian Moller. 1914. *The psychology of management.* New York: Sturgis and Walton.

Hartness, James. 1912. *The human factor in works management.* New York: McGraw-Hill.

Hoxie, R. F. 1915. *Scientific management and labor.* New York: D. Appleton and Co.

———. [1917] 1966. *Trade unionism in the United States.* Reprint. New York: Russell and Russell.

Jacoby, Robin Miller. 1976. Feminism and class consciousness in the British and American women's trade union leagues, 1890–1925. In *Liberating women's history: Theoretical and critical essays,* ed. Bernice Carroll. Urbana, Ill.: University of Illinois Press.

Kanter, Rosabeth Moss. 1983. *The changemasters.* New York: Schocken.

Kessler-Harris, Alice. 1982. *Out to work: A history of wage-earning women in the United States.* New York: Oxford University Press.

Kuhn, Thomas S. 1970. *The structure of scientific revolutions.* Chicago: University of Chicago Press.

Levine, Louis. 1924. *The women's garment workers: A history of the ILGWU.* New York: B. W. Huebsch.

McFeely, Mary Drake, ed. 1982. *Women's work in Britain and America from the nineties to World War I: An annotated bibliography.* New York: G. K. Hall.

MacGregor, Douglas. 1960. *The human side of enterprise.* New York: McGraw-Hill.

Marot, Helen. 1899. *Handbook of labor literature: Being a classified and annotated list of the more important books and pamphlets in the English language.* Philadelphia: Free Library of Economics and Political Science.

———. 1903. *The makers of men's clothing: Report of an investigation made in Philadelphia.* With Caroline Pratt. Philadelphia: Philadelphia Branch of Consumer's League, Members of Octavia Hill Association, United Garment Workers of America, and Philadelphia Union of Journeymen Tailors.

———. 1910. A women's strike: An appreciation of the shirtwaist makers of New York. *Proceedings of the Academy of Political Science in the City of New York* 1:119–28.

———. 1914. *American labor unions: By a member.* New York: Henry Holt and Co.

———. 1916. Revolution in the garment trades. *Masses,* Aug., 29.

———. 1918. *The creative impulse in industry: A proposition for educators.* New York: E. P. Dutton and Co.

———. 1919a. Labor at the crossways. *Dial,* Feb. 22, 165–68.

———. 1919b. Responsible unionism. *Dial,* Aug. 23, 131–33.

———. 1919c. Why reform is futile. *Dial,* Mar. 22, 293–96.

Mason, Otis. 1910. *The origins of invention.* New York: Scribner's.

Merchant, Carolyn. 1980. *The death of nature: Women, ecology, and the scientific revolution.* San Francisco: Harper and Row.

Mumford, Lewis. 1934. *Technics and civilization.* New York: Harcourt, Brace and Co.

———. 1967. *The myth of the machine: Technics and human development.* London: Secker and Warberg.

———. 1972a. Authoritarian and democratic technics. In *Technology and culture: An anthology,* ed. Melvin Kranzberg and W. H. Davenport. New York: Schocken.

———. 1972b. Technology and the nature of man. In *Technology and culture:*

An anthology, ed. Melvin Kranzberg and W. H. Davenport. New York; Schocken.

————. 1979. *Works and days: A personal chronicle.* New York: Harcourt, Brace and Co.

Noble, David F. 1983. *Forces of production: A social history of industrial automation.* New York: Knopf.

O'Neill, William L. [1969] 1971. *Everyone was brave: A history of feminism in America.* Reprint. Chicago: Quadrangle.

O'Sullivan, Judith, and Rosemary Gallick, eds. 1975. *Workers and allies: Female participation in the American trade union movement, 1824–1976.* Washington, D.C.: Smithsonian Institution Press.

O'Toole, Patricia. 1983. *Corporate messiah: The hiring and firing of million-dollar managers.* New York: Morrow.

Peters, Thomas J., and Robert H. Waterman, Jr. 1982. *In search of excellence: Lessons from America's best-run companies.* New York: Harper and Row.

Radcliffe College. 1973. *Schlesinger Library inventory, Arthur and Elizabeth Schlesinger Library on the History of Women in America.* 3 vols. Boston: G. K. Hall.

Reiter, Rayna. 1975. *Toward an anthropology of women.* New York: Monthly Review Press.

Rogers, Everett M. 1983. *Diffusion of innovations.* 3d ed. New York: Free Press.

Rothschild, Joan, ed. 1983. *Machina ex dea: Feminist perspectives on technology.* New York: Pergamon Press.

Soltow, Martha Jane, Carolyn Forché, and Murray Massre, eds. 1972. *Women in American labor history, 1825–1935: An annotated bibliography.* East Lansing, Mich.: School of Labor and Industrial Relations and the Library, Michigan State University.

Tead, Ordway. 1918. *Instincts in industry.* Boston: Houghton Mifflin.

————. 1939. *New adventures in democracy.* New York: McGraw-Hill, Whittlesey House.

Trescott, Martha Moore. 1983. Lillian Moller Gilbreth and the founding of modern industrial engineering. In *Machina ex dea,* 23–37. *See* Rothschild 1983.

Veblen, Thorstein. 1914. *The instinct of workmanship and the state of the industrial arts.* New York: Viking.

Woloch, Nancy. 1984. *Women and the American experience.* New York: Knopf.

Females and Computers: Fostering Involvement

Linda H. Lewis

The U.S. Department of Labor predicts that by 1995 at least 2 million people will be employed in occupations directly related to computers, while millions of others will have to use computers as a routine part of jobs that do not presently require them.[1] Such projections, taken at face value, suggest a future in which computers and computer-related careers will be commonplace. However, current statistics reflecting sex-specific disparities in computer usage, class enrollment patterns, and high-tech careers forebode neither equal participation nor equity in the new technologies.

In 1981, white males comprised 67 percent of the computer specialists in the United States.[2] Only 26 percent of the master's degrees and 8.4 percent of the doctorates granted in computers and information sciences in 1983 by American colleges and universities were awarded to women.[3] Nationally, males outnumber females two to one in computer classes in secondary schools.[4] Such differences in the acquisition of computer proficiency tend to increase the gender and socioeconomic inequities that already exist in the labor market.

Numerous nationwide studies further underscore the seriousness of the skills gap. EQUALS in Computer Technology, a computer equity training program at the University of California, Berkeley, found girls comprised only 29 percent of the enrollment in high school computer classes. Even more discouraging was the fact that this percentage dropped, and the proportion of males increased, as the courses became more advanced.[5] Similar findings are reported by the Project on Equal Education Rights (PEER). According to independent studies in California, Maryland, and Michigan, PEER found boys outnumbering girls two to one in academic-based courses in computer programming.[6]

The literature on participation in the new technologies is replete with research probing the variables related to the underrepresentation of females and minorities. The evidence consistently suggests that girls, influenced by sex role stereotypes and the expectations of teachers, friends, and parents, often perceive computers as too difficult. These perceptions are exacerbated as children advance within the educational system. The Johns Hopkins University Center for Social Organization of Schools found that first-grade girls were as interested as boys in learning to program computers. By the sixth grade, however, boys' interest surpassed girls' by a two-to-one ratio, and by the ninth grade more than four-fifths of all interested students surveyed were males.[7]

This article examines a variety of factors that contribute to disparities in computer use and participation and suggests ways for developing sex equity in computer education and training. Various psychosocial processes, from the influence of visual depictions in the media to lack of support or encouragement from significant others, can have long-term effects on young women's decisions to engage in the new technologies. In addition to discussing these factors, I will examine environmental variables such as classroom interactions, and incorrect assumptions regarding the mathematical basis of computers that act to inhibit female participation. The objective is to call attention to the myriad influences that often go unnoticed but that play a pivotal role in determining both the kinds of computer training females receive and the decisions they subsequently make about computer use and careers.

To encourage female participation in computer education, this article argues for an appreciation of sex-specific differences. Such differences, if meaningfully incorporated into computer education, require a change of perspective on the part of everyone from teachers and administrators to parents and friends. A careful evaluation and consideration of software, pedagogy, and interaction patterns suggests specific strategies that have the potential to humanize and restructure computer education.

The Environment: Friendly or Hostile?

The Media: Sending Subliminal Messages

The fact that most computer labs and courses are taught by men serves to reinforce the idea that the new technologies are part of the male domain. Not only is there a dearth of female role models, but textbooks, advertisements and magazines perpetuate the stereotype. An analysis of four large-circulation computer magazines (*Compute, Popular Computing, Info World,* and *Personal Computing*) by the Women's Action Alliance revealed the following:

1. In 28 photos depicting passive involvement with a computer (watching other people use computers or demonstrate computer products), 30 percent of those portrayed were women.
2. In 144 photos demonstrating active computer involvement (using or demonstrating computers), 17 percent of those portrayed were women.

3. Of ninety-one articles featured in the volumes surveyed, 70 percent were written by men; 12 percent were written by women. (In 12 percent of the cases, the sex of the author could not be determined, and 6 percent were coauthored by both men and women.)[8]

Thus the media, by depicting a world in which it is primarily men who sell, use, and write about computers, do little to counter the female's tendency to view computers as a "male thing."

The Myth of Computers as Mathematical

What on the surface seems nothing more than a simple administrative decision to locate computers in a particular environment or classroom can actually become a powerful factor influencing computer use. For example, placement of terminals in the math department sends forth the message that computer proficiency is related to mathematical competence. While there are those who believe that sex differences in mathematical aptitude and learning are largely responsible for the differing responses of men and women to computers, the fact remains that most computer applications are nonnumeric. Simply by locating computers in music, language, and arts classrooms, in media centers and libraries, educators could move the technology into an atmosphere that deters stereotypic thinking and debunks the myth of requisite competencies.

Despite the fact that more females than males say they are afraid of mathematics and technology, there is evidence suggesting that such anxiety is a learned response that is internalized more by women than men because of a pervasive popular belief that science and technology are male domains.[9] A study by the National Assessment for Educational Progress indicates that although girls are doing slightly less well on programming tests nationwide, when given good exposure to computers they perform as well as or better than boys.[10]

An Issue of Support

Peer approval, interpersonal support, and peer culture, especially during the formative years, all have a significant effect on the participation of females in educational programs. At a time when social interests come to the fore, females often back away from competition and are reluctant to skip grades or participate in advanced placement classes for fear of peer rejection.

One of the most poignant examples of females' need for interpersonal relationships and support is evidenced in requests by high-achievement girls to return to lower grades because they had no one with whom to eat lunch. For them, having friends was more desirable than participation in advanced classes.[11]

In addition, the issue of participation may be compounded by reluctance of school girls to compete with boys for access to the hardware. At one U.S. high school, the Educational Testing Service found teenage boys harassing girls by telling them they were stupid, in order to dissuade them from registering for after-school computer courses.[12] Exclusive male after-school clubs have become a favorite pastime for "computer jocks" who rally around the hardware. Such male networks have been euphemistically referred to as the intellectual equivalent of sports.[13]

The offering of same-sex learning opportunities has been explored recently as a way of encouraging females to use computers more often. The development of programs targeted for "girls only" is predicated on the assumption that with a sex-specific learning opportunity, preadolescent girls in particular would not be discouraged by males, who might challenge their participation. However, a survey of New Jersey and Oregon students by the Computer Equity Training Project of the Women's Action Alliance revealed that while the presence of female friends was more encouraging than the presence of males, a subgroup responded that the presence of male friends was encouraging as well.[14] When asked about factors that discouraged computer use, the absence of friends, either male or female, was by far the most important factor for girls.[15]

A Wisconsin study of fifty-eight seventh- and eighth-grade girls further underscores the importance of peer support. Seeing one's friends use computers, having a girls' computer lunch period, and watching girls use computers were found to be the three highest motivators for computer use.[16] The study did not distinguish between male and female friends, but clearly the variable that was important was the availability of friendship groups, which made computer use more enjoyable.

The Parental Prototype: Discouraging High Tech

From studies of home computer use, it is clear that the issue of computer equity extends beyond the classroom. Stanford University researchers surveyed 87 middle- and upper-income students in grades five through eight and found all of the 13 percent who reported owning home microcomputers were boys.[17] This result was unexpected in a population evenly divided between boys and girls who had equal exposure to computers in school. Moreover, home interviews with typical computer-owning families revealed that the amount of time spent using computers also differed by sex.[18] Similar findings are confirmed by a Computer

Equity Training Project study of 459 seventh and eighth graders. Boys were found to be more than three times as likely as girls to say they used their home computers (67 percent versus 21 percent). Boys also reported much heavier use exclusively by other males in the home than did girls for exclusively female use.[19]

The influence of the home becomes apparent again in studies of computer camp enrollments. Miura and Hess, in a nationwide survey of over 55,000 students participating in 132 different programs conducted by 23 sponsors of computer camps, report enrollments favoring boys (74 percent males, 26 percent females).[20] In addition, beginning and intermediate classes were 28 percent female, but female enrollment dropped to 14 percent in advanced classes, and to a meager 5 percent in assembly languages. Thus as the difficulty of the curriculum increased, female enrollment declined. This same relationship was observed when female participation was plotted against the variable of cost. As camps became more expensive, female enrollments diminished from 32 percent for sessions under $100 to 15 percent for those over $1,000.[21] Such data suggest that parents are more willing to expend larger sums of money to support their sons' involvement with computer technology than they are their daughters'.

Finding a Mentor

Research on successful professionals in science and math demonstrates that supportive individuals are critical to career choice. Female college-bound seniors participating in a National Science Foundation program designed to stimulate interest in science and math cited lack of encouragement from both counselors and teachers as one of the major factors that reduced their own interest in scientific and technological careers.[22] Biased behaviors, although often unintentional and unwitting, frequently discourage enrollment and achievement in high-tech fields. Observational studies reveal that teachers, often unknowingly, discourage girls from using computers by asking boys to move equipment and demonstrate programs. Girls, as well as minority males, get less actual performing experience, take fewer field trips, and have less hands-on opportunity than Anglo males who take the same course.[23]

Transforming Our Perspectives

In an attempt to account for sex differences in computer use and participation in the new technologies, there are those who advance explanations ranging from biologically based differences in mathematical aptitude to the sex typing of computers as part of the male domain. Although biological factors cannot be ruled out, to date no single explanation to account for gender differences has emerged with unequivocal support. While thus far we have focused on the attitudes, policies, and practices that work to impede female participation, an alternate view of sex-specific differences, based on syllogistic reasoning, deserves attention.

There are those who believe that males and females are essentially the same since they share the same human nature. For those who are essentially the same, education should be essentially the same. However, one can work from another assumption—namely, that males and females, for whatever reason, are significantly different. For those who are different, a strategic differentiation of educational practice is required. Based on this logic, it would follow that because males and females qualify the meaning of things in different fashions, the same teaching strategy will in fact have different meanings for females and males in the same situation. Unless these differences are acknowledged and respected, many individuals will consistently be at a disadvantage in the learning environment.

Carol Gilligan, in her book *In a Different Voice,* provides a strong foundation for the development of alternate teaching and learning strategies founded on the premise that women and men have differential access to certain understandings.[24] Gilligan's writings challenge us to reshape our concept of human experience rather than continuing to train for new technologies using the same model that has heretofore served as the educational standard.

Based on her research into women's reasoning and the imagery of female thought, Gilligan has been able to establish a worthy argument for women's tendency to view the world in terms of connectedness and relationship. By asking questions that are sensitive to differences between the sexes, she establishes the tendency of males to be comfortable operating in autonomous situations, whereas females tend to feel threatened by isolation. Gilligan also demonstrates important differences in the responses of both sexes to violence and intimacy. Men tend to project more violence into intimate situations; women, comfortable with intimacy, perceive competitive success as threatening.

> For boys and men, separation and individuation are critically tied to gender identity since separation from the mother is essential for the development of masculinity. For girls and women, however, issues of femininity and feminine identity do not depend on the achievement of separation from the

mother but are defined through attachment. Thus, males tend to have difficulty with relationships, while females, who are threatened by separation, tend to have problems with individuation.[25]

It is important to emphasize that Gilligan's findings are based primarily on white, middle-class women; nevertheless, the intuitive "fit" of her assertions for all women cannot be denied. Clearly her claims demand that further empirical testing be conducted with disparate samples drawn by social class, generation, and education; however, her work does provide a basis for rethinking the manner in which both females and males respond to the new technologies. By applying Gilligan's work to the world of computers, a different understanding of the underrepresentation of females emerges. If men tend to see the world in terms of their autonomy, then males may more readily embrace computer technology because they view it as enhancing autonomy and power. Women, on the other hand, may display ambivalence or reluctance because they view the technology as distancing them from others.

Shotton reports that "computer junkies," who are mostly male, talk about their love of the machine by saying, e.g., "It's not going to be rude to you or criticize you. You don't have to worry about it as you do humans."[26] Conversely, females, with a humanistic perspective, attempt to make the computer user-friendly and work toward changing the nonhuman, depersonalized image associated with the technology. According to Genevieve Cerf of Columbia University, women programmers are much more verbal in their choice of descriptors, choose easily identifiable variable names, and are more likely to write programs with the user in mind.[27]

Given the "different voices" of men and women, it appears that one of the first priorities when attempting to increase female representation in the new technologies should be to create a positive learning environment that will avoid isolating students and simultaneously pitting "human" against "machine." For example, it has been common practice to place students in rows with individual computers; an alternative strategy would call for computer networks and cooperative activities, circular seating arrangements, and team projects to encourage communication among participants. Traditionally, math, and now computer science, have been taught in a hierarchical setting. The alternative is to create a supportive context for learning through the development of team approaches, partnerships, and cooperative work groups, where nurturance and encouragement become the predominant characteristics of the learning environment. In such an atmosphere, preferences for interconnectedness and sharing can be capitalized upon to promote further learning and continued participation.

Innovative programs for encouraging equal participation are developing nationwide, and the results are heartening. In Palo Alto, California, the computer abilities of both girls and boys improved dramatically when students were given their initial training by a peer.[28] This is but one example of the many models that could be developed to foster interpersonal support and to increase female participation.

Software Reconsidered

In addition to modifying classroom environments and teaching strategies to promote involvement with the technology, we must shift from our current preoccupation with violent and destructive computer games. As long as software is being utilized that violates an ethic of caretaking and harmony, females will spend less hands-on time using computers. Many classroom teachers who enthusiastically promoted the use of computer games as a major means to achieve computer literacy are now finding that such games "tend to be designed by boys, for boys, and that stereotypical masculine values are powerfully reinforced in boys."[29] Thus many girls are discouraged from using computers, while those with antisocial predispositions are encouraged to become involved with the technology.

In considering the issue of software, serious questions emerge concerning how biased programs contribute to the gender gap. In many software programs, the language and sex roles are stereotyped and the main characters are male. Recreational software in particular is continually criticized for its role in perpetuating racist and sexist attitudes that alienate females. Violence, aggression, war, and competitive sports, the central themes of many recreational and educational programs, are often antithetical to females' socialization and ethic of nonviolence. Significant efforts were made in the 1970s to produce teaching materials that were sexually and racially nonbiased; now these efforts must be extended to the new medium of software.

Numerous studies have been conducted to chronicle software preferences. Findings validate the assumption that girls are more likely to get involved with software they find emotionally or intellectually meaningful and generally select programs that involve writing (story programs) or music. Boys, on the other hand, are more attracted to action-oriented, competitive games and software requiring hand-eye coordination.[30] Moreover, while males are often interested in computer manipulation and graphics in themselves, females tend to view the computer more as a tool—a means to an end rather than an end in itself.[31] At issue is the fact that the programs that appeal strongly to females are less widely used and less frequently available than programs that appeal to males. In addition, there are many indicators that the computer language LOGO is more interesting to girls than boys due to its pictorial and graphic nature; however, the algebraic language BASIC is the one taught in the schools.[32]

In a recent study by the Women's Action Alliance, the belief that females are repelled by violence in computer programs was not entirely borne out. Through viewing the reactions of students to an action and shooting program, Mastertype, researchers found that both males and females responded favorably to the software.[33] It may be, however, that the redeeming feature of the program was that it taught typing, and that this side benefit is what increased girls' favorable reaction. Clearly more research using extreme examples of educational and recreational programs that lack such redeeming features is necessary before significant statements can be made. Perhaps the question that needs to be asked is not whether male-biased content with a destructive bent discourages females, but rather whether such software has redeeming value for either sex. By continuing to teach deductive reasoning and problem-solving by using "search and destroy" tactics, we are supporting the very paradigm feminists are working hard to change. When we continue to use strategies and classroom techniques predicated on competition rather than cooperation, we preserve a macho perspective and fail to view females on their own terms.

A Matter of Style

Any proposal for changing the way one introduces and teaches computers is incomplete without some consideration of cognitive learning style. Even though scientists suggest that cognitive style does not predict aptitude, females' cognitive style preferences can be easily capitalized upon to promote involvement in the new technologies. For example, most females show early superiority in language skills. Certainly, the ability to master languages can include computer languages that are now being expressed more and more frequently in words.

Women's tendency to ignore extraneous factors and concentrate on the task at hand is another factor that stands them in good stead as programmers. Numerous personality studies have shown that while boys tend to be more curious and take risks, girls are better able to screen out irrelevancies, carry out tasks, and solve problems under stress. Women's plight, however, is that these positive attributes, and others such as

motor skill proficiency and the ability to carry out rapid sequential movements, are used as the basis for relegating monotonous tasks to females.
Instead of being viewed as a promise of success with computers, these
strengths are deemphasized and females' work is deskilled, while male
qualities are more highly valued.[34]

Sherry Turkle, author of *The Second Self: Computers and the Human Spirit,* defines two distinctive styles of computing.[35] The "hard"
style (overwhelmingly male) involves mastering and manipulating computers, as is taught in traditional programming courses. The "soft" style
(mostly female) involves a more intuitive and personalized approach to
what is on the screen. It is Turkle's belief that such disparate approaches
are the result of a culture that socializes girls to the practice of "give and
take" and boys to the "imposition of will."[36] Whatever the origins of the
stylistic differences, the problem is that for the most part only the hard
style is respected in computer classes, while the soft style is not taken
seriously.

While theories of cognitive style emphasize the importance of individual differences, they do not suggest that one style is best. Instead,
diversity should be celebrated. Thus it behooves educators and trainers
to offer an array of learning experiences so that individuals will have an
opportunity to capitalize on their own distinctive learning preferences.
By varying teaching methods to accommodate individual differences,
one not only ensures that the learning environment will not be biased;
one can also minimize the growing gender gap in computer access, interest, and use.

If indeed each person's learning style is unique, it follows that it is
the distinctive contributions of both males and females that will enrich
the technology and make it adaptive. At long last, differing modes of
reasoning and expression, which for females have been merely descriptive differences and developmental liabilities, can become the basis for
women's inclusion in the new technologies.

Changing the Paradigm

This examination of female involvement in computer usage has indicated
a need for families, schools, and communities to rectify sex-specific imbalances. Several specific steps to promote equity can be derived from the
factors already cited. For example, through staff development workshops
and educational programs, parents, teachers, counselors, and administrators can become sensitive to inappropriate behaviors and unfair educational practices. Collecting and analyzing participation data by course,
level, and sex can serve not only to document inequities but also to

provide the impetus for establishing norms and standards that guarantee adequate preparation for both males and females.

It is important that experimental programs and curricular reforms be initiated in traditional learning environments in order to assess the efficacy of alternative strategies such as same-sex programming, mentorships, and field-based experiences on participation patterns and success ratios. Cooperative ventures with business and industry need to be developed to ensure a joint commitment to eliminating gender disparities. For example, through on-site seminars, career days, and exposure to female and minority role models in high-tech professions, young adults can see for themselves the array of employment opportunities that are available.

Women must not become the "techno-peasants" of today's or tomorrow's labor market. It is essential that we make equal participation a priority issue. This means that educational decision makers, as well as parents, concerned citizens, and business leaders, must be alert to male predominance in computer use and high-tech careers and take firm actions to help overcome the imbalances. Only by highlighting this issue and educating individuals about the severity of the disparities will interventions follow that can lead to significant changes in the future.

As we progress through decades of rapid technological change, there are some who question the ways in which this new technology is being utilized, its side effects, and its potential consequences. For those concerned with the militarism so commonly linked with technological development today, there is no better argument for why we should ensure the participation of females in this high-tech world than the one so persuasively stated by Dorothy Austin, lecturer in psychiatry at Harvard Medical School: "No longer is woman's moral reasoning viewed as less developed or simply a different style: it has become a political necessity for the preservation of the world."[37]

NOTES

1. Lindsy Van Gelder, "Help for Technophobes," *Ms.*, Jan., 1985.
2. U.S. Department of Labor, Bureau of Labor Statistics, *Current Population Survey* (Washington, D.C., 1981).
3. U.S. Department of Education, "Earned Degrees Conferred," (National Center for Educational Statistics, Higher Education General Information Survey, updated tabulations, Oct., 1983).
4. Kay Gilliland, "Equals—Computers in Education," *Math/Science Network Broadcast* (Berkeley) 2, no. 1 (Fall, 1981): 1–3.
5. Ibid.

6. Project on Equal Education Rights, *Are Girls Getting an Even Break?* (Washington, D.C., 1983).
7. Center for Social Organization of Schools, Johns Hopkins University, *School Uses of Microcomputers* (Baltimore, 1983).
8. Women's Action Alliance, Inc., "Making the Computer Neutral," chapter 1, in Draft Manual (New York, 1985).
9. Lynn H. Fox, *The Problem of Women and Mathematics.* Report of the Ford Foundation (New York, 1981).
10. R. Anderson, D. Klassen, K. Krohn, and P. Smith-Cunien, *Assessing Computer Literacy: An Empirical Assessment* (St. Paul, 1982).
11. M. F. Angel. "A Study in Precocious Math Ability and Education: Wolfson I" (Master's thesis, Johns Hopkins University, 1974).
12. Phyllis Rossen, "Do Schools Teach Computer Anxiety?" *Ms.,* Dec., 1982.
13. Project on Equal Education Rights, *Sex Bias at the Computer Terminal: How Schools Program Girls* (Washington, D.C., 1984).
14. Jo Shuchats Sanders, "Making the Computer Neutral," *Computing Teacher,* Apr., 1985, 23–27.
15. Ibid.
16. Ibid., 13.
17. Irene Miura and Robert D. Hess, "Sex Differences in Computer Access, Interest and Usage" (Paper presented at the 91st annual APA convention, Anaheim, Calif., Aug., 1983).
18. Ibid., 4.
19. Sanders, "Making the Computer Neutral," 5.
20. Irene T. Miura and Robert D. Hess, "Enrollment Differences in Computer Camps and Summer Classes," *Computing Teacher,* Apr., 1984.
21. Ibid.
22. G. T. McLure and E. Piel, "College Bound Girls and Science Careers," *Journal of Vocational Behavior* 12, no. 2 (Apr., 1978): 129–39.
23. Peggy Caldwell, "A Damning Set of Data: Subtle Differential Treatment of Girls and Blacks," *Education Week,* July 27, 1983.
24. Carol Gilligan, *In a Different Voice* (Cambridge, Mass., 1983).
25. Ibid., 8.
26. Cited in P. Lange, "Compulsive Computing," *Manchester Guardian,* June 7, 1984.
27. Ellen McClain, "Do Women Resist Computers?" *Popular Computing,* Jan., 1983.
28. Van Gelder, "Help for Technophobes," 89.
29. D. Chandler, *Young Learners and the Micro Computer* (Milton Keynes, U.K., 1984).
30. I. Miura, "Differential Attitudes toward the Microcomputer in Middle School Age Range" (Manuscript, Stanford University, 1982).
31. McClain, "Do Women Resist Computers?"
32. Maryann Marrapoli, "Females and Computers? Absolutely!" *Computing Teacher,* Apr., 1984.
33. Sanders, "Making the Computer Neutral," 8.

34. Eleanor Maccoby, "Sex Differences in Intellectual Functioning," in *The Development of Sex Differences*, ed. E. Maccoby (Stanford, 1966).
35. Sherry Turkle, *The Second Self: Computers and the Human Spirit* (New York, 1984).
36. Ibid.
37. Lindsy Van Gelder, "Carol Gilligan: Leader for a Different Kind of Future," *Ms.*, Jan., 1984.

Expanding Access to Technology:
Computer Equity for Women

Sandy Weinberg

In August of 1984 the media overflowed with stories about the Summer Olympic Games. Particularly in live television coverage, so-called color commentators filled in the time between scheduled events by discussing a wide range of semirelated topics. In one such discussion, broadcast internationally on ABC, adlibbing commentators decried the proliferation of what they smugly described as "nonsporting sports." They suggested that the new synchronized swimming event was an artificial creation added to appease women, who would never be on the same performance level as men in the more traditional sports like javelin throwing and wrestling.

It does not take a great deal of sports expertise, or much of a background in formal logic, to see the flaw in this argument. As similar as the sexes may be in important ways (other than reproduction), there are obvious physical differences. These differences do not provide one sex with natural superiority over the other, but they do suggest that in certain activities, specifically those designed around inherent physical differences, one sex will have a natural advantage. Conversely, sports designed to test the limits of the inherent physical characteristics of the other sex would reverse that advantage. Obviously, if one sex designs the contests, which are selected for the degree to which they showcase certain skills, then that sex will tend to excel in those contests. Males are likely to outperform females in strength sports, while females (with equal training opportunities) may well pull ahead of males in endurance events. The addition of new sports that capitalize on skills more common in female bodies simply represents correction of a long-standing bias.

An analogy can be drawn from sports to other fields. Because sporting events are largely tests of physical skill, the division into two groups on the basis of sex is largely reasonable.[1] In activities that are less dependent on physical ability, however, such a division becomes problematic. Even biological categorization by sex is perhaps more accurately viewed as a continuum than as a simple division.[2] When cultural, social, and psychological factors are considered, their categorization as characteristically "male" or "female" becomes meaningless. The macho-male world discourages most females and also many androgynous males, who may not be able or may not choose to claw their way through an environment defined by aggression and power.

The fast-lane computer world is just such an artificially "male" environment. As such, it has traditionally forced potential players in that world either to conform to the macho-aggressive image it thrives upon, or opt not to play. That choice puts most females at a real disadvantage, for they are forced to compete in an economic event designed specifically for the characteristics of the males currently in control. More androgynous males find themselves similarly disadvantaged, though with a greater chance to succeed if they are willing to compromise on life-style and goals. In some environments, one can argue, the circumstances favoring a given sex or philosophy are inherent, and while everyone should have a chance to cope, it is unreasonable to expect the environment to be modified to meet individual needs. The barriers in place in the computer field, however, are purely artificial; they were added solely as screening mechanisms at a time when the characteristics important to success were misunderstood by those who controlled the field.

The goal of this article is *not* to suggest that tactics be developed and implemented to help females (and others) move into the fast lane of the computer world. Some females, thriving on the excitement of that environment, will do well there as long as impediments to equal opportunity are removed. No doubt they should be removed. Certainly equity should exist in that high-tech world of engineers, mathematicians, and technomanagers, but that is not the focus here. An equal or greater necessity is the development of strategies for modifying the computer world to become one in which computers are preprogrammed with all the math, engineering, and analysis systems required, so that the broadest possible range of users can effectively control and utilize the new technology. In such an environment, equity in computer access will be achieved "for the rest of us."

Present educational requirements, job descriptions, and experiential opportunities do not accurately reflect the reality of skill expectations or needs. The development of strategies for overcoming these now antiquated barriers will help open up career opportunities—not by forcing round pegs into the square holes of the current environment, but by redrilling those holes. And because those holes have been so artificially shaped, the change can be accomplished without weakening the structure for which the holes have been designed.

Problem Definition

Today's computer environment is dominated by programmers, engineers, systems analysts, and designers.[3] Traditionally raised males have a natural advantage in these areas. From birth they were supplied with toys that required action, control, and direction.[4] The games they were encouraged to play involved acting in roles of leadership, command, and decision making. In such activities, the emergent (dominant) leader is encouraged to make decisions unilaterally.[5] Those who supply the information upon which decisions are made have relatively low status. And the decisions made are judged on the basis of their capacity to generate excitement: males are consistently encouraged to modify the rules of their reality to meet their desires.[6]

Most children today are first exposed to computers in the form of video games.[7] Many of the most popular games are simply programmed versions of traditionally male noncomputer games. With the exception of a small amount of excellent nonsexist software,[8] most games involve shooting, blowing up, speeding, or zapping in some way or another. Not surprisingly, those games often frustrate or bore the nonmacho players exposed to them. As a result, macho males often have a positive first experience with the computer; others have a negative initial experience.

Recent research with individuals who exhibit a high level of anxiety when dealing with computers has shown that the single most powerful predictor of such resistance is an initial negative experience.[9] Most computerphobics report a prior incident in which a computer made them feel frustrated, confused, or denigrated. Even an interaction with a video game in which the participant was forced to fire when he or she was more inclined to negotiate can be sufficiently negative to lead to a negative attitude and continued anxiety in the future. Incidentally, computerphobics are not disproportionately female.[10] However, those fields in which females have traditionally been encouraged to seek employment—teaching, child care, nursing—are only now beginning to take advantage of the power of computers. As a result we are seeing more women who have to deal with computers.

The phobic or frustration reaction becomes critical when the individual begins to make career decisions. At an early age, often around puberty, students are asked to opt for either "people-oriented" careers or "object-oriented" careers. Males with high-level math or science aptitudes are likely to be steered toward the "object" fields, while males lacking such ability, males in whom the ability or interest has yet to emerge, and most females are encouraged to pursue so-called people fields.

The problem with this "choice" is that it is based on two faulty assumptions: (1) that persons are wholly or largely oriented in one direction or the other rather than both; and (2) that occupational fields including engineering, psychotherapy, nursing, woodworking, or any other eventual career, do not require a mixture of both skills. The carpenter unable to effectively manage fellow workers, or the teacher unable to cope with mechanical problems, is doomed to high frustration and low productivity.

The problem becomes more acute when the individual enters serious career training and observes the role models available in the computer field. The majority of computer professors are practitioners who (regardless of sex) embody traditional male values and approaches. Many managers report that their most serious problems arise from trying to get programmers and analysts to cooperate on teams: they are too competitive to work well together.[11]

The training, too, is rife with artificial barriers. In the educational environment, computer courses have usually been introduced and taught either by engineering or mathematics departments. In each case, the plan of study necessary to earn a degree may include unnecessary courses included from the "parent" discipline in a political compromise. There is little regard for what topics are necessary or valuable for the computing field itself. The recommended curriculum developed by the Data Processing Management Association (the data processing professional organization) has been accepted in only a very small minority of schools.[12]

Similarly, initial job entrance requirements often reflect artificial barriers. In a recent survey, forty-two college graduates of a business information systems undergraduate program reported that COBOL programming knowledge was a prerequisite for obtaining even an interview for the jobs they eventually secured. Yet only three of those persons reported that they were asked to do any programming on the job: COBOL was an entrance barrier, not a job requirement.[13]

Clearly, then, unnecessary and probably unintentional barriers steer people uninterested in the highly competitive aspects of programming away from the computer field entirely. Only those students excited by the challenge of head-to-head battle are encouraged to pursue computer careers, even though that battlefield does not actually exist, even though that attitude is counterproductive, and despite the necessity of a cooperative attitude for success in the real computer environment.

How Closed Doors Can Begin to Open

In the wake of new technology there always seems to come a period of assessment and evaluation in which people-oriented concerns surface. As the computer revolution has reached a popular audience, it has brought such a period: doors, once closed and avoided because of the apparent expertise required, are inevitably being opened, simply because less and less expertise is required.

Modern information systems can be effectively utilized without years of programming experience, without engineering training, and without any special technological expertise. Menu-driven systems, in which the computer asks the user what function is desired, make it possible to use highly sophisticated computers effectively without knowing much more than how to turn them on.

For example, millions of Americans have mastered the automated teller machines (ATMs) that are changing banking habits. These micro-computer-based robotic devices can accept deposits, transfer funds, and hand out cash to persons who have never had an hour of computer training. After inserting a coded identification card, the user simply answers the questions appearing in English on a small screen. The computer uses those responses to activate preprogrammed instruction modules and performs the desired tasks. The skills a human user requires to be an expert-level user of sophisticated systems have thus been adjusted downward by the technology itself.

Unfortunately, society has not kept up with technological progress. User-oriented career opportunities and training programs still parallel the requirements of programming and systems design positions, using mastery of these skills, which are not relevant for the user positions, as screening devices. In fact, the skills of programming and technical design may be more than irrelevant, they may be actually counterproductive. A user trained in the technical skills may have inadequately developed the more humanistic skills that computer applications now require.

Before discussing specific tactics for opening doors and keeping them open, it may be valuable to specifically state the three underlying givens that will make those tactics functional. First, and perhaps most obviously, it is necessary to remove through enforced regulatory action any artificial and *de facto* discriminatory barriers that exclude persons on the basis of any factor other than relevant ability. Historical forces have often encouraged the evolution of job specifications, educational admissions requirements, or instructional objectives that subtly discourage individuals who may in fact possess all the skills relevant to success. For example, most computer science college degree programs require several semesters of advanced calculus.[14] There is, of course, no inherent reason why females should not do as well as males in a calculus course. However, females may have been discouraged from obtaining a strong high school mathematics background and hence may shy away from a demanding mathematics requirement. In reality, calculus is simply not a relevant prerequisite for most computer-related disciplines. Similarly, all traditional job specifications should be reviewed to determine whether or not they are in fact relevant to performance.

Second, a nonsexist environment is essential for the development of any sort of equal opportunity in the computer field. As long as women are underpaid overall, are at a disadvantage in terms of child care, and must deal with society's lower expectations for them, true equity will remain elusive. Role models will be lacking; opportunities for informal experience will be few; and subtle discouragements will be everpresent.

Finally, successes should be publicized as much as possible, with the media used to document and hence multiply progress. Publicity that increases the visibility of valuable role models will encourage others to pursue related goals. Females who have achieved success in the computer field should seek recognition for those accomplishments; enlightened males should also provide positive images. For the females, the mere fact of success may be sufficient. Males might more creatively and subtly portray an androgynous image of their work in computing ("a program my daughter helped me with"; "a problem referred to me by my wife's consulting firm"; "I asked my neighbor for advice, and she suggested . . .").

These givens provide a context for specific tactics that can lead to greater equity in the computer field.

Tactical Approaches

The development of specific tactics and approaches to accomplish this goal is an individual process, dependent largely upon the interests, resources, and opportunities available. Nevertheless, the following case study may prove helpful as an illustration and a model.

This study originated at St. Joseph's University in Philadelphia, and the work described here continues today both there and at Drexel University. In developing an information systems program for a business college, faculty wanted to offer students an opportunity for experiential learning. Such an opportunity not only provides a very useful occasion to apply learned skills; it also serves as an object lesson in the real-world problems that never seem to be addressed in the artificial environment of the classroom.

Significant pedagogical problems arise from that artificiality. If an instructor simply provides students with a project to program, they miss the challenge of determining how a program can be used to solve a complex practical problem. If you ask them to review software, they miss the opportunity to define the subtle prejudices, design preferences, and phobic reactions that have a significant impact on real software decisions. All the important human conflicts of the computer world are filtered out. A classroom experience teaches theory, but applications function atheoretically.

As an alternative, the faculty supervisor of the program sent a letter to all human services organizations in the metropolitan area offering free consultation on acquisition of computers, implementation of systems, training of personnel, development of software, or evaluation and purchase of equipment. As the major project of the course, students were assigned to a particular organization, generally in teams of three. Each team was responsible for the analysis and solution of the computer-related problem of the human services organization. Faculty provided support, guidance, and in-house consulting to the project groups.

It may be helpful to add a few specific notes for those who may use this description as a model. First, in the project described, client organizations were screened according to three criteria: (1) they had to be charitable, nonprofit organizations (this is a matter of letting the IRS screen out groups with questionable reputations); (2) the organization could not have plans to put the same project out for commercial bid (this criterion prevented any alienation of private consulting firms in the area); and (3) requests for help were not accepted from organizations whose expressed purpose was in conflict with the goals of the sponsoring university. This last criterion was used to placate a Catholic university in the case of a request from a Planned Parenthood group. It was successfully argued that though the Planned Parenthood center did perform procedures contrary to those approved by the Catholic Church, the organization's goals were not in conflict with the educational goals of the university. Individual students had the option, of course, of not participating in a specific project.

The class itself was structured like a consulting organization. A student-led team was assigned to each project and drew on faculty as consulting advisors. The supervising faculty member met regularly with all team leaders as well as with individual teams, to help with technical matters and keep the project on track.

The program has been extremely successful on a number of levels.

Students have enjoyed an excellent educational experience. Local nonprofit human services agencies have gained access to free computer consulting. And, in a subtle but nonetheless meaningful way, the cause of computer equity has been advanced. The design, structure, and implementation of the program has led to an appreciation of the importance of humanistic skills in the computer fields, while humanistic organizations have been able to use computers to further their own important ends.

The project also produced a number of specific benefits. The students learned to cope with clients who were not quite certain of their needs and may have had a number of misconceptions about computers; they also were able to add this practical experience to their résumés. The universities involved received very favorable publicity in the community for providing help to social service groups with important problems.

The agencies were able to computerize their budgeting, training, record-keeping, and other functions without taxing their already tight budgets to pay for the advice they required. In effect, computers were brought into a sphere in which they otherwise would have been unobtainable. And human services managers, traditionally in the backwater of new technology, were provided with an opportunity to move into the mainstream.

But it is another, more subtle benefit that is of the greatest interest here. Both male and female students in the program began to appreciate the importance of "people" skills in dealing with even the most technological of computer problems. If such appreciation became widespread, it could eventually lead to a reduction of the macho-mystique of the machines and open up the field to humanized technocrats. Often women (and less traditional males) who had been aiming at careers in education, personnel, or other "people-related" fields came to see through this consulting project the potential for a career in computers and thereby increased their personal options and flexibility. And the purely machine-oriented, fast-track technicians in the program were shown the value of expanding their training to include interpersonal skills.

At the same time, the program and the media attention it attracted provided an opportunity to create positive role models for other students and potential students. The appointed team leader of each project naturally became a media spokesperson, and it was not difficult to ensure representation of females in the ranks of project team leaders. Although the faculty advisors did not discriminate in favor of women, the establishment of logical selection criteria (previous experience, leadership, and academic background) led naturally to a large number of female team leaders.

Finally, it should be noted that the project had a valuable tertiary effect. The service organizations that received assistance with computerization tended to be staffed by women. Clients included museums, rape counseling centers, schools, senior citizen centers, and day-care organizations. The management staffs of these organizations found themselves acquiring a new set of valuable and marketable skills as they worked with the project teams. While it is to be hoped that this improvement in their credentials will not result in a bleeding of human service organization staff to fill better-paying positions in the corporate sector, the new expertise does provide greater flexibility for the people employed in those organizations. Some may well decide to make a career change to areas previously closed to them for lack of computer-related experience; others may force an upgrading of salary scales to prevent major recruitment problems.

Conclusions

Projects like the St. Joseph's program can help bring us closer to achieving equal opportunity in the computer field. Inherent in this approach is a belief in evolutionary change: a conviction that even small changes, influencing only a few individuals, are worth pursuing. In effect, even these small steps become magnified as they minutely modify the existing climate. As the computer field becomes less restrictive and more humanized, it will be open to and will attract more humanizing people.

The likelihood of our achieving computer equity is good, for demand is high while the supply of macho-male technocrats is relatively small and dwindling. A computerized society requires a large number of qualified professionals; it cannot afford to discriminate according to arbitrary factors that may restrict the pool of applicants. This pressure is helping to develop rational entrance criteria, reasonable promotional policies, and adequate training opportunities. As these vectors mature, the field may well emerge as the first major equal-opportunity discipline.

NOTES

1. The gap between performance levels in sports attracting both males and females will probably shrink, however, as a generation matures in which members of both sexes receive equal training and encouragement.
2. See Herb Goldberg, *The Hazards of Being Male* (New York: New American Library, 1976).

3. S. Weinberg and M. Fuerst, *Computer Phobia* (New York: Banbury Books, 1984).
4. Mary J. Collier and Eugene L. Gaier, "The Hero in the Preferred Childhood Stories of College Men," *American Image* 16, no. 2 (1956): 177–94.
5. See R. D. Middlemist and M. A. Hitt, *Organizational Behavior* (Chicago: SRA, Inc., 1981), sec. 1.
6. David B. Lynn, "The Process of Learning Parental and Sex-Role Identification," in *Sex Differences in Personality,* ed. D. L. Schaeffer (Belmont, Calif.: Wadsworth, 1971), 41–49.
7. See Henry Horenstein and Eliot Tarlin, *Computerwise* (New York: Random House, 1983).
8. "New Tech Times," interview and demonstration with S. Weinberg (broadcast no. 7, taped Nov., 1983).
9. See Weinberg and Fuerst, *Computer Phobia.*
10. S. Weinberg, "Cyberphobia," *Impact,* May, 1983.
11. R. Murdick, J. Ross, and J. Claggett, *Information Systems for Modern Management* (Englewood Cliffs, N.J.: Prentice-Hall, 1984).
12. See Data Processing Management Association, *CIS* [Computer Information Systems] *'86—The DPMA Model Curriculum for Undergraduate Computer Information Systems* (Santa Cruz, Calif.: Mitchell Publishing Co., 1986).
13. In-house Placement Report, College of Business and Administration, St. Joseph's University, 1983.
14. See Data Processing Management Association, *CIS '86.*

Gender and Earnings Inequality among Computer Specialists

Katharine M. Donato and Patricia A. Roos

The most salient feature of occupational segregation by sex is its persistence over time. Measures of sex segregation show that women work in substantially different occupations from men and that this differentiation has existed at essentially the same level throughout much of this century (Blau and Hendricks 1979; Reskin and Hartmann 1985). Recently, women have made some progress integrating occupations traditionally held by men, with the aggregate measure of occupational sex segregation declining by approximately 10 percent between 1970 and 1980 (Beller 1984). Coexisting with this modest decline in occupational segregation by sex is the persistence of a substantial amount of segregation at both the occupation and job level (Bielby and Baron 1984).

Findings such as these suggest that although some traditionally male occupations are opening up to women, most remain closed. One set of occupations in which women have made modest inroads is computer specialties, a field that has grown dramatically over the past decade. In 1970, women accounted for 13.6 percent of all systems analysts; by 1980 that figure had increased to 22.5 percent. During the same period, women increased their representation as operations and systems researchers (from 11.1 to 27.7 percent) and as computer programmers (24.2 to 31.2 percent) (U.S. Bureau of the Census 1984a).

This article results from a larger project investigating the determinants of changing sex composition between 1970 and 1980 (Reskin and Roos 1985). Our aim is to investigate whether computer specialties, as representatives of new occupations in the rapidly developing high technology fields, offer greater access and better opportunities and rewards for women workers than do older, more established occupations. More specifically, using 1980 census data for California (a leading center for high technology jobs), we examine gender differences in earnings for three computer specialties: systems analysts, operations and systems researchers, and computer programmers.[1]

291

Historical Context: Technological Change and Women Programmers

Computer occupations are a very recent phenomenon, with modern programming being introduced just forty years ago (Kraft 1977).[2] Programming, in turn, spawned new computer specialties, most notably systems analysis. As a preliminary to our empirical investigation, we present a historical overview of how these relatively young occupations have changed. We pay particular attention to how factors external to the occupations, such as technological change, affected the nature of the work, since they may have important implications for women's access to these jobs as well as for the opportunities available to men and women currently working in the computer field.

Since the introduction of the computer, the relevant technology has changed dramatically (Greenbaum 1979). In the beginning, programming computers was a slow, tedious job that consisted of rewiring circuits for each new calculation entered into the machine. The computer's hardware consisted mostly of vacuum tubes that required constant maintenance by programmers. Although the labor intensiveness of these early machines may have been a drawback for users, the concurrent development of the first stored program computer that could change programs and instructions without rewiring enhanced the adaptability of these early computers for a variety of commercial uses.

The vacuum tube computers, known as first-generation machines, were replaced in 1958 by computers with solid state transistor hardware. Transistors offered users the benefits of speed, smaller size, and enhanced reliability, advantages considered very important to encouraging the acceptance of computers in the business community. With expanding business markets in the 1960s, the success of early computers, and efforts to find inexpensive and more reliable hardware, the third computer generation was born. The important technological breakthrough during this period was the introduction of integrated circuit components that promoted a "general-purpose" computer, allowing for compatibility between business and scientific applications and interchangeability between operating and programming software (Greenbaum 1979, 28). Integrated circuits composed of transistors further enhanced computer speed and reliability and lowered consumer prices. Continued advances in microelectronics have led to the large-scale combination of integrated circuit components, in which thousands of transistors are packed onto tiny chips that can store data or process thousands of instructions per second.

In addition to changes in computer hardware, systems software has changed markedly since the early days. In first-generation machines, there were no operating systems or any other support programs. Each time a program was run, workers had to load the program and start up the hardware. Thus, early programmers were fairly eclectic—their tasks included anything that was necessary to ensure the efficient operation of the computer. Whether it was problem analysis or hardware maintenance, programmers acted independently on the job, with management understanding little about their work (Greenbaum 1979).

Operating systems and other support programs first appeared in second-generation machines. Although these programs offered greater machine and labor efficiency, users still complained. First, most programs required too much memory to run efficiently, leaving little or no room for user programs. Second, many new operating systems were incompatible with other computers, whether run in different models of the same computer or in computers manufactured by competitors. Hence the development of software support systems lagged behind new hardware development throughout the 1960s (Greenbaum 1979).

Amid these rapidly occurring changes in computer hardware and software, managers implemented an authority hierarchy that subdivided programming labor into three suboccupations: coders, programmers, and systems analysts (Kraft 1977), a division that remains to the present day. As the most skilled programming workers, systems analysts are responsible for "designing whole, complex data processing systems rather than parts of larger ones as programmers do" (Kraft 1977, 16). Programmers solve specific data processing problems through the design, debugging, or documentation of programs. The least skilled coders, who are now essentially clerical workers, take programs prepared by systems analysts and programmers and translate the symbols of these programs into computer language. By 1970, programming had been redefined and split into relatively more and less skilled subspecialties.

Women's involvement in computer work began with the first computer, the ENIAC (Electronic Numerical Integrator and Computer). In fact, the first programmers were women college graduates with a background in math or science, who did hand calculations and developed software during the postwar period to help predict ballistic trajectories (Kraft 1977; Greenbaum 1979). Women were initially hired because it was assumed that programming would be similar to clerical work. Employers learned early on, however, that programming demanded more complex skills, including abstract logic, mathematics, electrical circuitry, and machinery, all of which the ENIAC women used to perform their work. With the realization that the programming required more skills than originally predicted, employers began to hire more men, and the sex composition of programming shifted (Kraft 1977). Although many of the early pioneers remained, few new women were recruited. Greenbaum (1979, 87) speculated that some women were denied access to programming because of employer prejudice, while others may have self-selected themselves out because of the field's mathematical and scientific image.

By the mid-1960s, the outlook for women in programming changed again. With an increase in the demand for computer personnel, women were again recruited into programming occupations. Also changing during this period, as described above, was the division of labor in the computer field as a whole (Greenbaum 1979). As the field of programming became subdivided and the duties of programmers and operators became more narrowly defined to comprise a smaller number of tasks, women began to reenter computer occupations. Although the direction of causality is far from clear, it may well be that the field opened up to women again precisely because the occupation was undergoing deskilling.

Occupational Growth and Job Opportunities in the Computer Field

There is no doubt that computer occupations have sustained rapid growth in recent years. From 1970 to 1980, there was a 94 percent increase in the number of computer programmers, an 88 percent increase in systems analysts, and a more modest 24 percent increase in operations researchers and analysts (U.S. Bureau of the Census 1984a). Projections for job opportunities in the computer field indicate that these occupations are expected to continue to increase dramatically. As reported in the *New York Times* (1984), between 1982 and 1995 new systems analysis jobs are expected to increase by 85 percent. A similar increase of 77 percent is expected in computer programming. In addition to the growth predicted for these particular occupations, employment in high technology industries as a whole increased faster than all wage and salary employment between 1972 and 1982 (Riche, Hecker, and Burgan 1983). Despite the recent slump in American manufacturing of silicon chips (*New York Times* 1985), employment opportunities in computer occupations outside of the manufacturing industry are likely to continue to expand.

While it is clear that growth has occurred in computer specialties, it is less evident that this growth has benefited women. Certainly, as we noted earlier, women have begun to move into these occupations in larger numbers, providing further documentation that women's opportunities for moving into traditionally male occupations are greatest in those job sectors experiencing rapid growth (O'Farrell and Harlan 1984; Bielby and Baron 1984). Moreover, Dubnoff and Kraft (1984) found that women in computer programming are better paid relative to women in other occupations, and that there is also less income inequality between the sexes (see also Strober and Arnold 1987, table 7). In 1981, for example, the earnings of female programming specialists averaged 70 percent of men's, a wage gap less than the male-female wage differential for all occupations (Kraft and Dubnoff 1983).

Although women apparently benefit monetarily from working in computer occupations, at least relative to other women, indications are that their status is not yet comparable to that of their male coworkers. Male computer specialists are better represented in the higher-paid and higher-prestige systems analysis and programming jobs than in other computer occupations. A 1974 *Computerworld* magazine survey cited by Greenbaum (1979) found that women constituted 13 and 20 percent of business systems analysts and programmers, respectively. During the same year, they represented 20 and 99 percent of computer operators and keypunchers, respectively. More recent data provide even better documentation for the general finding that the lower the status and pay of the occupation, the greater the representation of women (Strober and Arnold 1987). Data from the 1980 census show that women are currently 22 percent of systems analysts and 31 percent of computer programmers. Women now predominate as computer operators (59 percent female), an occupation classified as an "administrative support, including clerical occupation" by the U.S. Census, and remain vastly overrepresented as data entry workers (92 percent) (U.S. Bureau of the Census 1984a; see also Strober and Arnold 1987).

There is also evidence that male and female computer specialists work on different job tasks, which has important implications for their potential earnings. Dubnoff and Kraft (1984) found a strong negative association between the percentage of females and the average pay of programming specializations. Moreover, they found that women in high-paid specializations, such as management, earn less relative to men (60 percent), than women in low-paid specializations such as maintenance and documentation (85 percent).

Industrial Location, Local Labor Market, and Wages

Recent literature on earnings differences has focused on the explanatory effects of structural characteristics on earnings attainment (e.g., Stolzenberg 1975; Bibb and Form 1974; Talbert and Bose 1983; Roos 1981; Parcel and Mueller 1983; Hodson 1983; Hodson and England 1986; for a review, see Kalleberg and Sorensen 1979). We build on this literature by assessing for computer specialists the impact on earnings of industrial and local labor market factors, in addition to traditional ascriptive and achievement factors.

Previous research suggests that one reason for women's lower earnings relative to men's is their concentration in lower-paying or "peripheral" industries (Bibb and Form 1974; Beck, Horan, and Tolbert 1978; Hodson 1983). Increases in the percentage of women within an industry may result in competition for jobs between men and women, which may lead to lower wages for all incumbents, or to the segregation of women into low-paying industries (Parcel and Mueller 1983, 25). Strober and Arnold (1987) found that women computer specialists tend to be employed in lower-paid, end-user industries that use computers and software, rather than in the computer industry itself, where computers and/or their software are designed and developed. They also found that men were somewhat more likely than women to work in high-tech jobs, which they speculated might enhance men's earnings opportunities.

In addition to industrial characteristics, previous research suggests that features of local markets affect earnings (Parcel and Mueller 1983). We define local labor market as the setting in which workers offer their labor in return for wages, status, and other rewards of the job (Kalleberg and Sorensen 1979), and we investigate whether variation across markets affects the microlevel distribution of rewards. Initial support for this can be found in research documenting variation in rewards for computer specialists by geographic region (U.S. Department of Labor 1984; Marion 1984).

Methods

Data

The data we use are from the 5 percent sample of the 1980 census microdata for California (U.S. Bureau of the Census 1983a). We chose California because it is one of the major centers for growth in high technology employment. Using Riche, Hecker, and Burgan's (1983) definition of high technology industries,[3] California is the largest U.S. employer of high-tech workers, employing 933,100 workers in 1982. These workers represented 9.5 percent of the state's total nonagricultural labor force (Riche, Hecker, and Burgan 1983, 57). A second reason for choosing state, rather than national, data was to enable us to concentrate on developing indicators for local labor markets, which we measured as the "county group" where the respondent lived.[4] California has several well-known local centers of high-tech development: the Los Angeles area, which has the highest level of high technology employment in the state, and the San Jose area in Santa Clara county (containing the well-known "Silicon Valley"), where one-third of the jobs are in high-tech industries (Riche, Hecker, and Burgan 1983, 56). Our interest in developing a measure of the local labor market is based on the assumption that the greatest earnings will accrue to workers in areas with the greatest concentration of high-tech employment, since demand for skilled labor would be highest there.

We include in our sample workers between the ages of twenty-five and sixty-four in three computer specialties: computer systems analysts and scientists, operations and systems researchers and analysts, and computer programmers. These three detailed occupations were the professional and technical computer specialties identified in the 1980 census occupational classification. The age restriction selects for a more occupationally and financially stable portion of the population. For the regression analyses, we further select only those who indicated they worked in 1979. Given our restrictions, our working sample for the regression analyses includes 2,618 male and 974 female computer specialists.

Measurement of Variables

The basic variables we use in our analyses are those identified as important in previous analyses of earnings attainment.[5] We focus on one dependent and two sets of independent variables, namely individual and structural factors. We are particularly interested in the explanatory power of the structural variables, which estimate the effects of industrial location and the local labor market on individual earnings.

Dependent Variable
Our dependent variable is earnings of the respondent, which we measure as the sum of wage or salary income and net self-employment income from farm and nonfarm sources in 1979, with the data coded as the midpoints of $10 intervals up to $75,000 a year. "Earnings" includes those sources of income most often used with labor force characteristics such as occupation and hours and weeks worked in 1979 (U.S. Bureau of the Census 1983b, app. K, 23).

Individual Factors
Age refers to age at last birthday, coded in years. Education is the number of years of school completed.[6] We expect positive relationships between both these variables and earnings.

Because of its demonstrated importance for women's labor force behavior (Roos 1983), we include marital status as a set of dummy variables. "Currently married," the omitted category, includes only those who are presently married; "formerly married" refers to those who are currently separated, divorced, or widowed; the "never married" category includes those who have never married.

We calculated an hours-worked-per-year variable by multiplying the usual hours worked per week in 1979 by the number of weeks in 1979 in which the respondent worked for pay or profit.[7] Inclusion of this variable is particularly important in comparing the attainment processes of women and men, given women's lesser likelihood of working full-time (Treiman and Terrell 1975; Roos 1981). In table 1 only, we present data separately for the two original categorical variables, usual hours worked per week in 1979 and weeks worked in 1979.

We include class of worker as a set of dummy variables, distinguishing between "private wage and salary" (the omitted category), "government," and "self-employed." Our class of worker indicator is a collapsed version of the original census variable.[8]

Structural Factors

We specify several different types of variables to tap industrial location. First, each of the fifty-two categories of the Census Bureau's intermediate industrial classification (U.S. Bureau of the Census 1984c, app. A, list B) was recoded to equal the mean annual earnings in 1979 of employed men sixteen years and older (U.S. Bureau of the Census 1984c, table 2). We chose this measure to determine whether, as Strober and Arnold (1987) have speculated, the earnings gap between male and female computer specialists is attributable in part to their concentration in industries that pay men less. Unfortunately, earnings data were not available for the more detailed industry classification. Hence our measure is a conservative one, since it is unable to tap gender differences *within* the broader fifty-two industry categories. This is important given Strober and Arnold's (1987) finding that women computer specialists also earn less than men within industries.

While industrial earnings were not available for the more detailed three-digit industrial classification, our second industry variable was. We use percent female as an alternative measure of the differential distribution of men and women across industries. For this variable, each of the more than 230 detailed industry codes was recoded to the percent female of each industrial category (calculated from U.S. Bureau of the Census 1984c, table 4). Following Kraft and Dubnoff (1983) and Strober and Arnold (1987), our expectation is that sex differences in earnings are due in part to the concentration of women in difficient and lower-paying industries.

Another indicator of industry refers to whether the industry is recognized as a high technology industry. We used Riche, Hecker, and Burgan's group III designation (see note 3 below) to compile a list of the twenty-eight Standard Industrial Classification (SIC) codes designated as high-tech (see Strober and Arnold 1987, which used the same indicator). After translating the SIC codes into 1980 census industrial codes, we created a dummy variable with "1" indicating high-tech industry, and zero otherwise. Following Strober and Arnold (1987), we expect that being in a high technology industry will increase the earnings of computer specialists.

Our final measure of industrial location is based on Hodson's (1983) sectoral model of economic segmentation. We use the six-sector industrial classification (a collapsed version of his sixteen-sector classification), which we updated for use with the 1980 census industrial classification. Because Hodson developed his classification for private wage and salary employees only (Randy Hodson, personal communication, Dec., 1985), we added a seventh sector to account for those computer specialists who work in public administration and the postal service.

To include these industrial sectors, we added a set of dummy variables. "*Oligopoly*" (the omitted category) includes industries that rank highest in size, concentration, foreign involvement, profits, and employee wages. Included in this sector are the largest and most concentrated multinational corporations. The "*core*" sector is dominated mostly by large manufacturing industries with a high degree of unionization, foreign involvement, and profits. Workers in this sector can earn as much as those in the oligopoly sector. The "*periphery*" sector refers to industries dominated by local and regional establishments with limited capital, a nonunion labor force, and little foreign involvement. Included in this sector are service industries, several durable and nondurable manufacturing industries, retail chain stores, and offices of physicians and dentists, settings where earnings are usually low. "*Core utilities*" is typified by industries with high foreign dividends and high assets but low profits, such as electric and gas utilities, radio and television broadcasting, finance industries, brokerage houses, and railroad, bus, air, and water transport services. The "*periphery utilities*" sector is comprised of industries that rank lower on size and foreign involvement than those in core utilities (miscellaneous utilities, and trucking, warehousing, and pipeline transport industries). The final sector Hodson (1983) identifies is *"trades,"* which is composed of industries that rank lowest on assets, concentration, and foreign involvement and that are located in local labor markets (educational institutions, nonprofit and agricultural services, and hospitals). As noted above, we include a seventh sector to account for computer specialists in *public administration and the U.S. Postal Service.* Hodson (1983) reports that women occupy few positions in the core industry sector and many positions in periphery and trades sectors. We thus expect sex differences in earnings to be attributable in part to the concentration of women in the periphery and trades sectors.

Our final structural variable is a measure of the local labor market, measured as the county group of the respondent's place of residence. The variable refers to the percentage of the county group's *establishments* that are high tech.[9] This variable was calculated from published census data (U.S. Bureau of the Census 1982) by taking the number of jobs designated as high tech (using Riche, Hecker, and Burgan's [1983] group III definition) in a county group relative to the total number of establishments in that county group. Our expectation is that computer specialists working in areas where demand for their services is great (i.e., county groups with a high concentration of high-tech establishments) are likely to have higher earnings than their fellow workers not working in such areas.

Earnings Attainment of Male and Female Computer Specialists

Our major goal in this section is to investigate explanations for gender differences in the earnings attainment of computer specialists. Before proceeding to those analyses, however, we first examine the labor force characteristics of incumbents of our three computer occupations. We then move to a different level of analysis, that of comparing *occupational* characteristics, as opposed to labor force attributes. We present these descriptive statistics to provide a fuller description of the occupations themselves, as well as of the people who work in them. To more directly assess how women fare in these rapidly developing occupations, and to take account of gender differences in background factors, we then estimate a regression model of earnings. By directly comparing the metric regression coefficients for men and women, we identify differences in the labor market benefits men and women accrue from the variables we include in our model. We conclude with a decomposition of the earnings differential between men and women, to determine how much of the earnings gap can be attributed to individual and structural factors.

Labor Force Characteristics

Table 1 presents data on selected *labor force* characteristics by occupation and sex. We concentrate in our discussion on identifying those
background characteristics that may negatively affect women's earnings
relative to men's. With respect to educational achievement, in each
occupation women are significantly less likely than men to have at least
graduated from college. Approximately 62 percent of male, and 51 percent of female, systems analysts have at least one college degree; the
comparable figures for operations researchers and programmers are 50
versus 39 percent and 57 versus 52 percent, respectively. As is true for
many other professional occupations, men in computer occupations are
more likely to be married than their female coworkers, suggesting that
marriage and professional work are not as easily compatible for women
as for men.

Sex differences in the extent of labor force participation are consistent with previous research on other occupations. Not only are males in
all three occupations slightly more likely to have worked in 1979, but
they are also significantly more likely to work full-time (thirty-five or
more hours per week) and year-round (at least fifty weeks in 1979).

With respect to class of worker, most computer specialists work
primarily in private wage and salary employment, and there are no significant sex differences across the categories in any occupation. Operations
research is the only occupation with a sizable group in government work,
and it also has correspondingly fewer self-employed workers.

These results indicate that part of the earnings gap between men
and women should be attributable to women's lower values on traditional human capital variables, education and labor force participation.
We investigate this further in a subsequent section.

Occupational Characteristics

In Table 2, we present data on *occupational* characteristics for our three
computer occupations. The data for California come from our census
microdata, while the figures for the United States were calculated from
published census data (U.S. Bureau of the Census 1984b, table 1) and
presented for comparison purposes. With respect to occupational characteristics, we find that in California women represent just over one-
quarter of the incumbents in each occupation, with slightly fewer women
systems analysts, proportionately, than operations researchers or programmers. Interestingly, there are more women systems analysts proportionately in California than in the United States as a whole. This finding

TABLE 1. Labor Force Characteristics of Computer Specialists, Ages 25–64, by Occupation and Sex, California, 1980, in Percentage

	Systems Analysts		Operations Researchers		Programmers	
	Men	Women	Men	Women	Men	Women
Education						
0–8 years	0.3	0.3*	1.5	0.0*	0.2	0.8*
9–11 years	0.8	2.2	1.5	0.0	0.6	1.3
12 years (H.S. degree)	9.0	19.0	18.4	21.2	9.5	13.6
13–15 years	28.3	27.2	28.2	40.1	32.6	32.1
16 years (B.S./B.A. degree)	25.2	30.0	23.4	19.7	31.6	28.4
17 years or more	36.4	21.3	27.0	19.0	25.5	23.8
Total	100.0	100.0	100.0	100.0	100.0	100.0
Marital Status						
Currently married	67.0	48.7*	71.8	51.8*	61.6	56.9*
Formerly married	14.8	26.3	12.5	28.5	12.8	19.7
Never married	18.2	24.9	15.7	19.7	25.6	23.4
Total	100.0	99.9	100.0	100.0	100.0	100.0
Percent Who Worked in 1979	98.6	96.4*	97.0	94.9	97.7	95.3*
Usual Hours Worked per Week in 1979						
Less than 35	3.7	11.2*	4.8	11.7*	6.9	16.0*
35–40	74.1	71.1	75.1	80.3	73.1	74.7
41 or more	22.2	17.6	20.2	8.0	20.1	9.3
Total	100.0	99.9	100.1	100.0	100.1	100.0
Weeks Worked in 1979						
Did not work	1.4	3.6*	3.0	5.1*	2.3	4.7*
1–39	5.1	7.6	6.8	7.3	6.6	14.4
40–49	5.5	10.6	6.5	18.2	8.8	11.0
50–52	88.0	78.2	83.7	69.3	82.3	69.9
Total	100.0	100.0	100.0	99.9	100.0	100.0
Class of Worker[a]						
Private wage and salary	83.5	82.0	77.2	72.3	80.0	81.6
Government	11.5	14.1	21.1	27.7	14.5	15.5
Self-employed	4.9	3.9	1.8	0.0	5.6	2.8
Total	99.9	100.0	100.1	100.0	100.1	99.9
N	1,013	357	337	137	1,327	529

[a]Three unpaid family workers were deleted from these percentages. Therefore class of worker percentages for female systems analysts and female computer programmers are based on $N = 355$ and 528, respectively.

*Chi-square for sex differences within each occupational group is significant ($p < .05$).

might indicate that opportunities for women in systems analysis are greater in states such as California where demand for computer specialists is higher.

Systems analysts in California are on average better educated than other computer specialists, followed closely by programmers and then operations researchers (15.6 years of schooling compared with 15.3 and 15.0, respectively). This finding supports Kraft's (1979) claim that an educational hierarchy produces different levels of skilled workers for employment in the computer industry. A similar hierarchy exists for each occupation's representation in California's high-tech industries: 54 percent of systems analysts work in high-tech industries, compared with 53 and 40 percent of programmers and operations researchers, respectively.

Perhaps attributable to their higher average education and greater representation in high-tech industries, systems analysts in California are the highest paid of all three computer specialties. Interestingly, even though they have on average less education and are less likely to work in high-tech industries than programmers, operations researchers actually earn slightly more than programmers. Incumbents of both occupations, however, earn less than systems analysts (operations researchers earn 92, and programmers 88, percent of the systems analyst wage). Computer specialists in California, when viewed as a group, earn slightly more than their U.S. counterparts, although when the earnings variable is broken down by occupation we find that this holds true only for programmers.

The figures broken down by sex for the occupational characteristics data for California show some interesting variations. Whereas male systems analysts are somewhat better educated than their male coworkers in other computer occupations, the best-educated female computer specialists are programmers. Similarly, while male systems analysts are the most likely to work in high-tech employment, female programmers are more likely to be high-tech workers than are female systems analysts or operations researchers. Like men, however, women systems analysts are still the best paid of the female computer specialists. Finally, women earn less than men in all computer specialties. In each occupation, women earn approximately 72 percent of the male wage, a finding that replicates estimates made by Kraft and Dubnoff (1983) and Strober and Arnold (1987). In a subsequent section, we correct these estimates to take account of gender differences in background factors (see table 5).

Distribution of Variables by Sex

We turn in this and later sections to an analysis of the earnings attainment of computer specialists. We estimate a regression model of earn-

TABLE 2. Occupational Characteristics for Three Computer Occupations, for California and Total United States, Ages 25–64, 1980

Occupational Characteristics

| | Percent Female | | California | | Mean Earnings (in dollars) | |
	United States[a]	California	Mean Education (in years)	Percent in High Technology Industry[b]	United States[a]	California
Systems analysts	21.0	26.1	15.6	54.1	23,069	22,863
Operations researchers	26.7	28.9	15.0	39.9	22,282	21,122
Programmers	28.9	28.5	15.3	52.6	18,549	20,156
Total[c]	25.7	27.6	15.4	51.5	20,747	21,289

Occupational Characteristics by Sex, California

| | Mean Education (in years) | | Percent in High Technology Industry[b] | | Mean Earnings (in dollars) | |
	Men	Women	Men	Women	Men	Women
Systems analysts	15.8	14.9	57.5	44.5	24,586	17,823
Operations researchers	15.1	14.8	43.3	31.4	22,975	16,459
Programmers	15.5	15.1	55.1	46.5	21,840	15,811
Total[c]	15.5	15.0	54.5	43.8	23,029	16,604

Note: Percent female and the education and high technology means for California are based on 1,370 systems analysts (1,013 men and 357 women), 474 operations researchers (337 men and 137 women), and 1,856 computer programmers (1,327 men and 529 women). For earnings only, there are 104 missing values.

[a]Calculated for the 25–64-year-old population from U.S. Bureau of the Census 1984b, table 1. Note that these figures differ slightly from those presented in the beginning of the article because the latter refer to all age groups.

[b]See text for description of high technology industry.

[c]Weighted mean.

TABLE 3. Means and Standard Deviations for a Model of Earnings Attainment, Employed Male and Female Computer Specialists, Ages 25–64, California, 1980

Variable	Mean		Standard Deviation	
	Men	Women	Men	Women
Age (in years)	37.4	35.5	9.08	8.64
Education (in years)	15.5	15.0	2.33	2.28
Currently married	0.650	0.517	0.477	0.500
Formerly married	0.134	0.240	0.341	0.427
Never married	0.215	0.242	0.411	0.429
Systems analysts	0.381	0.351	0.486	0.478
Operations researchers	0.125	0.133	0.330	0.340
Computer programmers	0.495	0.515	0.500	0.500
Private wage and salary workers	0.811	0.806	0.391	0.396
Government workers	0.140	0.164	0.347	0.371
Self-employed workers	0.049	0.030	0.216	0.170
Hours worked per year	2,056	1,888	455	560
Industry				
Industry earnings (in dollars)	18,467	18,597	2,795	2,986
Industry percent female	38.1	41.4	14.3	16.3
High technology industry	0.548	0.445	0.498	0.497
Industry sector				
Oligopoly	0.142	0.095	0.350	0.294
Core	0.235	0.223	0.424	0.416
Periphery	0.347	0.307	0.476	0.461
Core utilities	0.111	0.175	0.314	0.380
Periphery utilities	0.005	0.004	0.073	0.064
Trades	0.078	0.095	0.269	0.294
Public administration/U.S.				
Postal Service	0.081	0.101	0.273	0.301
Local Labor Market				
Percent high-tech establishments				
in county group	2.16	2.10	1.19	1.18
Earnings (in dollars)	23,054	16,604	9,889	7,362
N	2,618	974		

ings separately by sex.[10] For the regression analyses, we incorporate occupation into the analysis as a dummy variable, with systems analyst as the omitted category. Table 3 presents the means and standard deviations for all the variables.

Table 1 indicated that women computer specialists are somewhat less educated, and work fewer hours, than their male counterparts; these findings are reaffirmed in table 3. In addition, men are also somewhat better represented in higher-paying systems analyst positions, while women are most likely to be programmers. Table 3 also shows,

contrary to our expectation, that men are in slightly lower-paying industries than women. As noted above, our estimate of industrial earnings is
a crude one, since it is based on the earnings of men in only fifty-two
industrial categories. There are probably gender differences in earnings
within these broader categories, as Strober and Arnold (1987) suggest.

As noted above, men and women also differ notably in their concentration in high technology industries: 55 percent of the men and 44
percent of the women work in high technology industries. Men and
women also differ somewhat in the *types* of industrial sectors in which
they work. Men are somewhat better represented in the oligopoly and
core sectors, where wages are high, while women are better represented
in the low-profit core utilities and trades sectors.

Earnings Attainment

Table 4 presents the regression results separately by sex. We view earnings as a function of age, education, marital status, occupation, class of
worker, hours worked per year, industry earnings, industry percent female, high technology industry, industry sector, and the percent high
technology establishments in the respondent's county group place of
residence. The R^2 values indicate that we have done better predicting
the earnings of female computer specialists than those of males (36
versus 28 percent).

An examination of the standardized regression coefficients reveals
that the number of hours worked is the most important factor affecting
the earnings attainments of both male and female computer specialists.
For both sexes, age and education are the next best predictors. For men
only, the percent high-tech establishments in their county group's place
of residence is a significant predictor of earnings, while for women,
industry percent female is a significant predictor.

Turning to the unstandardized coefficients, we note that men benefit more from their education and age than women, although only the
age coefficient is significantly different. Men earn $663 for each addi-
tional year of education, and $294 for each year of age, compared with
the $520 and $186 earned by women, respectively. While not significantly different by gender, the two coefficients for hours worked are in
the expected direction: men benefit more from the hours they work,
earning $7.77 for each additional hour worked, compared with $7.00 for
women.

While marital status has no significant effect on the average earnings of female computer specialists, never marrying significantly de-

TABLE 4. Regression Coefficients for a Model of Earnings Attainment, Employed Male and Female Computer Specialists, Ages 25-64, California, 1980

	Earnings (dependent variable)	
Variable	Men	Women
	Unstandardized Coefficients[a]	
Age[b]	294*	186*
Education	663*	520*
Formerly married	44.4	−528
Never married[b]	−2,325*	594
Operations researchers	−2,271*	−1,318*
Computer programmers	−1,257*	−759
Government workers	−1,386	−493
Self-employed workers	765	2,424*
Hours worked per year	7.77*	7.00*
Industry earnings	0.0397	−0.00923
Industry percent female	−21.8	−34.8*
High technology industry	599	−440
Core	−7.88	−1,594*
Periphery	−366	−422
Core Utilities	−300	322
Periphery Utilities	730	−1,378
Trades	−1,379	−1,996
Public Administration/U.S. Postal Service	182	211
Percent high-tech establishments in county group	437*	316
Intercept	−13,588	−8,712
R^2	0.280	0.365
	Standardized Coefficients[c]	
Age[b]	0.270*	0.218*
Education	0.157*	0.161*
Hours worked per year	0.357*	0.533*
Industry earnings	0.0112	−0.00374
Industry percent female	−0.0316	−0.0769*
High technology industry	0.0301	−0.0297
Percent high-tech establishments in county group	0.0525*	0.0507

[a]Omitted categories for dummy variables are: marital status (currently married), occupation (systems analyst), class of worker (private wage and salary), industry sector (oligopoly).

[b]Male and female slopes significantly different ($p < .05$)

[c]Since standardized coefficients for dummy variables with greater than two groups lack substantive interest, they are not included in the table.

*Coefficient significant ($p < .05$)

presses the earnings of men by $2,325, a finding consistent with other analyses of gender differences in earnings (e.g., Roos 1981). This provides additional evidence for the assertion that men benefit more from marriage than women, reflecting the likelihood that their wives assume the primary caretaker role for their households (Walker and Woods 1976; Pleck 1983). Men's greater earnings benefit from marriage may also be due to their greater tendency to maximize their earnings given the financial burden of maintaining a family (Oppenheimer 1974).

Both male and female operations researchers earn significantly less than their counterparts in systems analysis, even controlling for differences in educational preparation. While male programmers also earn significantly less than male systems analysts, no such difference exists for women.

The metric coefficients for class of worker show that being self-employed represents a substantial advantage for women but that no significant effect exists for men. Self-employed women earn on average $2,424 more than their counterparts in wage and salary work.

With respect to industry characteristics, we find that larger numbers of women in an industry decrease the earnings of both men and women, but only the latter significantly so. For each 10 percent increase in percent female, women's earnings decrease by approximately $350. Contrary to our expectation, neither industry earnings nor high-tech employment significantly affect the earnings of male or female computer specialists. One reason for this, as noted above, is our inability to code industrial earnings at the most detailed level, and thus we were unable to tap gender differences *within* the fifty-two broad industry categories. Economic segmentation, as measured by the seven-sector industrial classification, also has little explanatory potential. The only significant effect is for women: women computer specialists in the core sector earn $1,594 less than women in the oligopoly sector.

Finally, with respect to the local labor market variable we see that men gain signficantly from working in county groups with large numbers of high-tech establishments, whereas women are not able to realize this advantage.

Gender Gap in Earnings

In this final analytic section, we turn to an investigation of the extent to which the gender gap in earnings can be accounted for by differences in composition on the individual and structural variables we have identified. We employ a regression standardization procedure described by Duncan (1969, 100–102), substituting the generally lower female mean

TABLE 5. Decomposition of Earnings Gap, Employed
Computer Specialists, Ages 25-64, California, 1300

Variable	Percentage of Male-Female Earnings Gap Attributable to Variable[a]
Individual Factors	
Age	9.6
Education	5.6
Marital status	0.6
Occupation	0.8
Class of worker	1.4
Hours worked per year	20.3
Structural Factors	
Industry earnings	−0.2
Industry percent female	1.7
High technology industry	0.6
Industry sectors	−0.0
Percent high technology establishments in county group	−0.4
Total Percentage Explained by Gender Differences in Background Factors	40.0
Total Percentage Left Unexplained	60.0
Total	100.0
Total Earnings Gap[b]	$6,450

[a]The decomposition of the male-female earnings gap was accomplished by substituting the means for women on the background factors into successive male regression equations of earnings on a sequentially ordered set of independent variables. See text for details.

[b]The earnings gap is based on mean values of $23,054 for men and $16,604 for women (see table 3).

values on the independent variables into successive regression equations of earnings on a sequentially ordered set of independent variables.[11]

We know from table 3 that women computer specialists earn 72 percent as much as their male coworkers, which represents an earnings gap of $6,450. The question we pursue in this section is how much of this gap can be explained by compositional differences (i.e., gender differences in mean background and locational factors), and how much by differences in rates of return from these variables (i.e., gender differences in the unstandardized regression coefficients). The results presented in table 5 suggest that gender differences in composition on the individual variables are an important explanation for the earnings gap. Women in computer specialties would apparently enhance their earnings, relative to men, if they increased the hours they worked and completed more schooling. Approximately 20 percent of the earnings gap is attributable to gender differences in the number of hours men and women work each year, and another 6 percent to gender differences in achieved education. In addition, women are at a disadvantage with respect to earnings since they are slightly younger than their male coworkers, and greater seniority (for which age is a crude proxy) is associated with higher earnings.

Contrary to our expectation, sex differences in composition on the structural variables are evidently not an important explanation for women's lower earnings in computer work. Only gender differences in industry percent female and working in a high technology industry account for any of the gender gap, and these effects are quite small. Almost 2.0 percent of the earnings gap is attributable to women's concentration in different and apparently lower-paying industries than the ones in which men work. In addition, another 0.6 percent is due to gender differences in working in a high-tech industry.

The major conclusion that can be drawn from table 5 is that a large part of the earnings gap is attributable to women's receiving lower earnings returns from important background factors, such as age, education, and hours worked. Fully 60 percent of the earnings gap between male and female computer specialists remains unaccounted for by gender differences in the background and locational variables we were able to identify for our analysis.

An alternative way to think about these results is to ask what women's earnings would be if they had their own background and locational characteristics, but the same rate of return men enjoy. Looking at our results this way we find that adding all the individual and structural factors to the model increases women's relative earnings from 72 percent to approximately 89 percent of men's, a finding roughly comparable to Kraft and Dubnoff's (1983) figure of 85 percent. The residual 11 percent indicates that gender differences in rates of return remain an important explanation for the gender gap in earnings in computer specialties, as in other occupations.

Discussion

What do these data tell us about the relative economic position of women computer specialists? Our interest throughout has been in how female computer workers fare, relative to men, in their occupational and earnings opportunities. We know from Strober and Arnold (1987) and Dubnoff and Kraft (1984) that women do benefit monetarily from working in computer occupations, at least relative to other women, and our findings confirm this advantage. However, our research also suggests that for a variety of reasons, some attributable to their lower levels of human capital (over which they have some control) and some to lower labor market benefits they receive for their investments (over which they have little control), women computer workers do not fare as well as their male coworkers. These findings are noteworthy because computer occupations have experienced, and will continue to experience, rapid growth, and hence could provide substantial future job opportunities for women as well as men. In addition, such occupations do not have the legacy of sex segregation that exists in other more well-established occupations, and hence one might expect the problems of gender inequality that exist in other occupations to be mitigated in the computer field.

Our analysis confirms past work showing that women computer specialists do better economically than their female counterparts in other occupations. Relative to the well-known 62 percent earnings ratio for the average woman and man in the U.S. labor market (U.S. Bureau of the Census 1984d), women computer workers earn 72 percent as much as their male coworkers. Moreover, women in these occupations could theoretically improve their earnings potential if they worked more hours and completed additional schooling. In addition, part of the difference between men's and women's earnings in this field is attributable to women's lower average age, a factor that can only be remedied with time. If women achieved parity with men on these three factors, they could reduce the earnings gap by 36 percent.

While these results suggest that women's prognosis is good, there are important factors that limit our optimism regarding the opportunities existing for women in the computer field. Part of the earnings gap, albeit a small part, is due to men's and women's different industry distribution: women work in different industries that are apparently lower-paying than those men work in, and men are also somewhat more likely to work in high-tech industries. These results suggest that women's economic opportunities will continue to be limited because of their differing industrial distribution.

Additional evidence that limits our optimism derives from our investigation of the *process* of earnings attainment for the two sexes. The factors we identify as important for explaining earnings affect men and women differently. While age, education, and hours worked are important factors enhancing the earnings of both male and female computer specialists, males also benefit substantially from residing in areas with a large concentration of high-tech employment. Women have not realized this advantage. In addition, women lose earnings by working in industries with large numbers of women (while the coefficient is also negative for men, it is not significant). Thus, as noted above, movement into the industries in which men predominate is required before women's earnings can reach parity with men's.

While education and hours worked enhance the earnings of both women and men, these factors are more important for men. For each variable, men enjoy a greater benefit for their investments. They also receive greater earnings returns from age. These gender differences in rates of return are important, since they represent a significant portion of that part of the earnings gap not accounted for by gender differences in compositional factors. From table 5 we found that taking into account gender differences in all the background and locational variables reduced the earnings gap by 40 percent. According to these results, women with backgrounds equivalent to those of men would earn 89 percent as much as their male coworkers. What remains to be explained, however, is the 60 percent of the earnings gap that cannot be explained by the factors we have included in the model.

This 60 percent figure represents several components. First, an unspecified part of this remaining gap is probably due to *intraoccupational* gender differences in specific job tasks. Bielby and Baron (1986) found, for their sample of California firms, that even a three-digit occupational classification scheme, similar to the one we use here, fails to tap sex segregation existing at the level of the organization. By comparing segregation indices across major occupational groups, detailed occupations, and jobs, the authors found that occupational measures of sex segregation substantially understate the degree to which sex segregation exists in the workplace. Unfortunately, data limitations do not permit us to explore this issue here. However, there is evidence that within-occupation gender differences are important in understanding the opportunities and rewards of computer workers. Dubnoff and Kraft (1984) found that male and female computer workers report different job tasks, with women more likely to specialize in maintenance and documentation work and men in management. Assuming that intraoccupational job segregation exists in computer work, and that this job differentiation is associated with earnings, measuring sex segregation at the job level would allow us to reduce the earnings gap somewhat.

Second, the remaining portion of the earnings gap is attributable to differences in the labor market benefits women and men receive for their investments in education and hours worked, and for all the additional factors we identify. This part of the gap, often labeled discrimination, is more difficult to change. Changing it relies not on the characteristics of individual workers, but on altering the way labor market institutions reward workers. Such changes must be accomplished before the computer field offers women opportunities equal to men's.

NOTES

This article is a revised version of a paper presented at the annual meetings of the American Sociological Association, Aug., 1985. We thank Veronica Abjornson, Lee Clarke, Myra Marx Ferree, Polly Phipps, Barbara Reskin, Judith Tanur, Sen-Yuan Wu, and the editors for their helpful advice on an earlier version.

1. These three occupations represent the two professional and one technical computer occupations defined in the 1980 detailed census occupational classification (U.S. Bureau of the Census 1983b). We focus on these three in our discussion and analyses. See Strober and Arnold (1987) for a similar analysis of these and other computer occupations (e.g., computer operators and data entry keyers).

2. See Donato (1986) for more details on the history of programming occupations.

3. We use the Riche, Hecker, and Burgan (1983) group III definition of high technology industry ($N=28$): manufacturing industries with a proportion of technology-oriented workers equal to or greater than the average for all manufacturing industries, and a ratio of R&D expenditures to sales close to or above the average for all industries; the defintion also includes two nonmanufacturing industries that provide technical support to high-tech manufacturing industries (computer and data processing services and R&D laboratories).

4. "County group" as used by the census is not equivalent to county. For California there are fifty-two county group codes, which refer in some cases to several small (and generally contiguous) counties collapsed into one county group code and in other cases to subdivisions within counties. The Census Bureau's criterion for grouping counties is an area with a population of 100,000 or more (U.S. Bureau of the Census 1983b, app. K, 12). By way of example, Napa and Solano are two counties collapsed into one county group code; similarly, Del Norte, Mendocino, Trinity, and Lake counties form another county group. Los Angeles County, on the other hand, is subdivided into Los Angeles City, Long Beach City, and the balance of the county; similarly, Santa Clara County is divided into San Jose City and the balance of Santa Clara County. Because published census data (U.S. Bureau of the Census 1982) were available only for actual counties, and not county groups, we were unable to use the additional detail provided by the county subdivisions. This brought the number of unique county codes down to thirty-six. In addition, because some of the county group codes consisted of more than one county (up to seven counties in one case), we computed weighted means for each county group code containing more than one county.

5. For additional information on the coding of variables, see U.S. Bureau of the Census 1983b.

6. This variable was calculated from two census variables. First, the "grade"

variable (highest year of school attended) was recoded so that the metric equaled the grade specified (i.e., "11," referring to ninth grade, was recoded to "9"). Second, to adjust for nonfinishers, we subtracted 1 for all those who had not finished the grade they specified in the "grade" variable (using the information provided by the "fingrade" variable).

7. These variables (earnings and hours worked per year) depend on the accurate recall of census respondents. Since the accuracy of retrospective data is imperfect, readers should bear in mind these limitations when generalizing from our study.

8. The original "class of worker" variable included: last worked before 1975 or never worked, private wage and salary, federal government, state government, local government, self-employed worker with unincorporated business, employee of own corporation, and unpaid family worker. Because there were only three unpaid family workers, we eliminated these workers from the analyses.

9. In earlier drafts of this paper, we included a second local labor market variable, the county group's percent *residents* working in high technology employment. Because this variable was highly collinear ($r=.96$) with the county group's percent high-tech *establishments,* we chose only the latter to tap the availability of high technology employment in local labor markets.

10. To test whether separate models of earnings attainment for male and female computer specialists were justified, sex was treated as a dummy variable and all interactions between sex and the other independent variables were computed. Adding sex and then the interactions over our basic model significantly incremented R^2, thereby justifying separate equations for men and women.

11. Our choice to substitute the female means into the male regression equations is more conservative than the alternative, which substitutes the male means into the female regression equations. It asks, more realistically for our purposes, what women's earnings would be if they had their own background and locational characteristics, but the rate of return from these characteristics that men enjoy. Our choice reflects our assumption that regardless of their differing background characteristics, women should receive equal "returns" from the characteristics they do bring to the labor market. Thus, for example, in a gender-neutral labor market one would expect that women would receive an earnings return equivalent to that men receive for each year of education or each hour worked.

REFERENCES

Beck, E. M., Patrick M. Horan, and Charles M. Tolbert. 1978. Stratification in a dual economy: Sectoral model of earnings determination. *American Sociological Review* 43:704–20.

Beller, Andrea H. 1984. Trends in occupational segregation by sex, 1960–1981. In *Sex segregation in the workplace,* ed. Barbara F. Reskin, 11–26. Washington, D.C.: National Academy Press.

Bibb, Robert, and William H. Form. 1974. The effects of industrial, occupational, and sex stratification on wages in blue-collar markets. *Social Forces* 55:974–96.

Bielby, William T., and James N. Baron. 1984. A woman's place is with other women: Sex segregation within organizations. In *Sex segregation in the workplace,* ed. Barbara F. Reskin, 27–55. Washington, D.C.: National Academy Press.

———. 1986. Men and women at work: Sex segregation and statistical discrimination. *American Journal of Sociology* 91:751–99.

Blau, Francine D., and Wallace E. Hendricks. 1979. Occupational segregation by sex. *Journal of Human Resources* 14:197–210.

Donato, Katharine M. 1986. Social and economic factors governing the changing composition of computer specialties. Paper prepared for the annual meetings of the American Sociological Association, New York.

Dubnoff, Steven, and Philip Kraft. 1984. Gender stratification in computer programming. Paper presented at the Eastern Sociological Society meetings, Mar.

Duncan, Otis Dudley. 1969. Inheritance of poverty or inheritance of race. In *On understanding poverty,* ed. Daniel P. Moynihan, 85–110. New York: Basic Books.

Greenbaum, Joan. 1979. *In the name of efficiency: Management theory and shopfloor practice in data processing work.* Philadelphia: Temple University Press.

Hodson, Randy. 1983. *Workers' earnings and corporate economic structure.* New York: Academic Press.

Hodson, Randy, and Paula England. 1986. Industrial structure and sex differences in earnings. *Industrial Relations* 25:16–32.

Kalleberg, Arne L., and Aage B. Sorensen. 1979. The sociology of labor markets. *Annual Review of Sociology* 5:351–79.

Kraft, Philip. 1977. *Programmers and managers: The routinization of computer programming in the United States.* New York: Springer-Verlag.

———. 1979. The industrialization of computer programming: From programming to software production. In *Case studies on the labor process,* ed. Andrew Zimbalist, 1–17. New York: Monthly Review Press.

Kraft, Philip, and Steven Dubnoff. 1983. Software workers survey. *Computerworld,* Nov. 14.

Marion, Larry. 1984. The big wallet era. *Datamation* 30:77–78.

New York Times. 1984. Occupational outlooks: Where tomorrow's jobs will be. Oct. 14.

———. 1985. Pushing America out of chips. June 16.

O'Farrell, Brigid, and Sharon L. Harlan. 1984. Job integration strategies: Today's programs and tomorrow's needs. In *Sex segregation in the workplace,* ed. Barbara F. Reskin, 267–91. Washington, D.C.: National Academy Press.

Oppenheimer, Valerie K. 1974. The life-cycle squeeze: The interaction of men's occupational and family life cycles. *Demography* 11:227–45.

Parcel, Toby L., and Charles W. Mueller. 1983. *Ascription and labor markets: Race and sex differences in earnings.* New York: Academic Press.

Pleck, Joseph H. 1983. Husband's paid work and family roles: Current research issues. In *Research in the interweave of social roles,* ed. Helena Z. Lopata and Joseph H. Pleck, 251–333. Greenwich, Conn.: JAI Press.

Reskin, Barbara F., and Heidi I. Hartmann. 1985. *Women's work, men's work: Sex segregation on the job.* Washington, D.C.: National Academy Press.

Reskin, Barbara F., and Patricia A. Roos. 1985. Collaborative research on the determinants of changes in occupations' sex composition between 1970 and 1980. Grant proposal submitted to the National Science Foundation, Feb.

Riche, Richard W., Daniel E. Hecker, and John U. Burgan. 1983. High technology today and tomorrow: A small slice of the employment pie. *Monthly Labor Review* 106, no. 11 (Nov.): 50–58.

Roos, Patricia A. 1981. Sex stratification in the workplace: Male-female differences in economic returns to occupation. *Social Science Research* 10:195–224.

———. 1983. Marriage and women's occupational attainment in cross-cultural perspective. *American Sociological Review* 48:852–64.

Stolzenberg, Ross M. 1975. Occupations, labor markets and the process of wage attainment. *American Sociological Review* 40:645–65.

Strober, Myra H., and Carolyn L. Arnold. 1987. Integrated circuits/segregated labor: Women in computer-related occupations and high-tech industries. In *Computer chips and paper clips: Technology and women's employment,* ed. Heidi I. Hartmann, Robert E. Kraut, and Louise A. Tilly, 2:136–82. Washington, D.C.: National Academy Press.

Talbert, Joan, and Christine E. Bose. 1983. Wage-attainment processes: The retail clerk case. *American Journal of Sociology* 83:403–24.

Treiman, Donald J., and Kermit Terrell. 1975. Sex and the process of status attainment: Comparison of working women and men. *American Sociological Review* 40:174–200.

U.S. Bureau of the Census. 1982. *County business patterns 1980, California.* CBP-80-6. Washington, D.C.: GPO.

———. 1983a. *Census of population and housing, 1980: Public-use microdata sample A, California.* Washington, D.C.

———. 1983b. *Census of population and housing, 1980: Public-use microdata samples, technical documentation.* Washington, D.C.

———. 1984a. *Detailed occupation of the experienced civilian labor force by sex for the United States and regions: 1980 and 1970.* Supplementary Report PC80-S1-15. Washington, D.C.: GPO.

———. 1984b. *Earnings by occupation and education.* Washington, D.C.: GPO.

———. 1984c. *Occupation by industry*. Washington, D.C.: GPO.

———. 1984d. *Statistical abstract of the United States 1985*. Washington, D.C.. GPO.

U.S. Department of Labor. 1984. *Occupational outlook handbook*. Bulletin no. 2205, 1984–85 ed. Washington, D.C.: Bureau of Labor Statistics.

Walker, Kathryn E. and Margaret E. Woods. 1976. *Time use: A measure of household production of family goods and services*. Washington, D.C.: American Home Economics Association Center for the Family.

Technology and Emerging Patterns of Stratification for Women of Color: Race and Gender Segregation in Computer Occupations

Evelyn Nakano Glenn and Charles M. Tolbert II

The spread of computer technology is fundamentally transforming the nature of work and the shape of the labor market in the twentieth century. Work processes are changed, some jobs are eliminated, new ones are created, and different groups of workers are hired into jobs that are new or transformed. As the transformation accelerates, social scientists, journalists, policymakers, and union leaders have become concerned about understanding the changes that are taking place and predicting their future consequences for American workers. In this article, we focus on the particular implications of changing technology for women and their work. In considering this issue it is important to remember that women are not an undifferentiated mass: they belong to different racial and ethnic groups and occupy different positions in the class structure. Technological change can be expected to have different consequences for these different segments.

Race and Gender Differences in Relation to Technology

Historically women's relationship to technology has differed from that of men because their work has differed from that of men. Similarly, women of color—black, latina, and Asian-American—have had a distinctive relationship to technology because their role in processes of production and their position in the labor market have differed from those of white women and of both white and racial ethnic men. The work of racial ethnic[1] women has been shaped by a labor system stratified by both race and gender.

Blacks, latinos, and Asian-Americans were initially incorporated into the United States as a source of cheap and malleable labor.[2] Their labor was exploited to build the economic infrastructures of the less-developed south, southwest, and far west regions of the country.[3] Within these regional economies, dual labor systems operated to keep racial ethnic workers subordinated and to prevent competition with native white workers.[4] Blacks, Chicanos, Chinese, and other Asians were

318

confined to the lower tier of jobs in industries and firms that used low-level technology and therefore relied on labor-intensive methods. They were also paid on a separate, lower wage scale.[5] Men of color were concentrated in agriculture, mining, and service occupations, holding jobs that were considered too low paying, insecure, dangerous, or degraded for U.S.-born white men.

Similarly, women of color were confined to the lowest rungs of female-typed occupations. Outside of agriculture, women of color were limited to the least desirable women's jobs and were paid less than white women. They were overwhelmingly concentrated in private household work or other service employment, typically the most technologically backward sector. When employed in industries that also employed whites, women of color performed the tasks that were considered too dirty, arduous, or demeaning for women of the dominant culture. These were also the jobs that were the least connected to advanced technology. In southern tobacco factories, for example, black women were employed to perform the dirty work of stripping tobacco leaves to prepare them for processing, while the actual machine-processing jobs were reserved for white women.[6] In Texas, Chicanas were employed in the lower-level manual jobs in laundries, while the skilled positions as sorters, checkers, supervisors, and office assistants were reserved for Anglo women. Not so coincidentally, Chicanas earned less than half the average wages of white workers, i.e., $6.00 a week compared with $16.55 in 1919.[7]

This pattern of race and gender segregation in employment was clear through World War II. We review this history in order to underscore the way in which men and women of color were associated historically with labor-intensive, low-technology work. In particular, high technology and racial ethnic women were seen as mutually exclusive and contradictory categories.

Desegregation and Resegregation of Occupations

Since World War II, older, seemingly impervious color barriers have been breached, especially since the civil rights era of the 1960s. The occupational distribution of black, Chicana, and Asian-American women has become much more similar to that of white women. They have broken through in two areas that were previously barred to them, clerical and sales occupations, and they have dramatically increased their proportion in the professional technical fields.

The growing similarity in the distributions of majority and minority women among broad occupational categories, however, disguises the continuing differences among groups at the finer level of specific occupations.[8] Broad occupational categories, such as clerical work, are made up of jobs differing in skill, discretion, authority, and relation to technology. If we look at the distribution of racial ethnic women in specific clerical specialties, we see that they are concentrated in more routine, largely manual jobs. Moreover, the jobs that racial ethnic women have entered tend to be those which are being negatively affected by office technology—jobs that are being deskilled by automation (e.g., filing) or reduced in number by more advanced systems (e.g., keypunching.)[9]

Conversely, racial ethnic women are underrepresented in jobs that involve greater discretion, contact with the public, and interaction with management. For example, although blacks constitute 10.8 percent of all clerical workers, they make up over 15 percent of file clerks, mail handlers, keypunchers, and office machine operators but constitute less than 6 percent of secretaries, receptionists, bank tellers, and bookkeepers.[10]

What this means is that even though racial ethnic women have moved into white-collar work, they are nonetheless ghettoized within it. In effect there is now a racial stratification of jobs within the office. Thus the overall trend, at least in the clerical area, has been to desegregate at the broad occupational level and to resegregate at the narrower level of specific occupations.

This raises the question whether the desegregation-resegregation trend applies to the most technologically advanced areas of employment: Will the reorganization of the occupational structure resulting from the spread of computer technology facilitate the further breakdown of stratification of jobs by race, ethnicity, and gender? Or will the realignment of the occupational structure reproduce existing patterns of inequality in only slightly changed forms, perhaps leading to different, more subtle forms of inequality?

We will address this issue by examining patterns of occupational and earnings stratification in the central core of jobs created by the new technology: that is, the computer-related occupations, such as programmers and computer operators. These computer occupations vary widely in skill, prestige, and pay. The Census Bureau and the Department of Labor classify computer-related jobs into several major categories that can be ranked from high to low. At the top are the computer scientists, including systems analysts, and next are computer programmers; below them are, in descending order, computer service technicians, computer operators and peripheral equipment operators, and data entry keyers. If the trend toward resegregation applies to computer occupations, we would expect that racial ethnic women have not been excluded altogether from these "advanced technology" occupations, but that they are not equally integrated into all types and levels of computer-related jobs.

Data

The data for our analysis are drawn from one of the only data sets large enough to allow us to count and compute the percentage of race and gender segments in specific computer occupations—the Current Population Survey (CPS) conducted monthly by the U.S. Bureau of the Census. This article presents results from the descriptive stage of a longer-term project that will entail a more elaborate time series analysis of trends over the last fifteen years. Our analysis here is based on the March, 1983, survey, which contains information on 162,635 individuals. Computer workers were included in our subsample if they were employed full-time or part-time at the time of the CPS interview *and* if they had worked during 1982 as well. Applying these criteria, we extracted 1,072 computer workers for analysis purposes. CPS March supplement sampling weights were used, resulting in a weighted sample of 1.6 million persons or roughly 2 percent of the civilian labor force.

Stratification of Computer Occupations

Table 1 lists the five computer-related occupations on which we base our analysis. The occupation titles are associated with the Standard Occupational Classification (SOC) codes listed in the second column of the table.[11] The third column of table 1 lists the number of workers in each occupation weighted to approximate actual counts in the 1983 U.S. labor force. Computer operators is the largest occupation with nearly 600,000 workers. Computer scientist, computer programmer, and data entry keyer occupations each employ between 260,000 and 360,000 persons. Computer equipment repairers is by far the smallest of the computer-related occupations with a weighted total of less than 80,000.

The remaining columns in table 1 reveal substantial socioeconomic differentials between the occupations. The "adjusted annual earnings" variable reflects income from wages, salary, and self-employment in 1982. Following Beck, Horan, and Tolbert, the reported total earnings figures were adjusted to reflect weeks worked in 1982.[12] The earnings figures indicate substantial disparities among computer workers, as computer scientists, programmers, and equipment repairers average at least

TABLE 1. Descriptive Statistics for Computer-Related Occupations in the March, 1983, *Current Population Survey*

| Occupation | SOC Code | Weighted N | Adjusted Annual Earnings | | High School | Some College | College Graduate |
			Mean	SD			
Computer scientist	64	264,918	$28,383	$10,930	13.3%	25.0%	61.7%
Computer programmer	229	357,111	21,946	10,495	13.3	30.6	56.1
Computer equipment repairer	525	77,261	23,575	10,808	50.5	40.7	8.7
Computer equipment operator	304, 308, 309	598,560	14,245	7,606	52.1	32.0	15.9
Data entry keyer	385	303,505	11,700	5,919	75.4	20.5	4.1

$7,700 more than computer operators and data entry keyers. The last three columns of table 1 describe educational levels associated with computer-related occupations. The "high school" category indicates the percentage of persons who completed twelve or fewer years of schooling. The percentages of persons completing thirteen to fifteen years of schooling are represented in the "some college" category, and percentages for sixteen or more years are listed in the "college graduate" column. One-fourth to one-half of computer equipment repairers, operators, and data entry keyers have no more than a high school education. On the other educational extreme, a large proportion of computer scientists and programmers are college graduates.

These data on education and earnings suggest sharp socioeconomic differences among workers in the five computer-related occupations. Indeed, the apparent hierarchy of occupations resembles stratification elsewhere in the occupational structure. Does the stratification evident in these data also lead to the reproduction of institutionalized inequality for racial ethnic women? Are racial ethnic women segregated into the lower tier of computer occupations? Within those occupations, are racial ethnic women the victims of substantial earnings discrimination? These issues are the subject of the further analysis that follows.

Occupational Segregation

We focus here on four gender and racial ethnic groups: white males, white females, racial ethnic males, and racial ethnic females. Those respondents indicating Hispanic ethnicity and those reporting race as "black" or "other" are classified in our scheme as racial ethnic. The distribution of the four groups across computer-related occupations is given in table 2. In the table, the distributions of the four race/gender/ethnicity segments are strikingly different: 60 percent of white males in computer occupations are located in the top two occupations (computer scientist and programmer). In sharp contrast, only 23 percent of the women of color are employed in these top occupations; instead, they are overwhelmingly concentrated (77 percent) in the lower-level computer operator and data entry occupations. White women do not fare much better than their racial ethnic counterparts, but white men have a considerable advantage over racial ethnic men, among whom only 42 percent are in the computer scientist and computer programmer occupations. Hence, the data in table 2 suggest a definite pattern of occupational segregation in which racial ethnic women are allocated to low-paying and low-skill computer jobs.

The chi-square value indicates that these results clearly depart from

TABLE 2. Percentage Distribution of Workers in Computer-Related Occupations by Race, Gender, and Ethnicity

	Weighted N	Computer Scientist	Computer Programmer	Computer Repairer	Computer Operator	Data Entry Keyer
White males	638,868	27.8	32.1	10.3	27.3	2.5
White females	666,003	8.1	14.9	0.6	44.0	32.4
Racial ethnic males	94,410	21.1	21.4	7.3	46.1	4.1
Racial ethnic females	202,433	6.7	16.0	0.5	43.3	33.5

Notes: Chi-square = 279.72, df = 12, $p < .001$, PRU = .103.

the distribution across occupations that would be expected by chance alone.[13] The information-theoretic proportional reduction in uncertainty (PRU) measure means that knowledge of an individual's race/ gender/ethnicity improves our ability to predict his/her occupation by 10.3 percent.[14] By comparison, the PRU measure for a cross-classification of educational attainment and occupation results in a 12.1 percent reduction in uncertainty about occupational allocation. Since our race/gender/ethnicity categories may be strongly associated with education, we also computed a PRU measure for the joint effects of the two variables on occupational allocation.[15] The resulting PRU measure (.208) indicates that even when educational attainment is taken into account there remains a substantial influence of race/gender/ethnicity on placement in the hierarchy of computer-related occupations.

We can conclude from this portion of the analysis that racial ethnic women are segregated into low-paying, low-skill computer occupations. The next issue is how they fare economically once employed in computer-related occupations. We turn now to an analysis of earnings inequality among computer workers and the extent to which that inequality is attributable to race, gender, or ethnicity.

Earnings Inequality

If earnings inequality based on race, gender, or ethnicity exists among computer workers, it should be evident in a comparison of earnings of various groups to earnings of white males. Table 3 contains information on white males' earnings (adjusted for weeks worked per year) in each of the five computer-related occupations. The table also reports ratios of other race/gender/ethnic groups' adjusted earnings to those of white males. The ratios clearly indicate a substantial differential between male and female earnings within each occupation. Moreover, in two of the three high-paying occupations (computer scientists and repairers), white females earn substantially more than racial ethnic women. Interestingly, racial ethnic males earn the same or more than white males in three occupations. Further analysis of these data will be carried out to determine the factors accounting for this finding. In any case, the information in table 3 suggests important earnings disparities for racial ethnic women that do not occur with racial ethnic men.

Of course, it could be argued that the earnings inequality stems from variations in levels of human capital to which different race, gender, and ethnic groups have unequal access. In our final analysis, we sought to determine the influence of various factors (including race/

TABLE 3. Earnings Ratios by Computer-Related Occupation

Occupation	Mean Earnings of White Males	White Females	Racial Ethnic Males	Racial Ethnic Females
Computer scientist	$29,725.00	.82	1.12	.67
Computer programmer	24,545.00	.70	1.02	.75
Computer repairer	24,311.00	.76	0.87	.51
Computer operator	18,487.00	.65	0.76	.73
Data entry keyer	16,556.00	.66	1.00	.76

gender/ethnicity) on the earnings inequality evident among computer workers. To do this, we turned to work by the economist Henri Theil in which he introduces an information-theoretic measure of inequality in an earnings distribution.[16] Allison[17] gives the formula for the inequality measure T as follows:

$$T = \frac{\frac{1}{n} \sum_{i=1}^{n} X_i \log X_i - \mu \log \mu}{\mu}$$

where X_i = earnings of the ith person and μ = the mean of the distribution.

An important feature of the Theil measure is that it can be decomposed into within-group and between-group components. Allison provides a formula for the decomposition of T:

$$T = \sum_{j=1}^{j} \left(\frac{p_j \overline{X_j}}{\overline{X}}\right) \left(\frac{\overline{X_j}}{\overline{X}}\right) + \sum_{j=1}^{j} \left(\frac{p_j \overline{X_j}}{\overline{X}}\right) T_j$$

where p_j = the proportion of the population in group j, $\overline{X}$ = the grand mean, $\overline{X_j}$ = mean for group j, and T_j = inequality for group j.[18] The decomposibility of T means that we can determine the relative effects on inequality of key factors such as race, gender, and ethnicity.

Results of our application of the Theil measure appear in table 4. Even though Theil notes that T varies from zero to log N, the computed value (.171) is not particularly informative without a benchmark for comparison. But the value of T does gives us a basis for determining how much inequality is due to various factors listed in the first column of the table. The first decomposition reported is for our four-category race/gender/ethnicity variable. The between-group inequality calculated at

TABLE 4. Decomposition of Earnings Inequality

Component	Between Group	Percentage	Within Group	Percentage
Race/ethnic/gender group	.038	22.1	.133	77.9
Occupation	.049	28.8	.121	71.2
Education	.024	14.1	.147	85.9
Occupation–race/ethnic/gender group	.061	35.9	.109	64.1
Education–race/ethnic/gender group	.050	29.1	.121	70.9
Education-occupation	.055	32.1	.116	67.9
Race/ethnic/gender group–occupation–education	.067	39.3	.104	60.7

Note: Total inequality T = .171.

.038. Likewise, the within-group inequality was computed to be .133, and the two figures sum to the computed overall value of T. Since the between-group inequality (.038) is 22.1 percent of .171, we can conclude that gender/race/ethnicity accounts for about 22 percent of the inequality in earnings among computer workers.

The next two decompositions indicate that occupation (measured by the five computer-related occupations) accounts for 28.8 percent of the inequality. The three categories of education introduced in table 1 account for 14.1 percent of the earnings inequality. The next set of decomposition results are for the joint effects of the three variables. The largest percentage of inequality is accounted for by the combination of occupation and race/gender/ethnicity. The final decomposition suggests that the variables taken together account for 39.3 percent of the inequality in earnings of workers in computer-related occupations. Most notably, the role of the race/gender/ethnicity variable in determining earnings inequality remains apparent even after occupation and education are taken into account.

We conclude our analysis of earnings inequality with three observations: (1) women of color experience earnings inequality in computer-related occupations, (2) some degree of earnings disparity persists even when educational or occupational levels are taken into account, and (3) the greater part of the unequal earnings stems from occupational level and is therefore attributable to labor market segregation. The implications of these patterns of stratification and the issues that they raise are our next concern.

Discussion

At first blush, the spread of computer technology might appear to provide great new labor market opportunities for women of color by creating new jobs. In several specific instances in the past, the expansion of a new field, one that did not exist before or was very small, opened opportunities to groups that had previously been excluded. When industries or occupations expand rapidly enough, the demand for labor outstrips the primary source of labor, usually white men, and employers are forced to turn to other pools of workers. This is essentially what happened with the growth of clerical occupations in the late nineteenth and early twentieth centuries: it led to the widespread recruitment of women, which culminated in the feminization of clerical work.[19] Sometimes the rise of a new field that is not gender-typed will lead to its being designated for usually less favored groups. The pioneers in computer technology apparently assumed that programming would involve primarily clerical tasks, and they recruited women for these positions.[20] Thus, at least at the beginning, women were able to get a foot in the door, even though subsequently it was decided the job was more complex than originally thought.

Computer occupations seem to fit both models, that is, they did not exist before and were not therefore monopolized by a particular race/gender segment, and they are undergoing rapid expansion. According to the U.S. Department of Labor, computer occupations are expected to be the most rapidly growing in the economy over the next decade. The department projects that employment will rise from 1.455 million in 1980 to 2.140 million by 1990, including a 65 percent increase in systems analysts, 47 percent in programmers, 63 percent in computer and peripheral equipment operators, and 93 percent in computer service technicians; the only computer occupation expected to decline is keypunching (by 14 percent).[21] Of course, it is important to keep this growth in perspective by noting that although the rate of growth will be high, the absolute number of new jobs is relatively small. Slower growing but currently large occupations are expected to provide the lion's share of new jobs; these occupations are for the most part low-status, low-wage service jobs, such as building custodians, waiters and waitresses, and clerical positions. For every computer service technician job there will be fourteen jobs for custodians; for every programmer, three clerical jobs. Thus the computer field will not provide a great deal of employment for racial ethnic women, who will continue to find most of their employment in the labor-intensive service occupations or in deskilled clerical work.

As our analysis shows, even if racial ethnic women get into computer occupations, they are more likely to enter the lowest ranks of the computer hierarchy and to experience wage discrimination. Their earnings disadvantage is at least partly attributable to race and gender discrimination within occupations. Yet a larger portion of racial ethnic women's earnings disadvantage in the computer field is due to their concentration in lower-level occupations. Hence, moving them into the higher ranks of computer scientists, analysts, and programmers would go a long way toward improving their economic situation.

How likely is it for this to occur? At least part of the answer lies in the kind of access racial ethnic women will have to training and experience in computer science. As with other resources, access to computers and computer education is not equitably distributed. More affluent school districts, i.e., those with fewer than 5 percent of their students living under the poverty line and presumably predominantly white, had computers earlier and in greater numbers than less affluent school districts.[22] A survey conducted by Johns Hopkins University in 1983 found that while two-thirds of the schools in the most affluent school districts had microcomputers, only 41 percent of those in less wealthy districts had them.[23] At least initially, then, it appears that inequities in the education system have widened the gap between whites and racial ethnics.

In the meantime, however, microcomputers in school have become nearly universal. Market Data Retrieval of Connecticut reported that 86 percent of all school districts in the United States began the 1983 school year with microcomputers.[24] It was reported that in the fall of 1984 many inner city schools districts, such as Philadelphia's, were putting a large part of their scarce resources into microcomputers and forgoing purchases of books and supplies. The Philadelphia school authorities are banking on computers as a way of motivating students. Yet many educational experts contend that not enough quality software is available to make effective use of computer hardware.[25] Furthermore, it has been observed that computers in economically disadvantaged schools tend to be used as high-tech flash cards to run students through rote drills rather than to expose them to programming, simulation, and other high-level skills that would outfit them for the job market.[26] In such cases computers are being used as a substitute for effective teaching.

It would be a double tragedy if computers were seen as a panacea for educational problems in the ghetto, deflecting demands for more basic reforms and raising false hopes that they will provide pathways for large numbers of racial ethnic men and women to enter high technology occupations. Given past patterns and current trends, it seems more likely that even if minorities manage to get into computer-related employment, their jobs will be at the bottom of the hierarchy and most subject to rationalization.

NOTES

We thank Ada Haynes for her assistance in library research and Barbara Wright and the editorial board for their comments and suggestions.

1. The term "racial ethnic" is used to refer to groups that are simultaneously racial and ethnic minorities; specifically, we use this term to refer collectively to blacks, Hispanics, and Asian Americans. We avoid using the more common terms "nonwhite" and "women of color" because of their implication that white is the norm and because "racial ethnic" carries positive connotations of collective cultural identity.

2. Native Americans can be considered a colonized minority, but they are not included in this analysis because they were not incorporated into the labor force to the degree that the other groups were.

3. Robert Blauner, *Racial Oppression in America* (New York; Harper and Row, 1972) notes that recruitment into less developed regions was one characteristic that distinguished the labor market experience of racial ethnic workers from that of European immigrants.

4. For a discussion of the concept of dual or colonial labor systems, see Mario Barrera, *Race and Class in the Southwest* (Notre Dame, Ind.: University of Notre Dame Press, 1979).

5. See Barrera, *Race and Class in the Southwest,* and also Lucie Cheng and Edna Bonacich, *Labor Immigration under Capitalism: Asian Immigrant Workers in the United States before World War II* (Berkeley: University of California Press, 1984), for discussion of black and Asian labor in the nineteenth century.

6. Gerda Lerner's *Black Women in White America* (New York: Pantheon, 1972) contains contemporary descriptions of the conditions black women faced in industry.

7. Mario T. Garcia, "The Chicana in American History: The Mexican Women of El Paso, 1880–1920—A Case Study," *Pacific Historical Review* 44 (May, 1980): 315–38.

8. Segregation also takes the form of allocation to different industries. Racial ethnic women in the professions and in clerical occupations are overrepresented in government and underrepresented in private industry. See, for example, Patrica A. Roos and Joyce F. Hennessy, "Assimilation or Exclusion? Attainment Processes of Japanese, Mexican Americans and Anglos in California" (Paper presented at the meetings of the American Sociological Association, San Antonio, Texas, Aug., 1984).

9. Roslyn L. Feldberg and Evelyn Nakano Glenn, "Technology and Work Degradation: The Effects of Office Automation on Women Clerical Work-

ers," in *Machina Ex Dea,* ed. Joan Rothschild (New York: Pergamon Press, 1983), 59–78.

10. Diane Nilsen Westcott, "Blacks in the 1970's: Did They Scale the Job Ladder?" *Monthly Labor Review* 105, no. 6 (June, 1982): 29–38.

11. There are three occupation titles for computer operators: supervisors, computer equipment operators (304); computer operators (308); and peripheral equipment operators (309). The first and last of these contained so few persons that we collapsed the categories into a single computer operator occupation. For further information, see the *Standard Occupational Classification Manual, 1980* (Washington, D.C.: U.S. Department of Commerce, 1980).

12. The adjustment procedure used by Beck, Horan, and Tolbert simply expresses annual earnings as a function of the proportion of weeks worked during the year. It is a conservative treatment of the labor supply issue in that it does not take into account discouraged workers or other forms of hidden unemployment. (E. M. Beck, Patrick M. Horan, and Charles M. Tolbert II, "Industrial Segmentation and Labor Market Discrimination," *Social Problems* 28, no. 2 [Dec., 1980]: 113–30.)

13. The chi-square value was calculated with a normalized version of the sampling weight so as not to inflate the N in the statistical test.

14. See Patrick M. Horan, "Information Theoretic Measures and the Analysis of Social Structures," *Sociological Methods and Research* 3 (1975): 321–40.

15. For brevity these latter contingency tables are only summarized here. The education variable employed in the unreported tables is the same as in table 1. The detailed results are available from the authors.

16. Henri Theil, *Economics and Information Theory* (Chicago: Rand McNally, 1967).

17. Paul D. Allison, "Measures of Inequality," *American Sociological Review* 43 (Dec., 1978): 865–80.

18. Ibid.

19. Evelyn Nakano Glenn and Roslyn L. Feldberg, "Degraded and Deskilled: The Proletarianization of Clerical Work," *Social Problems* 25, no. 1 (Oct., 1977): 52–64.

20. Phil Kraft, *Programmers and Managers: The Routinization of Computer Programming in the United States* (New York: Springer-Verlag, 1977).

21. U.S. Department of Labor, *Employment Trends in Computer Occupations* (Washington, D.C.: GPO, 1981).

22. *Education Week,* Apr. 18, 1983.

23. *School Use of Microcomputers,* 1 (Apr., 1983). Publication of the Center for Social Organization of Schools, Johns Hopkins University.

24. *Education Week,* Apr. 18, 1983.

25. Paul Bonner, "Computers in Education: Promise and Reality," *Personal Computing,* Sept., 1984, 64–77.

26. Ibid.

A Comparative Survey of Responses to Office Technology in the United States and Western Europe

Maria-Luz Daza Samper

In today's office there is a convergence of what has been called a techno-logical trinity: electronics, computing, and telecommunications technolo-gies. They have all been developed to handle information, and thus the term "information technology" has been used interchangeably with the term "office technology" to describe them. In the last few years, informa-tion technology has been increasingly applied to everyday office activi-ties in pursuit of the "automated" or "paperless" office. It has been projected that this transformation will eventually affect about two-thirds of the U.S. white-collar work force.

This trend is now being studied intensively, both in this country and abroad. The purpose of this article is to review the effects of information technology and responses to it, both in Western Europe and in the United States, in the hope that this knowledge will provide guidelines for a humanization of technological applications. By looking beyond the U.S. context, much can be learned about the stages that are likely to occur in the introduction of new technologies, about the ways in which workers can participate in the implementation of new technology, and the means other countries have employed to deal with negative effects of new technology.

This article first describes office technology and examines its effect on workers' well-being and security; second, it reviews reactions to the implementation of new technology in a variety of Western European nations; and finally, it suggests policy implications for the United States. While it would be interesting to consider the social and political contexts that have led to very different responses in the United States and West-ern Europe, such an analysis lies beyond the scope of this article.

The Automation of Office Work

Computerization has already affected repetitive office tasks such as bill-ing, accounting, and routine clerical and data processing work. The typewriter has been replaced by a variety of word processors ranging from the memory typewriter that can be used on its own to shared-logic word processing systems in which several peripherals make use of the same computer. Rada (1980) argues that information technology has come to the office relatively quickly for the following reasons: (1) rising labor costs, (2) low growth in the productivity of traditional office workers as compared to industrial workers, and (3) low cost (an office worker currently requires about $2,000 worth of equipment, while a factory worker needs $30,000 to $40,000 worth).

Obviously, the introduction of information technology affects both office workers and the organization of the office in which they are employed. Ultimately, new office technology may affect nearly all elements of the white-collar work force. However, just as clearly, new technology does not affect all white-collar workers in the same way, and different technologies have different effects.

At the outset, it is essential for us to differentiate office workers by gender. First, in the United States, a significantly greater proportion of women than men work in office jobs of all kinds: in 1981, it was 66 percent of women versus 43 percent of men (U.S. Department of Labor 1983). Within the office setting, women are strongly concentrated in clerical occupations; they comprise, for example, 88.2 percent of billing clerks, 91.1 percent of bookkeepers, 93.5 percent of bank tellers, 93.5 percent of keypunch operators, 96.3 percent of typists, and fully 99.1 percent of secretaries. The above-named occupations alone accounted in 1981 for approximately 7.56 million office positions filled by women. In professional and technical areas, by way of contrast, women are less well represented both in percentages and in raw numbers. For example, women comprise 18.8 percent of engineering and science technicians, 27.1 percent of computer specialists, and 38.5 percent of accountants, and these occupations accounted for approximately 820,000 of the positions held by women in the U.S. labor force in 1981. In the same year, women represented 23.9 percent of insurance agents, brokers, and underwriters. The proportion of female managers and administrators has posted a sizeable gain in recent years, reaching 27.5 percent, but women remain concentrated in the lower echelons.

Elsewhere in this volume, Eileen Appelbaum examines the insurance industry in some detail. Her table 2 projects the composition of the insurance industry in 1990. According to a U.S. Department of Labor estimate, in 1990 managers and officers will account for 14.8 percent of those employed in the industry, professional and technical workers will account for 5.5 percent, and sales personnel will account for 33.8 percent, while clerical workers will account for 44.3 percent. Whereas females may represent one-quarter to one-third of the first three groups, the clerical group is likely to remain overwhelmingly female. In this way, insurance, like other "office industries," will continue its traditional dependence upon a cadre of support personnel that is overwhelmingly female; this group, in turn, is likely to continue to be supervised by and serve groups of workers who are predominantly male.

Both here and abroad, many service industries that employ large numbers of white-collar workers have adopted information technology. This is the case, for example, in communications, banking, and retailing, as well as in insurance. The governments of industrialized nations are also using word processing and automating many services. Although levels of female participation in the paid labor force vary from country to country in Western Europe, astonishingly similar patterns of occupational sex segregation prevail—along with the lower earnings relative to educational achievement that we are familiar with for women workers in the United States (Roos 1985). Thus when the effects of office automation, including fragmentation and job displacement, are described below, we must bear in mind that it is overwhelmingly women workers who are being affected, here and abroad, both by reason of their sex and by reason of the position they occupy in the labor process. Clerical workers, women workers, are the backbone of the so-called information society.

Whether an individual occupies a professional/managerial or clerical position can be of crucial importance when new technology is introduced into the office. Gutek (1983) has identified six factors that determine whether a person's work will be enriched or impoverished as a result of using computers in the office. They are:

1. The purpose of the terminal. Data entry and telephone operators are hired to work at terminals; professionals and managers, in contrast, use the terminal at their own discretion to access information or to communicate with others in the organization.
2. The kind of terminal the person uses and the kinds of tasks performed. Clerical workers, for example, are more likely to use simple systems and the transferability of their training is limited.
3. The "user-friendliness" of the system. This term usually refers to the ease with which an untrained user can learn to interact with the system. "User-friendly" may refer to software (computer programs that are easy to use), or the hardware (e.g., a nonglare screen or well-designed keyboard). A person hired to work at a terminal may well have a less friendly system than one who has the freedom to choose equipment or software.
4. Control of the equipment. Does the terminal control the worker or does the worker control the terminal? Control of the terminal by the

worker implies knowledge of the capabilities of the equipment. For some workers, computers facilitate access to data or enhance communications; for others, time at the terminal means pushing certain buttons to perform a specific operation without comprehension of the total process.

5. Monitoring of the workers. Is the computer used to monitor a worker's behavior? Some systems have built-in monitoring, so that the number of strokes or the number of calls is automatically recorded.
6. The kind of training the employee receives. Is the training geared to a fragmented part of the work process or to the whole process, thus providing transferability of skills?

Clearly, office work can be enhanced or degraded by computer technology. Neither outcome is inherent in the technology; rather, outcome is related to the organizational structure of the office and to the way the technology is incorporated into the system.

Effects of Information Technology on Workers' Well-being

One of the frequent, though not inevitable, outcomes of office automation is the fragmentation of jobs into discrete operations.[1] In the United States, office occupations are currently fragmented to the point that in 1985 the U.S. Bureau of Labor Statistics recognized thirty-six levels of selected office occupations with a range from key entry operators (Level I) to secretaries (Level V). There are three levels of key entry operators and three levels of word processors alone—and this was the first year that word processors had even been included at all.

The introduction of electronic data processing in European insurance companies proceeded well ahead of that in the United States. It led to a reorganization of basic internal administrative arrangements as well as to new methods of conducting business and processing insurance work (FIET 1980b). Among the functions affected by technology are drafting and storage of insurance policies and claims settlements; insurance brokering; actuarial research; underwriting; marketing and promotion; and premium billing and collection. With the equipment that is currently available in both the United States and Europe, an insurance worker whose job is coding does not need to make decisions or interpretations as often as before.

This fragmentation and routinization of work has also appeared in European banks since the early 1970s. The fundamental activities of banking include collection, verification, processing, and storage of information about monetary transactions. In the early 1970s the banking industry was labor intensive, generating vast amounts of information leading to the creation of "paper mountains." Since then, electronic data processing has allowed banks to reduce both the paper in circulation and their staffing requirements while increasing their capacity to handle data and offer new services. Competition among banks is based on things like twenty-four-hour automated banking service, immediate statements of account, improvements in account management, and international information networks. Accompanying changes in the organization of work and the structure of the banking work force have been described as a return to "strictly scientific management techniques," i.e., Taylorism or the breaking down of work processes into isolated, maximally time- and cost-efficient tasks (FIET 1980a).

Reacting to this trend, the International Federation of Commercial, Clerical, Professional and Technical Employees (FIET) conducted a survey on the effects of new technology in the banking industry. Responses were received from unions in Australia, Belgium, Denmark, West Germany, Austria, Great Britain, Italy, Sweden, Norway, France, and New Zealand. They all agreed that new office technology had led to a reduction in the skills required of retail bank staff, as well as to a strict division of tasks that produced monotony and boredom in all departments linked with the new technology. Employees enjoyed little knowledge of the overall production process. Moreover, many jobs had been redesigned (e.g., cashier, typist, standing order desk, foreign desk) and measurement of individual productivity had become more efficient. Small groups of experts had been developed in electronic data processing centers; at the same time less-qualified workers were now performing tasks that previously required specialized knowledge (FIET 1980a, 23).

Office technology has also had a noticeable effect on career ladders in clerical jobs. In the past, insurance companies were able to promote workers from within their own ranks. Appelbaum however, has described a new kind of highly skilled clerical worker, the "superclerical," who performs a variety of tasks formerly done by several workers (see Appelbaum in this volume). Since the superclerical is hired from outside, access to this type of job for workers within the firm is limited. The same situation has been observed in both insurance companies and banks in Western Europe, where these newly hired employees are called a "technological elite" (Dasey 1983). Both in Europe and in the United States, there seems to be a trend toward polarization of the work force between "experts" on one hand and a proletariat of data entry clerks on the other (Chamot 1985).

In the United States, Gutek and Bikson (1984) sought to determine whether technological innovation had a differential effect on male and female employees. They analyzed fifty-five offices in the private sector, using data from a multiple-instrument, multisite, two-wave study of the implementation of computerized procedures. They found that for men and women in computerized offices, differences in status and in the opportunity structure may be more important than the technology in accounting for different experiences. The organizations Gutek and Bikson studied have not used technology to break down traditional sex segregation. As a result, information technology has not served as a catalyst for progressive change, it has not improved the opportunity structure for women, and it has not ushered in new roles for women workers.

In summary, there is no magic ensuring that technology in and of itself will automatically enhance workers' well-being by providing them with jobs that require more skill, more integration of tasks, and more enjoyable work circumstances. While people in middle or upper management positions may well benefit from the availability of computers or other forms of office automation, this is by no means a foregone conclusion for the majority of clerical workers (Greenbaum 1983).

Effects of Information Technology on Workers' Job Security

In addition to looking at workers' well-being, it is important to consider the effect of information technology on the size of the office work force. Labor displacement appears to be one of the major problems caused by the introduction of this technology. The phenomenon may be observed in different countries and in a variety of industries. My examples are drawn mainly from the banking and insurance sectors in the United States and Western Europe.

In this connection, Greenbaum (1983) has identified two myths about technology and the job market. The first is that technology in the office of the future will create more jobs. In response to this myth, it is imperative to discuss trends in employment that have been observed both in Europe and in North America. When automation first comes to an industry, more workers are needed to input data; then the number becomes stabilized. Once automation is fully in place, however, a decline in employment may be observed.

The United Kingdom provides a concrete example. After rapid growth during the 1960s and early 1970s, employment in U.K. banks trailed off to a 2 to 3 percent increase in 1980–81. In the major British clearing banks, employment levels are now declining after rising for many years and then stabilizing. In 1981–82 the Midland Bank, one of the big four in Britain, made two thousand staff "redundant" (Dasey 1983, 51). Rapid automation of functions such as the sale, storage, publication, amendment, and research of insurance policies has affected staff in other countries, too. In Sweden, for example, it was noted that if technology had not been introduced, employment would have had to rise by thirty-five hundred during the late 1970s to cope with the increased workload.

Another trend that has contributed to job displacement and that has been aided by technology is the centralization of functions. A brokerage firm in Britain illustrates current operating methods.

> This company is transacting insurance business with brokers through a nationwide on-line network of display terminals which also provide for the composition or printing of policy documents and the automatic handling of premium payments. . . . The company's business is transacted with insurance brokers through its 24 branch offices staffed by inspectors and clerical staff, while administration is carried out from its headquarters. . . . It is expected that staff savings of up to 40% will result from these new procedures and that this will pay for the cost of installing the system. (FIET 1980b, 6)

Still another trend related to job displacement is the increase of part-time workers. In Great Britain, West Germany, the Netherlands, Norway, and Sweden, unions noted an increase in the use of part-time employees during the late 1970s.

With regard to the impact of technology on the number of office jobs overall, the Commission of the European Communities in 1980 estimated that by 1990, approximately 20 to 25 percent of the then current 15 million office jobs in the European community—i.e., 3 to 3.75 million jobs—were expected to be affected by the elimination of certain functions that fall in the unskilled category (Cammell 1983). Technology in the office of the future, far from creating more jobs, appears to be reducing the number of traditional office jobs.

According to a second popular myth, the number of high technology jobs is growing. The accuracy of this view is open to question on two grounds. First, high-tech jobs may not increase at a sufficient rate to offset the significant displacement created by technology; and second, the jobs now available in high-tech industries may not be available for those same workers displaced by information technology. Benston (1984) comments that the job of running automated equipment is increasingly subject to higher levels of automation. In the actual tending of the computers, as well as in the manufacture, repair, and maintenance of automated equipment, more and more functions are being handled by operating systems and automatic controls. Thus new jobs may disappear soon after they become available. Most of the new high-tech jobs in fact turn out to be assembly jobs, mostly part-time with low wages, and filled almost completely by female workers.

However, all of this is not to say that information technology produces no new jobs. It does create new jobs. Typically, two groups of workers enter the office work force upon the introduction of information technology. The first is a group of qualified technical specialists who design or adapt the computer programs necessary to automate the office (Feldberg and Glenn 1983a). The second group is composed of workers who are capable of performing a variety of skilled tasks, such as the production of letters, taking charge of customer services, bookkeeping, and related activities. These are the superclericals (Appelbaum in this volume; Kassalow 1985) or technological elite (Dasey 1983) referred to earlier. The appearance of these jobs, however, will not alleviate the problems of present clerical workers. The superclericals are hired from outside the companies, are generally college educated, and possess the necessary skills for the work. Displaced clerical workers are unlikely to be hired or promoted into these positions.

In summary, the introduction of information technology is having similar effects on the office work forces of a variety of Western countries. These effects differ according to where the individual worker is located in the organizational structure of the company. Clerical workers in particular seem to experience the most negative effects in terms of continuing occupational sex segregation, fragmentation, limited opportunities for promotion, and job displacement. Despite the strong similarities, however, the *response* to the situation has been quite different in different countries. Let us now consider these responses in the hope that they will suggest policy for the United States, where efforts to respond to the impact of office technology have been limited.

Responses to the Effects of Information Technology

The views of Cooley (1982), Wilkinson (1983), and Shaiken (1985) lead us to recognize that technology *can* be shaped and humanized. The responses to technology that I survey fall into three categories: (1) legislation and government policies; (2) workers' participation and unionization; and (3) training and research. All are important.

These categories are not mutually exclusive. On the contrary, there is considerable overlap in what governments, workers, and research institutions can do to cope with the effects outlined above. In this discussion, legislation and government policies will be treated separately because a number of Western European governments, being socialist or coming out of a socialist tradition, are more likely than the U.S. government to embrace policies that will protect workers. The section on workers' participation in general and unionization in particular demonstrates how workers can indeed change and monitor technology, rather than succumbing to a deterministic view of its impact. Finally, research and training are included in order to make the academic community aware of the contributions it can offer.

Legislation and Government Participation

In many Western European countries, governments have been involved in regulating the impact of technology in several ways: (1) they have passed legislation aimed at increased cooperation between labor and management in the hope that this will lead to humane implementation; (2) they have offered data on national planning and made projections on the country's needs, which have been used for mediation in national agreements bargained by labor and management; and (3) they have promoted research that supplies information on the likely impact of technology at the national level, thus providing a framework for discussion and negotiation.

Western European nations are examples of the most advanced forms of industrial democracy. Major pieces of labor legislation have contributed to this. For example, in West Germany, the Codetermination Law of 1976 (which superseded and updated a similar law passed in the early 1950s) mandates that stockholder companies with more than two thousand employees must give employees equal representation on the board of directors. The Amended Industrial Relations Act of 1972 gives employees of companies not covered by the Codetermination Law or its predecessor the right to one-third representation on the board of directors. For public employees, the Personnel Representation Act (revised in 1974) establishes joint labor-management personnel councils whose primary concern is working conditions and social issues as they relate to public workers. Presumably, labor representation on such boards helps safeguard workers' interests when the introduction of information technology is being contemplated.

Sweden, like West Germany, has very comprehensive labor legislation supplemented by a body of social welfare legislation without equal anywhere else in the world. With regard to technology, the Joint Regulation of Working Life Act guarantees unions full information about a given company, grants unions the right to approve organization of work and work assignments, and allows unions to veto subcontracting of work by the employer (Chamot and Dymmel 1981, 4).

Norway's labor legislation is also very comprehensive. The 1976 Law on Data Privacy establishes standards for the collection and use by firms of computerized personnel information. The 1977 Work Environment Act sets general principles that must be met in various areas affecting working life, and technology is one of the areas specifically covered. The first "Technology Agreement" was negotiated and signed by the Norwegian Employers Confederation and the Trade Union Congress in 1975. This agreement concerned computer-based personnel data systems only. The 1978 revision extended the agreement to cover those computer systems used for the planning and carrying out of work. And by 1982 the agreement covered all types of workplace technology, whether computer-based or not. It also includes the right of workers to hire outside technical experts at company expense.

In Norway, technology agreements can also be negotiated at the local level. A variety of technology-related rights in the workplace have been established through agreements that deal with issues such as information, training, participation, and bargaining. Workers are guaranteed both job-related training and general education about technical systems and their design. Negotiations by unions at the local level focus on their own workers' concerns and attempt to bring local practice into conformity with the general requirements of national agreements. Local unions also elect representatives known as data shop stewards[2] who are specifically responsible for technology-related issues.

Another function that Western European governments may perform is to serve as mediators between labor and management. The Austrian government, for example, plays a large and active role in national across-the-board wage negotiations. It contributes projections drawn from the input-output data bank of the country's bookkeeping system and links decisions affecting the industry in question to the situation of the country as a whole. Leontief (1982) demonstrates how the Austrian government participated in projecting the impact of new text-processing and printing technologies on the Austrian newspaper industry and worked out detailed plans that facilitated cooperation between labor and management. The Austrian Institute for Economic Research employed the country's input-output data bank to construct a model of the Austrian economy as of 1976. The model was then used to develop alternative scenarios to analyze in quantitative terms the impact of new technologies as well as the combined effects of economic, social, and educational policy measures (Leontief 1982, 105).

Western European governments have also been actively involved in promoting research. For example, the impact of microelectronic technology has been viewed by several governments as so significant that they have sponsored major research projects in order to provide general overviews of the situation created by the introduction of such technology. Among these reports are the Nora-Minc Report in France, the Siemens Report in Germany, the Rathenau Report in the Netherlands, the National Council for the Promotion of Sciences Report in Belgium, the National Board for Science and Technology Report in Ireland, and the ACARD Report in the United Kingdom.

Special concern has been shown by government agencies for the specific problems of women workers. The Commission of European Communities has published the *Community Action Programme on the Promotion of Equal Opportunities for Women, 1982–1985*. Meanwhile, members of the European Economic Community such as Italy, France, the United Kingdom, Belgium, and the Netherlands have been funded by the European Social Fund to conduct research on women's employment. One of the most interesting results was a conference organized in Belgium in 1981. The conference drew the following conclusions: (1) job loss resulting from the introduction of new technologies should not be dealt with by the introduction of part-time work but rather through a general reduction in working hours for all workers; (2) information technology should be included in the curriculum of all technical schools; (3) teacher training should be strengthened; and (4) it should be recognized that homeworking is neither a desirable nor an inevitable development, and the importance of human contact as an aspect of work life should not be overlooked (Zmroczek and Henwood 1983).

The United States presents a stark contrast. Labor legislation related to technology is nonexistent. Chamot (1985) states that the federal government has been conspicuous by its almost total lack of involvement, with the exception of some attempts at information gathering by committees of the House of Representatives. The Office of Technology Assessment of the U.S. Congress gathers information on current research on technology, and the Department of Labor, particularly the Women's Bureau, is concerned with the impact of technology on the American work force. Without appropriate legislation, however, their position is necessarily reactive rather than active. The executive branch has been more concerned with improvement of productivity and with the development and use of new technologies than with considering their impact on workers.

Workers' Participation

The participation of workers in the organization of their everyday work life is crucial if we are to moderate the negative effects of information technology. European workers have achieved this participation in large part through unionization. The proportion of workers in unions is 83 percent in Sweden, 71 percent in Belgium, 55 percent in the United Kingdom, and 42 percent in West Germany, to cite a few examples. In the United States, by comparison, it is 18 percent.

A high rate of unionization is important because it permits negotiation and allows management and labor to reach agreements that take into account the total economic and social picture. Chamot (1985) suggests that this high level of unionization, in Sweden, for example, has led both employers and government agencies to show concern for the human implications of technological change at the workplace.

Norway provides an example for the world. There unions, employers, and the state have together tried to influence the direction of technological change at work. Schneider (1984) conducted a study of eight Norwegian companies and analyzed them according to whether unions intervened in the introduction of new technology before the fact or after the fact. She found that many local unions chose the "after the fact" approach, preferring to negotiate with managment afterward on such issues as training or monitoring of individual performance. This approach allows workers to study the system before they intervene. Other unions prefer a before-the-fact approach so that they can have input into the system design itself. This approach demands more involvement and responsibility from the union. An emerging trend, however, is to place technology bargaining in a much broader field of intervention, one in which the impact of technology is viewed not merely on a local but on a national and international level.

Even though there are laws and regulations that protect Norwegian workers, influencing specific developments requires a strong commitment from workers. A case in point appears in Schneider's study (Schneider 1984). City government workers in Bergen, frustrated by the lack of training and lack of worker representation in the design of the new office technology system, demanded and won a moratorium on the development of all technical systems in the city of Bergen until management submitted a long-term plan for technological change. The Bergen union formed an alliance with the technical experts who actually designed the city government data systems, and together both groups opposed total control by the KDV, an external systems development agency for city governments whose philosophy was contrary to their own. The union then developed a Policy on Technological Change, which became the national union platform for technological change in the city government sector. This policy emphasizes the importance of grassroots local development and implementation of systems that take into account the interests of the union as well as quality of work life and relations between workers and management. The union is also presently involved in the planning of training programs, including one of three years' duration that offers courses in computer programming, project work methods, and organizational development.

In another study of work reorganization and worker participation, Schneider (1983) describes a program to engage workers in the automation of a teller system at a Norwegian bank. A technological change project turned into a total reorganization of work at the bank. The design, planning, and implementation of the system, as well as the redesign of jobs, were accomplished by a group composed almost entirely of tellers. A group composed of representatives from management and the union, meanwhile, studied the social and organizational consequences of the new system. This project stands in marked contrast to the way in which City Bank of New York automated its "back office" processing services. That project did include redesign of clerical work to promote integration of functions and potential for professional advancement with the support of computers. However, employee participation was limited to such activities as designing the work environment, testing office chairs, and picking color schemes. What technology would be used and how it would be used were determined by management. Thus City Bank's back office employees are currently monitored by computers that print out detailed daily records of their work performance.

When new technology is introduced into the workplace in West Germany, unions insist on the following points: (1) human and social needs must take priority over or at least be equal in importance to economic considerations; (2) wages, skills, and responsibility should at least be maintained, if not upgraded; (3) there should be no dismissals due to the introduction of the new technology; (4) health and safety issues related to the technology must be duly considered; (5) when work quotas are introduced into the office, agreements must be negotiated specifying the amount of work to be accomplished in a certain period; (6) there should be limitations and regulations on the collection of personal data; and (7) work should be organized to provide interesting, diversified jobs requiring skill and responsibility (Meyer 1983).

Nevertheless, trade unions throughout Western Europe have been frustrated in their attempts to deal with international corporations. The best and most ambitious example of work toward regional, national, and international solutions to the problems posed by new workplace technology is based in Sweden and is called the UTOPIA project. Through this project, graphics workers' unions throughout the Scandinavian countries have broadened the choice of production technologies by developing their own alternative software systems designed to meet trade union criteria for quality work and quality products. In other words, the project has empowered workers to choose their *own* software according to their *own* criteria.

In the United States, the role of the American union is essentially a reactive one, an "after the fact" approach. The "Technology Bill of Rights" of the International Association of Machinists (IAM)[3] has become a kind of landmark for union responses to technology and is frequently mentioned by other unions that are only now beginning to grapple with technology. The United Auto Workers, the United Steelworkers of America, and unions covering employees in the printing and textile industries have negotiated contract clauses on technological change. In fact, about 30 percent of major agreements surveyed recently had this type of clause (AFL-CIO Industrial Union Department 1982).

Some unions directly involved with the new information technology have also begun to negotiate clauses that deal with their concerns. For example, in 1980 the Communications Workers of America (CWA) negotiated with AT&T the establishment of a new Joint Technology Change Committee, which included equal representation from companies and from unions.[4] CWA also negotiated a "Supplementary Income Protection Program" for workers whose employment is affected by changes in equipment or methods, and monitoring of telephone workers has also been a subject of bargaining. The Service Employees International Union (SEIU) has negotiated a variety of clauses covering job classification, training, and leave of absence for retraining, as well as strong clauses on VDTs and health and safety issues. Locals of the American Federation of State, County and Municipal Employees (AFSCME) have negotiated agreements on wage rates, job security and training, advance notice, and consultation wages for word processing operations and work on VDTs. However, the general approach taken by unions has been to focus on the ways that existing language can be used to deal with new technology before introducing specific, new language.

The role of these unions is important and commendable, particularly in view of the limitations they face. For one thing, they are working at the local level with no possibility of regional or national bargaining. For another, there is no legislation to protect them or the workers they represent. And finally, they must negotiate on technological issues without benefit of professional or technical support that can help them to function at a level of expertise equal to that of management.

Research and Training

Everywhere, research plays a significant role in technological change. European workers and unions have access to research sponsored by their government offices or by public or private educational institutions. It was the Norwegian Computing Center, for example, that cooperated with the Iron and Metal Workers' Union in obtaining the first data agreement between the Norwegian Employer Federation and the Federation of Trade Unions. The Swedish Center for Working Life functions as a research institute for industrial relations and work life issues. West Germany has a federal agency, the Ministry of Technology and Research, that is charged with promoting development of new technology as well as conducting or promoting studies of ways to humanize new technologies. In addition, the German Metal Workers was funded to set up a nationwide system of "innovation advice bureaus" with ten full-time engineers, economists, and other technicians to help local unions evaluate and bargain over employers' plans for new technology. In Britain, the Microelectronics Application Program (MAP) is a division within the Department of Industry. Its functions are financial support, training, consulting, and development of new programs for managers and workers on the potentials of microelectronics. In addition, the European labor movement has pursued a second tactic to gain access to expert information on technological issues: unionization of professionals in technical fields.

U.S. workers and unions, on the other hand, are at a distinct disadvantage in their interactions with management. Although there is much research currently being conducted on technology, the results are not usually available or accessible to workers. Companies, meanwhile, hire specialists to do the type of research they wish to have. As for the second approach, unions in the United States are indeed focusing serious effort on the organization of more technical and professional workers knowledgeable about technology. For example, the Department for Professional Employees of the AFL-CIO, umbrella organization for twenty-seven national and international unions, is launching an organizing campaign aimed at such workers. American unions have a long way to go, however, to match the accomplishments of their European counterparts.

Training has been promoted at the national level in a number of countries. In Italy, France, and the United Kingdom, for example, there are projects to train women in computer skills, programming, and electronics (Zmroczek and Henwood 1983). In the United States, however, the Job Training Partnership Act, the successor to the Comprehensive Employment and Training Act, does not identify women as a group or attempt to address women's particular needs. Training and retraining have also been offered by private companies, both in Europe and in the United States. In Western Europe, training is a high priority that has come as an outgrowth of national policy, whereas in the United States training has largely come through the efforts of private advocacy organizations, informal labor and community coalitions, and women's groups.

Generally speaking, both in the United States and in Western Europe, training will have to meet two criteria in order to be truly successful. First, the programs that train people in the new skills must take into account the needs of specific groups of workers such as women and minorities. In both the United States and Western Europe, women need to be encouraged to enter nontraditional technical fields; there must be provision for special educational needs, such as language or math instruction; and there must be provision for special service needs such as child care or transportation.

Second, training cannot be seen as a panacea. It is not a cure for the problems caused by technological change. What are we training for? Will the jobs be there when the training is completed? How long can workers use that training before it becomes obsolete? An adequate response to the problems raised by technology must involve an examination of the very structures of society (Benston 1984). Because technology is a force that can produce social changes, it cannot be adequately met with individual survival strategies. Planning, legislation, and research—all are necessary to shape the context in which training will become meaningful.

Policy Implications for the United States

As we have seen, the effects of information technology differ depending upon the sex and position of the worker in the organizational structure of the office, and these differential effects appear to be remarkably consistent across a variety of Western countries. However, individual countries' responses to those effects differ considerably. The question now is which of these strategies would work in the United States if the appropriate vehicles existed. The answer is probably all of them.

The status of such vehicles as legislation and unionization in the United States can be summarized as follows: (1) there is an absence of legally mandated standards for the use of technological equipment as well as an absence of enforced regulations about the kinds of equipment that are to be used; (2) there is a lack of legislation that mandates worker or union participation in decisions about the introduction and use of technology; and (3) there is a low level of unionization, particularly in the service sectors; union representation in banking and insurance, for example, is virtually nonexistent.

It is also important to note that Western Europe experienced a recession during the first half of this decade that produced slow growth and rising unemployment. Information technology contributed to this situation, for when there is a threat of recession, companies automate to save the cost of labor. Problems associated with the introduction of new technology have appeared in Western Europe despite strong labor and social legislation, high levels of unionization, and workers' relatively easy access to technological research. In the United States, too, economic growth rates have slowed in recent times; in the absence of such safeguards as exist in Europe, the effects on U.S. workers could be all the more devastating unless preventive measures are taken. Therefore several suggestions and recommendations follow.

The response to technology cannot be an individual one. Workers have to find a common vehicle for their efforts, and unions appear to be the obvious choice. Though the climate in the United States for unions and unionization is not particularly favorable at present, workers can find unions helpful. However, to increase their effectiveness, unions will have to face a number of serious challenges.

First and foremost, unions must work to organize employees in the service sector. Unionization in this area is crucial because the service sector is growing at a tremendous rate, creating large numbers of new jobs. However, these jobs are for the most part low paid, low skilled— and going overwhelmingly to women workers. Second, unions need to become more sensitive and responsive than traditional male-dominated unions have been to the specific needs of women and minority workers. Third, unions must make a concerted effort to organize professional and technical employees. This will not only increase union membership and extend union solidarity across a broader spectrum of occupations; it will also provide unions with the expert information on technology that will enable negotiating teams to talk the same language as management at the bargaining table. Fourth, there needs to be union cooperation across national borders, in order to deal with automation in multinational enterprises. Looking beyond their immediate network, unions also need to develop coalitions with community agencies and social organizations, in recognition of the fact that ultimately technology is a social issue. And finally, using these coalitions, unions need to look for political allies. As Shaiken (1985) argues, the bottom line on technology is who winds up with power and control at the workplace. If unions can face these challenges successfully, then appropriate legislation will follow, along with more humanized applications of new technologies.

With respect to research and training, it is essential that government-sponsored as well as academic researchers focus on the problems of workers and that the information be made available to workers and communities. Beyond that, unions, community groups, and the research centers of universities need to form coalitions, so that together they can face and solve the problems posed by new technology. Training, too, must be offered by government-sponsored agencies, universities, unions, and companies as part of a total plan that takes into account workers' needs and the needs of the labor market as well as community goals and resources.

It would be impossible and probably undesirable for American workers simply to replicate the efforts of Western Europeans in their attempts to achieve equity in the technological workplace. Nevertheless, the societies surveyed here do provide challenging and inspiring models for change, which can perhaps be modified to the U.S. context.

NOTES

1. Fragmentation of work (which is also called rationalization) appeared first in the factory. Jobs were subdivided into various tasks. The worker learned only one task and performed it continuously without knowledge of the whole production process. The same tendency has reappeared with the application of information technology.
2. The data shop steward is an elected union individual whose main concern is to acquire information related to technology; the information is used to bargain with management as well as to educate the membership on technology issues.
3. The IAM developed its "Technology Bill of Rights" in 1981. It is based on the principle that the introduction of technology is not an automatic right of management but a process subject to bargaining. Special emphasis is placed upon the use of technologies that are socially beneficial.
4. The 1980 agreement between CWA and AT&T establishes a new Joint Technology Change Committee. Its task is to oversee problems and recommend solutions to problems in the area of job security affected by technological changes in equipment, organization, or methods of operation.

REFERENCES

AFL-CIO Industrial Union Department. 1982. Comparative survey of major collective bargaining agreements. Washington, D.C.

AFSCME (American Federation of State, County, and Municipal Employees). 1985. Facing the future: AFSCME's approach to technology. Washington, D.C.

Benston, Margaret Lowe. 1984. The chips are down. In *The technological woman: Interfacing with tomorrow,* ed. Jan Zimmerman, 44–54. New York: Praeger.

Braverman, Harry. 1974. *Labor and monopoly capital: The degradation of work in the twentieth century.* New York: Monthly Review Press.

Cammell, Helga. 1983. Women, technological change and employment levels: The role of trade union policies. In *Office automation: Jekyll or Hyde?* ed. D. Marschall and J. Gregory, 33–38. Cleveland: Working Women Education Fund.

Chamot, Dennis. 1985. Labor and technological change in Sweden. *Working Life in Sweden,* no. 29 (Feb., 1985).

Chamot, Dennis, and Michael D. Dymmel. 1981. *Cooperation or conflict: European experiences with technological change at the workplace.* Washington, D.C.: Department for Professional Employees, AFL-CIO.

Cooley, Mike. 1982. Design, technology and production for social needs. In *The right to useful work,* ed. Ken Coates, 195–211. London: Spokesman.

CWA (Communications Workers of America). 1984. Technological change: Challenges and choices. CWA Training Department field test, July.

Dasey, Robin. 1983. Training: The magic cure for all ills?" In *Office automation: Jekyll or Hyde?* ed. D. Marschall and J. Gregory, 50–58. Cleveland: Working Women Education Fund.

Feldberg, Roslyn, and Evelyn N. Glenn. 1983a. New technology and its implications in U.S. clerical work. In *Office automation: Jekyll or Hyde?* ed. D. Marschall and J. Gregory, 89–95. Cleveland: Working Women Education Fund.

———. 1983b. Technology and work degradation: Effects of office automation on women clerical workers. In *Machina ex dea,* ed. Joan Rothschild, 59–78. New York: Pergamon Press.

FIET (International Federation of Clerical, Technical and Professional Employees). 1980a. Bank workers and new technology. An International Trade Union Response. Geneva.

———. 1980b. Insurance and social insurance: Workers and new technology. An International Trade Union Response. Geneva.

Giuliano, Vincent E. 1982. The mechanization of office work. *Scientific American* 247, no. 3 (Sept.): 149–64.

Greenbaum, Joan. 1983. Assessing the myths of the job market. In *Office automation: Jekyll or Hyde?* ed. D. Marschall and J. Gregory, 69–72. Cleveland: Working Women Education Fund.

Gutek, Barbara. 1983. Women's work in the office of the future. In *The technological woman: Interfacing with tomorrow,* ed. Jan Zimmerman, 159–68. New York: Praeger.

Gutek, Barbara, and Tora K. Bikson. 1984. Differential experiences of men and women in computerized offices: Sex roles. Manuscript.

Hanisch, T. 1981. The impact of information technology on employment from the standpoint of labour market theory. In *Microelectronics, productivity and employment*, 63–74. Paris: Organization for Economic Cooperation and Development.

Kassalow, Everett M. 1985. Technological change and industrial relations in the U.S.: A survey of trends and practices. Paper presented at the ISVET (ENI) Conference, Rome, January. Mimeo.

Leontief, Wassily W. 1982. The distribution of work and income. *Scientific American* 247, no. 3 (Sept.): 100–109.

Meyer, Regina. 1983. Collective bargaining strategies on new technology: The experience of West German trade unions. In *Office automation: Jekyll or Hyde?* ed. D. Marschall and J. Gregory, 205–14. Cleveland: Working Women Education Fund.

Mosco, Vincent, and Andrew Herman. 1981. Critical theory and electronic media. *Theory and Society* 10:869–96.

Rada, J. 1980. *The impact of micro-electronics: A tentative appraisal of information technology.* Geneva: International Labour Office.

Roos, Patricia. 1985. *Gender and work.* Albany: State University of New York Press.

Rytina, Nancy, and Suzanne Bianchi. 1984. Occupational reclassification and changes in distribution by gender. *Monthly Labor Review* 107, no. 3 (Mar.): 11–17.

Schneider, Leslie. 1983. Alternative models of worker participation. In *Office automation: Jekyll or Hyde?* ed. D. Marschall and J. Gregory, 200–204. Cleveland: Working Women Education Fund.

———. 1984. *Technology bargaining in Norway: Technology and the need for new labor relations.* Discussion Paper Series, no. 129D. Cambridge, Mass.: John F. Kennedy School of Government, Harvard University.

Scott, Joan Wallach. 1982. The mechanization of women's work. *Scientific American* 247, no. 3 (Sept.): 166–87.

SEIU (Service Employees International Union). N.d. Technological change: Contract provisions. Washington, D.C.

Shaiken, Harley. 1985. *Work transformed: Automation and labor in the computer age.* New York: Holt, Rinehart and Winston.

U.S. Department of Labor. 1983. *Women's employment in occupations and industries.* Bulletin no. 298. In *Time of change: Handbook on women workers.* Washington, D.C.: GPO.

Wilkinson, Barry. 1983. *The shopfloor politics of new technology.* London: Heinemann Education Books.

Zmroczek, Christine, and Felicity Henwood. 1983. Government policies on new information technologies and their implications for employment: An overview of EEC countries, with particular reference to women. In *Office automation: Jekyll or Hyde?* ed. D. Marschall and J. Gregory, 39–49. Cleveland: Working Women Education Fund.

Women, Work, and the University-Affiliated Technology Park

Barbara Drygulski Wright

Clearly, technology is transforming the lives and work of millions of women in the United States and all over the world. Less clearly but just as significantly, technology is restructuring the economies of "developed" and "developing" countries alike and changing the face of the landscape. For those of us in academic life, this transformation may lie much closer to home than we have realized. For today, dozens of universities and colleges are developing their property holdings to create research and technology parks in which the tenants will be private business firms. It seems essential to ask what forces have led to the creation of such parks, what implications they hold for both business and universities, and where women are going to fit into this new trend, which has the potential to shape the national and international economy for decades to come.

At least one thing is certain, however: thus far, women and women's issues have not been adequately represented in the planning and debate that accompany the creation of technology parks. At a time when feminism, affirmative action, and women's studies have made the university somewhat more open to women, science and technology remain one of the last male preserves. The consulting team, the higher levels of university administration, and the disciplinary areas involved in planning a park are unlikely to include women or to consider the needs of women and minority males. Under those circumstances, the odds are good that traditional patterns of segregation and stratification according to race and gender (see, for example, Glenn and Tolbert and Donato and Roos in this volume) will reassert themselves in the new setting. Indeed, women's marginalization from control may well result in their being particularly hard hit by the costs of this new wave of economic development. And that is a turn of economic events that women, especially minority women, can ill afford.

Some Background

In 1948, Stanford University began to develop the first science- and technology-oriented park in the United States. The development of research parks gained momentum in the early 1960s, with more than fifty projects in progress during that decade, and twenty-five to thirty more were created in the early 1970s. In 1981 *Industrial Research Magazine* identified eighty-one restricted use parks with an emphasis on scientific activities in the United States; of that number, nineteen were affiliated with universities. Only three years later, in September, 1984, a telephone survey revealed forty university-affiliated research parks in the United States and another three in Canada either in the planning or development stages (Levitt 1984, 70, 75–81). Two years later, the number had more than doubled again: the International Association of University Research Parks, founded at Arizona State University Research Park in April, 1986, estimates the total number of university-affiliated parks now being planned or developed at just over one hundred. Obviously, this is a trend to be reckoned with—and one that doubtless has already reached the campuses of many readers of this volume.

To understand the research park phenomenon, it is necessary to place it in the larger context of emerging university-industry relations. A number of changes have occurred over the last ten years that make closer relations between business and research universities seem desirable to both parties and make the technology park seem an ideal physical location for those relations to be cultivated.

Universities find themselves facing financial, demographic, and structural problems. Over the past ten years, federal funding did not actually decline, but its rate of growth slowed to a crawl; figuring for inflation, the net effect was a loss. With implementation of the Gramm-Rudman Resolution in 1986, actual cuts are beginning. Meanwhile, the explosive growth of post-secondary education since the 1950s, which was fueled by the GI Bill and the high birth rates of the baby boom, has come to an end; many schools now find themselves with a larger faculty and a more extensive physical plant than they wish to maintain. Competition among universities for a leading position in high-tech research has been intensified by the realization that the revenues from the new technologies and from association with industry could prove significant. Responding to all these pressures, many colleges and universities have shifted from a conservative to an entrepreneurial posture toward their land holdings (Levitt 1984, 4–5).

The potential rewards to the institution from research park development are primarily financial; they include income from leased or purchased property and the chance to sell ideas to business in exchange for money to support research. Also important are increased opportunities for faculty research, for consulting, and for participation in the founding of new companies ("start-ups"), all of which may help a university to retain top researchers and attract others. In addition, a research park offers expanded employment for students and graduates, and the park can be planned to include facilities that the school needs but cannot afford to build on its own, such as a hotel, a conference center, or housing. All these benefits can help an institution remain competitive and keep its graduate programs viable during the current period of contracting student enrollment.

Businesses are attracted to university-affiliated technology parks for a different but related set of reasons. In the context of a U.S. economy that has been stagnating since the early 1970s, both business and government hope that technological breakthroughs will provide the impetus for another wave of economic expansion and improved competitiveness. High-tech industries, particularly information technologies and biotechnology, are becoming an increasingly important part of the U.S. industrial structure, and research and technological innovation are a crucial component of high-tech firms. Thus the U.S. economy is steadily becoming more dependent on research for economic growth, and this makes close ties with academe increasingly attractive.

Another reason for the interest of business in new technologies has to do with its reading of the current labor market—a reading that contradicts many of the findings in this book. According to this view, demographic changes are pushing business toward more advanced technologies. "The baby boom of the post-World War II period resulted in a labor force boom . . . but this surge in labor supply is over. The result is that the more labor-intensive technologies of the labor force boom years must be replaced with more capital-intensive methods of production" (Levitt 1984, 26). Of course, this diagnosis of a labor shortage jars with steadily rising unemployment rates and chronic underemployment in ever larger segments of the American work force, and it contradicts the findings of research presented in this volume (see Appelbaum, Glenn and Tolbert, and Samper). But it is an accurate reflection of American business's definition of "competitiveness"—a definition that excludes commitment to full employment in quality jobs.

There are other interested parties that stand to benefit from the university/business connection, including developers and federal, state, and local governments. For the developer, the most significant advantages beyond simple profit include access to property that would otherwise be unavailable for development, tax benefits through the tax-exempt status of the university as a non-profit organization, and the luster that the developer may acquire from association with a prestigious institution.

Towns, regions, and state governments have also begun to view the university as a key to economic growth. University-affiliated technology parks seem to offer high-income employment and high-quality, aesthetically appealing work environments, in contrast with traditional manufacturing industries. They promise increased job opportunities and an additional tax base, and they may contribute to the life of the local community by sharing facilities, sponsoring cultural events, or generally enhancing the prestige of the area as a place to live and work. Thus state and local governments have been willing to go to considerable lengths to attract the high-tech, high-growth businesses in which the most rapid job expansion is occurring (Levitt 1984, 25; Haemmerlie 1985, 42–49; Science Park Development Corporation 1984, 1985).

The emergence of ties between business and universities has also been encouraged by changes in public policies. These include national tax policies to promote research and development partnerships between industry and academe, more generous tax write-offs for businesses that make equipment grants to university laboratories, modification of anti-trust laws, and changes in patent policy that allow universities to keep the patent rights to new products and processes developed from federally funded research (Levitt 1984, 26).

The conjunction of all these changes—in business, at universities, and at the local, state, and federal levels—suggests that the move toward closer relations between business and academe is a long-term trend. The question is, who will ultimately benefit?

Technology Parks: The University's Perspective

What exactly are the implications of closer university-industry relations? And what kind of change from the past does this represent? The technology park is not the only or even the major form of relationship between academic research and industry, but rather an outgrowth of complex and changing research relations.[1]

From the end of the Second World War through the mid-1970s, the federal government was the major source of funding for basic scientific research in the United States. It channeled grant money particularly through the National Institutes of Health (NIH) and the National Science Foundation (NSF) to universities, which competed fiercely for funds and directed their research toward federally identified priorities. In this way an enormous structure for basic research was created on university campuses. Beginning in the mid-1970s, however, a number of important changes began to weaken this research structure. While public funding of research was not actually cut, the rate of its growth slackened, and at the same time NSF and NIH began to pressure universities to link with industry.[2] Meanwhile, private industry's interest in campus research soared, inspired by the realization that certain breakthroughs in basic science could have tremendous potential in commercial applications. In effect, private corporations began to lease the laboratories, staffs, and state-of-the-art expertise that had been developed with federal funding. When Ronald Reagan entered the White House in January, 1980, the political climate became even more sympathetic to private industry: "the new ideology was that any activity that could be privatized should be" (Kenney 1986, 29).

Since the mid-1970s, university-industry relations have expanded enormously in number and variety. There are two basic categories of relationships: those between industry and an institution, and those between industry and an individual faculty member. At the institutional level, contributions from companies have ranged from the relatively uncontroversial undirected grant through fellowships and targeted grants to contract research and industrial affiliate programs. Cooperative research centers or institutes have also been founded, some with support from NSF, some with multicorporate sponsorship, and some entirely dependent on a single funder, as is MIT's Whitehead Institute. The most interesting arrangements from a business point of view are those that provide the funder with some sort of competitive edge.

There have also been a few spectacular, multimillion-dollar long-term contracts, such as those between Monsanto and Harvard or MIT and Exxon. In this type of agreement large sums of money are directed to specific scientists, who continue their research while remaining at the university. Participating corporations insist they have no desire to influence the research process; they merely wish to benefit from its results. The high-water mark in long-term contracts was reached, according to Kenney, in about 1980; after that the rate of such contracts slowed down for the simple reason that the limited number of scientists and corporations interested and able to enter such relationships had already done so.

Still another means for a university to exploit its research is to create its own for-profit company. Harvard attempted this in 1980. The plan called for the university to supply patents, professors, and facilities, while venture capitalists would provide money and marketing know-how. The plan was greeted with a storm of criticism from students, faculty, alumni, and even the *New York Times*. They charged the university would lose its credibility and its professors would no longer be able to speak out on social issues as "impartial experts." Harvard president Derek Bok ultimately decided that the university should not participate directly in profit making, and the plan was scrapped. Harvard's action has not prevented less prestigious schools from launching for-profit companies, however.

Relationships between individual faculty members and private firms have also proliferated in the last five to ten years. Traditionally, professors have engaged in consulting, and the university administration has supported consulting as an enhancement of teaching and research. However, limits on consulting and provisions to prevent conflict of interest have been enforced loosely at best. In the last ten years, many professors have taken collaboration a step further and become involved in start-ups, new firms founded to take advantage of specific scientific breakthroughs. They are tempted by the opportunity to become principals and directors in these new companies, to receive an equity interest in the company, to be involved in the new company's research program, and to work for it as a consultant or member of a scientific advisory board. According to Kenney, most of these researchers, if given the chance, would refuse to work full-time in an industrial setting, because they would miss the freedom and creative stimulation of the academic research environment. However, combining the financial rewards of private industry with the security and advantages of an academic position seems to offer the best of both worlds.

For individuals as for institutions, the most powerful motivation for developing ties with industry is financial: for example, Nobel laureate Arthur Kornberg has said, "Understandably, the scientists that provided the ideas, techniques and practitioners of genetic chemistry are reluctant to be excluded from its financial rewards by entrepreneurs and venture capitalists" (quoted in Kenney 1986, 97). Conversely, Kenney observes, "the choice not to participate [is] also the choice to allow others to benefit from your research" (97). Leading research universities have tolerated extensive involvement of their faculty in private ventures for private gain because they fear restrictions will lead to a mass exodus of top personnel; less prestigious universities are actively encouraging their faculty to join the competition.

The university-affiliated research and technology park must be seen in this context of emerging university-industrial collaboration for financial gain. The park is designed to provide the physical space—a kind of middle ground between campus and factory—for development of the ambiguous relations described above. University-owned land is being sold or leased to companies that wish to locate close to the university campus. This marks a significant departure from traditional policies, which called for highly conservative management of land that the institution saw itself holding in trust for future generations. The push to develop research parks since 1983 may be viewed as an attempt on the part of many research universities to accomplish on a broad scale with many small companies what a handful of schools were able to accomplish on a very limited scale with a few large corporate contracts. Through the mechanism of a research park, universities can promote the formation of start-ups, facilitate faculty involvement in start-ups, and encourage the direction of research efforts on campus toward discoveries that will potentially be marketable and add to university income through patents and licensing fees.

At the same time that university-industry relations have been expanding, the ramifications of this development have become clearer. First, it is important to keep in mind that although the number and kinds of relationships between academe and business have increased, federal funds remain the basis of the U.S. research effort: whereas the federal government supplied 56.9 percent of the funds for basic research in 1953, in 1984 it supplied 66.5 percent; meanwhile, business's share has shrunk from 34.7 percent to 18.5 percent (Kenney 1986, 36). "The 'sophisticated' investor," as Kenney observes, "buys only what is economically valuable" (72). Kenney argues that this federal investment in research in fact represents an enormous subsidy to private enterprise, because the next wave of economic expansion will be information based and dependent on the expertise of university researchers.

What are the potential dangers and abuses from a further development of university-industry relations? First, there is the impairment of the university's perceived role as an independent and objective authority. The traditional, ideologically sanctioned conception of the university has been that of an independent institution whose faculty enjoyed the freedom to speak as impartial authorities on issues of concern to society. The university has been expected to devote its efforts to serving the public interest through unbiased teaching and research. Freedom in research and in expression of findings has been protected traditionally by the tenure system; the university's independence from economic pressures has been reflected in and protected by its tax-exempt status as a nonprofit institution. Of course, no university can be separated so cleanly from the values, biases, or political forces of the society in which it exists. Thus a feminist analysis reveals, for example, a distinct masculine bias in curriculum and research at American universities, a masculine bias that is also characteristic of American society as a whole. Universities have been careful, however, to avoid actions that would blatantly conflict with their traditional role and call their authority and credibility into question on a grand scale.

With the expansion of university-industrial collaboration for profit, however, an institution that was only imperfectly impartial and objective may become even less so. Greater corporate involvement is likely to mean a skewing of research toward work with probusiness implications and away from criticism or development of alternatives. While "directed autonomy" has been the effect of federal research funding, too, it has not been so consistently probusiness. While it may be desirable in some ways for the university's "objectivity" to be unmasked as a fiction, it is clearly dangerous for the university, with its considerable resources, to become the unapologetic servant of private industry and abandon its mission to serve other sectors of society. Concomitantly, it seems inevitable that individual faculty members will run into conflicts of interest. When professors hold an appointment from a university and at the same time work for or even own companies, they are working, as Kenney observes, for two entities with very different missions: one is to serve the public good, the other to serve the private corporate good. Monetary gain, and particularly personal monetary gain, was not originally part of the academic ethic (see also Ziman 1984, 145–47.)

Next, there is the problem of privatization and commodification of knowledge that was developed with public funds to serve the public good. This amounts to appropriation of public knowledge for corporate profit. Research that was intended to serve the interests of all—consumers, farmers, and workers as well as business—may become a source of profit to private industry and accessible only to those who can pay the price. Related to privatization is the danger that the free exchange of ideas that is supposed to characterize the academic community will be replaced by the secrecy characteristic of industry. While competition and rivalry in the scientific community have sometimes restricted the flow of information, this tendency has been offset in the past by the ideal of collegiality, as well as by the need to publish, by presentation of results at scientific meetings, and by peer review of research projects. According to Kenney, there is already evidence that in cases where discoveries appear to have commercial applications and the potential to earn a great deal of money, publication is being replaced by patenting and press conferences (1986, 130–31). Whereas the purpose of publication is to stimulate *further* research and testing, the effect of patents is to *limit* access and the effect of press conferences to enhance commercial value.

Finally, there is the danger that graduate and postdoctoral students will be exploited by professors seeking financial gain. Students provide labor that is both highly skilled and cheap; at the same time, students are dependent upon their faculty advisors for assistantships, fellowships, and eventually, jobs. Students may find themselves channeled into narrow specialties dictated by the research agenda of the private contracting firm, rather than pursuing research of more general academic merit. Students' ideas may be appropriated and they may become the victims of unfair patenting and copyright policies. There has always been an asymmetric power relationship between faculty and students, yet there were also traditional limits on what a professor could demand, and the relationship was supposed to be informed by trust and a set of mutual obligations. Those limits, Kenney charges, are now falling apart under the economic and competitive pressures emanating from close relationships to industry (cf. Ziman 1984, 178).

In sum, university-industry cooperation for financial gain raises a host of practical problems and ethical questions. Yet the university-affiliated technology park, apart from encouraging such cooperation, seems designed for the very purpose of blurring the distinction between public and private spheres and clouding the ethical issues rather than clarifying them. The comfortable, deliberately campuslike atmosphere, the proximity to campus, the sharing of personnel, the conduct of seminars and other forms of collaboration—all are promoted ostensibly to improve researchers' creativity and productivity and enhance the pursuit of knowledge. At the same time, however, intentionally or not, this environment serves to obscure the very real distinction between science for science's sake and science for profit's sake. It obscures for academics the problematic nature of collaboration and promotes instead a naive unself-consciousness and a simplistic sense that all research is somehow the same.

Technology Parks: The Business Perspective

Businesses seem eager to locate in university-affiliated technology parks, yet, paradoxically, proximity to university research capabilities is not the leading factor when businesses decide to locate there. In a survey of high-tech firms conducted by the Joint Economic Committee of the U.S. Congress in 1982 (Levitt 1984, 27), the quality and cost of the region's labor force and its tax and regulatory environment ranked ahead of proximity to a research university as key factors. The university itself also offered a number of attractions besides research: ranked first was the availability of a labor pool of college graduates; second was the availability of degree programs for employees, and third was access to the university's library and information systems. Cultural amenities available through the university also figured strongly. Of course, research counted for something: it was judged "somewhat important" but not as important as the preceding factors. Respondents also expressed preference for suburban over central city locations and cited good schools, cultural activities, and recreational facilities as additional important considerations. How can this contradiction be explained? There are perhaps two explanations, one of them ideological, the other practical.

First, the ideological. In the words of an international expert on attracting high-tech industry, "your research expenditure is your 'entry cost' into the 'club of high technology.' It shows you are a 'gentleman' and that you know how to do your research" (Haemmerlie 1985, 58). Teaming up with a university constitutes a relatively quick and inexpensive way for business to gain access not only to research itself, but also to the prestige of the gentlemen's club that research represents. By entering into partnership, both university and business appear to be trading on the prestige and power of science, as well as on the academic ethic of the pursuit of scientific knowledge for its own sake and not for profit. Is this pure vanity on the part of business? Not at all. For business, as I argued in the introduction to this volume, has profited enormously in the past from society's willingness to accept the consequences of science and technology as good or at least necessary; and business stands to profit handsomely in future if it can pull off the privatization of discoveries made at public expense. Maintaining those advantages may be more important than scientific research itself.

Prestige certainly figures strongly in the business-oriented literature describing technology parks. They are marketed as "high-quality," "sophisticated" settings "with a technical ambience" (Levitt 1984, 74). Developers are advised to create a "parklike" atmosphere through the use of plantings, sculptures, fountains, ponds, and green spaces, and to pay close attention to the design of buildings, roadways, and signs. The purpose of all this effort is twofold: the surroundings are intended to identify tenants of the park as successful and upscale (Levitt 1984, 81), and at the same time they are supposed to be campuslike, not only reflecting the economic and academic ties between the university and the industries housed in the park, but also suggesting a philosphical affinity. In other words, it appears that through the manipulation of imagery, business, too, wishes to blur the distinction between public and private and imply that it shares the traditional academic dedication to knowledge and the common weal rather than to profit.

Second, there is the practical advantage of locating in a university park. As mentioned above, labor is business's prime consideration in choosing a location. The most important factors regarding labor are its availability, its cost, and its level of technical training. What does this have to do with universities? Obviously, the local labor pool includes technicians, as well as the graduate students and postdoctoral students who train in university laboratories. But there is more. As a labor pool, the university community possesses many of the same attractions as the suburban locations preferred by many high-tech businesses (see, for example, Appelbaum and Samper in this volume), but it possesses these advantages to an even greater degree.

Universities have traditionally attracted a large community of hangers-on: graduates and others attracted to the amenities of the university setting, as well as spouses, significant others, children of faculty, and graduate students. Underemployment, however, is pervasive. These individuals often wish to remain in the area for personal reasons but have difficulty finding work commensurate with their abilities or training. Thus individuals are willing to work part-time for relatively low wages, often because they are subsidized by partners with better pay and benefits. These workers tend to be intelligent, college educated, and able to solve problems or perform complicated tasks with little or no training. They are also overwhelmingly female. The majority of faculty at U.S. universities are currently white heterosexual males; their spouses tend to be women who have subordinated their own careers to the relationship. And women, for a host of reasons discussed in this volume, have traditionally been paid less than males doing the same or comparable work. For business, in other words, university communities represent a vast untapped source of cheap, high-quality, disproportionately female labor.

A Feminist Perspective

Clearly, the development of university-industry relations in general and of research parks in particular has implications for women and minority communities. Yet these voices have been conspicuous by their absence from the discussion of these issues. The university presidents, the professors and corporate officials who have signed contracts, the participants in the Pajaro Dunes conference to set policy for university-industry relations, the consultants and scientific advisors (Kenney 1986, 86, 102–3)—the actors in this play have been almost without exception white males. Similarly, the literature on technology park development is geared toward business and university audiences, is promotional in purpose, and stresses potential advantages; it lacks any examination of the negative implications of this kind of economic development for society in general or for women and minorities in particular.

Women and minority communities today find themselves marginalized both from control of emerging technologies and from the debate surrounding their economic exploitation; yet women and minorities are hardly marginalized in terms of the impact these developments will have on them. Indeed, there may be a direct connection between the fact of their marginalization and the likelihood that these workers will enjoy fewer benefits while bearing a disproportionate share of the costs in the coming wave of technologically inspired economic expansion. As the articles in this volume have shown, there is often a considerable gap between the myth and the reality of new technology in the workplace. There is no reason why technologically inspired economic development should *not* benefit women and minority workers, but at the same time history gives us little reason to assume that it necessarily *will*. In a worst-case scenario, the next phase of economic expansion may actually serve to increase drastically the disparity in economic and political power between dominant and subordinate groups or classes.

Certainly, the shift in focus from federal funding of research to industry-funded, business-oriented research means that even more directly than before, research may serve the interests of male-dominated groups; their financial position may be strengthened, and their control of the economy may be increased at the cost of women, minority workers, the handicapped, consumers, and the general public. The university meanwhile, may be transformed from an implicit ally of the political and economic *status quo* with enough play in its system for dissenting voices, to an explicit extension of capitalist interests that do not share the academic ethic of open dissent and debate.

Large-scale privatization of public property by already dominant economic entities is a particularly ominous development. Like the seizing of agricultural land, fens, and forests by European nobility in the seventeenth century (Merchant 1980), the appropriation of common resources by individuals or corporations in the Third World today (Fernandez-Kelly 1983; Haddad in this volume), and the patenting of commonly occurring varieties of food plants by multinational agricultural corporations (Doyle 1985), this new wave of privatization is likely to widen the gap between rich and poor, the powerful and the disempowered. Once again, those at the bottom of the economic pyramid—women, children, and other disadvantaged groups—may pay the biggest price in impoverishment, social dislocation, and forced dependency.

Exploitation of students in research laboratories is serious in any case; because of their outsider status, however, women and minority males are particularly vulnerable, not only to low pay, pressure, and theft of ideas, but also to sexual, gender, and racial harassment. If academic science was not a very hospitable environment for these nontraditional science students before, it is unlikely to become more so now. Similarly, exploitation of the university community's labor pool is a general concern, but it is women who will be particularly hard hit.

Many forces—economic, social, and philosophical—and many interests—federal, state, local, academic, and business—are currently pushing for further growth of university-industry relations and for development of university-affiliated research parks. Future scholarship would do well to submit these trends to careful critical examination in order to determine what the gains and losses will be if they continue and to devise strategies for changing their direction or even stopping them altogether. This, however, is an enormous and long-term undertaking; at the same time, the historical record suggests that it is extremely difficult to change the course of movements toward privatization and economic restructuring when they enjoy the support of both politically and economically dominant groups.

Given the enormity and complexity of the problem, it seems most advisable to think and work simultaneously in terms of both long- and short-term solutions. In the short term, if a technology park is going up next door, women on campus and in the community should consider what steps may make sense and lead to greater race and gender equity without undermining efforts toward more radical long-term change. At the least, policy discussions should be initiated that will consider the effect of university-industry relations not merely from a narrow economic or scientific point of view, but with an eye to larger social ramifications. Because the technology park is usually created as a separate legal entity from the university, these policy discussions are likely to fall into two broad categories: university policy and technology park policy.

With regard to the university, there should be open and frank discussion of the implications of collaboration with business for profit, including privatization, conflict of interest, restrictions on publication, exploitation of students, and damage to the university's status as an independent and objective authority. Special attention should be focused on the university's policy for technology transfer.

Technology transfer is the process whereby the discoveries or inventions growing out of university research are transferred to the private sector for development and marketing. In March of 1982, federal policy regarding the administration of inventions made with federal funding changed in an important way. Previously, the government had retained title, with the effect that inventions could not move from research to development and commercial application. Since 1982, it has been possible for universities and other nonprofit organizations to obtain patents and collect royalties and licensing fees on inventions made with federal funds, provided they follow federal guidelines for doing so. Implicit in this new arrangement are the practical and ethical problems outlined above, as well as clear benefits to the direct participants in the partnership: from the federal government's point of view, this action should help to keep the United States competitive in world markets; universities and nonprofit research organizations stand to make considerable amounts of money through patent fees and royalties; and business firms will enjoy new access to potentially profitable innovations.

What needs to be clearly recognized is the powerful economic role that has been assigned to a university's office of technology transfer in this process. Under the new regulations, this office has become responsible for deciding which firm will or will not have the opportunity to develop and market a given invention. Thus directly or indirectly, this office may affect the formation and growth of new firms, just as it may affect the market position, control, and competitiveness of established ones. Technology transfer can be used to promote economic diversity and equity, or it may serve to reinforce existing economic oligarchies. In any case, research universities should recognize the power that has been put in their hands, and then develop conscious policies for how they intend to use it. Women on campus and in the community may wish to push for a policy to ensure that small women- and minority-owned firms are the preferred recipients of development rights. There *is* a precedent for this kind of policy: until 1984, the federal government itself encouraged the awarding of licenses to small businesses, and some offices have continued that policy informally, although it is no longer the official one, simply because the directors are personally committed to the principle.

With regard to the technology park, strategists might pay particular attention to the following: formulation of a plan for park development that includes the economic needs of the town or region; adoption by park management and tenants of a wage policy based on comparable worth; encouragement of women and minority entrepreneurs; and avoidance of military contractors.

While this list by no means exhausts the possibilities, it does suggest some tangible and practical actions that could potentially benefit women as well as minority men in technology-related employment. First and foremost, a university that is developing a technology park can be pressured to plan not only for its own financial health but for that of the town or region as a whole. While this kind of consideration may seem self-evident, it cannot be taken for granted. Universities have demonstrated a variety of motivations for pursuing real estate ventures, and the economic welfare of the surrounding region is seldom a leading factor.

The University of Connecticut's development plan, for example, lists "economic development of the greater community, thereby offering employment and entrepreneurial opportunity to its members" in ninth place out of a total of twelve major goals; enhancement of the university's stature, research capabilities, and its own financial picture take precedence. This is fairly typical. In contrast, when Yale developed its science park, having "a positive effect on the Dixwell/Newhallville neighborhood, an economically distressed community adjacent to the park," ranked as one of the project's two major goals (Science Park Development Corporation 1984, 1). In order to achieve that goal, Yale Science Park has explicitly dedicated itself to hiring and training workers from the local community and to recruiting minority-owned businesses. At the opposite end of the spectrum, the Princeton Forrestal Center seems chiefly interested in creating a buffer between itself and the nearby community. Its list of major objectives includes the university's wish "to protect its research activities and ensure that adjacent development would be conducive to research"; its desire to "preserve the environmental qualities that distinguish the Princeton community from the uncoordinated, scattered development typical of the US 1 corridor"; and its ambition to "establish a level of quality for later regional development to uphold" (Levitt 1984, 8). Not coincidentally, the marketing of the center has been aimed primarily at blue-chip corporations from outside the local area that are looking for divisional or headquarter sites.

Clearly, a university's policy toward economic development of the surrounding region can have a profound effect on who will find work or otherwise benefit from the park and who will not. Women on campus and in the community who wish to influence the planning of a technology park can work to ensure that economic development is acknowledged as a high priority both of the university and the surrounding community wherever there is a pool of unemployed or underemployed workers, particularly women or minority men. This is the case for many inner-city campuses, but also for rural campuses where the university is the major employer and other opportunities are scarce. At the same time, it is essential to push for a policy of comparable worth to prevent exploitation of the captive labor market of students and faculty spouses characteristic of university communities.

One of the most interesting features of Yale Science Park is the fact that it not only attempts to offer employment to the neighboring minority community but also promotes formation of minority-owned businesses. One of the ways it does this is by providing an "incubator"—a nurturing environment in which small businesses can get started. Typically, incubators provide fledgling entrepreneurs with low-cost space and centralized administrative services (e.g., word processing or bookkeeping) as well as assistance in business management and access to financing. In this way, incubators increase the odds that a new business will survive and grow. Existing parks vary with respect to their inclusion of incubator facilities: for example, they are a prominent part of the

Yale Science Park but do not play a role at the Princeton Forrestal Center.

In the last five years or so incubator facilities have emerged as one of the most effective ways to promote economic development, but their advantages have been enjoyed primarily by more traditional, white male entrepreneurs. At present, both women and minority men are less well represented in scientific and technological fields than white men—not only as workers and researchers or faculty members, but also as executives or entrepreneurs in technology-related firms. This is a serious loss, not only for the women and men who possess the aptitude for such work, but also for science and technology, which could benefit from the contributions of individuals operating from a different set of social, political, and psychological assumptions. The incubator may provide an effective mechanism both for introducing more women and minorities into science and technology related business and for promoting economic equity.[3] This will only work, however, if park policy is explicit about its desire to recruit women- and minority-owned businesses, and if the management of the incubator is sensitive to the specific problems and needs of women and minority entrepreneurs. When nontraditional companies succeed, they in turn can have an influence on the employment rates and income of women and minority workers. If enough of them succeed, they may be able to alter the economic structure of a region in the direction of prosperity with equity.

Finally, no one concerned about economic development with equity can avoid the issue of dependence on military spending. At the federal level, a startling 75 percent of all the money that is invested in research and development of new technologies currently flows to defense-related projects. A cynical reading of the current rush to create research parks is to interpret it as universities' attempt to cash in on the national defense budget, now that other sources of research funding are declining. Universities today may not be eager to collaborate with the military, but apparently they are at least willing. This willingness—along with the utter lack of controversy around the development of technology parks or the courting of military business today—stands in sobering contrast to the mood on campuses just fifteen years ago. At the same time, the U.S. economy in general and the economies of high-tech states such as California, Massachusetts, and Connecticut in particular are already alarmingly dependent on military spending.

University-affiliated research and technology parks need to think carefully about their involvement with the military and set policies to control that involvement. Technology transfer to military contractors can be avoided, and the park, together with the region and the state, can encourage economic conversion. Doing so will not only make it easier for individual states to take a reasonable stand on peace issues; it will also provide alternative employment opportunities for women in technology who refuse to work on military projects.

In the coming decade, both new technologies and the research park setting in which they will be developed are likely to have a strong influence on the American economy and the job market. Those who presently stand to gain are principally the white middle- and upper-class males who traditionally have constituted the overwhelming majority of science and technology majors, faculty, professionals, executives, and entrepreneurs. It is their priorities and values, and not an anonymous technological determinism, that will influence not only the creation and implementation of new technologies, but also the environment of the technology park in which collaboration between the university and industry occurs.

While science and technology claim objectivity and distance from political or economic interests, at least in their popular representations, this distance is clearly an illusion. Equally inaccurate is a deterministic view that sees technology as unilaterally shaping either work or society. What the essays in this collection have documented, over and over again, is an interaction of technological change with social and economic restructuring, and a dynamic struggle of interests as women workers maneuver to improve their economic position, sometimes with the help of new technologies, sometimes in spite of new technologies and those who profit from them. Both changes and constants have emerged, in the definition of male as well as female gender, in gender-, race-, and class-based divisions of labor, and in the exclusion not only of women but also of men from certain kinds of work. The collection has highlighted the diversity among groups of women workers, as well as technology's diverse impacts on them; and finally, the collection has suggested strategies for achieving both stronger representation of women in technological fields and economic equity for women working with new technologies.

These technological, economic, and social interactions may be expected to continue as the next phase of technological development unfolds. Similarly, the mix of gains and losses—in human values, equity, and the well-being of all life on earth—will continue to shift. Because specific interests and not an anonymous determinism shape the course of technological development, it is essential for women to enter not only technological occupations but also the planning process. The academic and business communities, meanwhile, bear a special responsibility to sound more life-affirming and inclusive "subthemes" in the development and application of new technologies.

NOTES

I would like to thank Myra Ferree for suggestions and advice that greatly improved this article.

1. For much of the material and analysis in the following section I am indebted to Martin Kenney's recent book, *Biotechnology: The University-Industrial Complex* (1986).
2. The NSF's probusiness tilt has become even more pronounced since the Reagan administration's appointment of Erich Bloch as director. Under him, the orientation of the NSF has shifted markedly from basic to applied research. Bloch also encourages university research specifically for industry, and he urges university researchers to look for matching funds from industry. In the meantime, the NIH has opened its competition to for-profit organizations.
3. It has been shown (see, for example, Donato and Roos in this volume) that women's earnings are more likely to approach men's when women are self-employed and paying themselves; perhaps not coincidentally, women are currently founding their own businesses at five times the rate of men (Loden 1985, 39).

REFERENCES

Anderson, Marion. 1982. *Neither jobs nor security: Women's unemployment and the Pentagon budget.* Lansing, Mich.: Employment Research Associates.
Ben Franklin Partnership Consortium and Technology Center for the North East Tier Region of Pennsylvania. 1983. Bethlehem, Pa.: Lehigh University.
Buck, Alison M., Daryl J. Hobbs, Donald D. Myers, and Nancy C. Munshaw. 1984. *Feasibility of high-tech company incubation in rural university settings.* Rolla, Mo: Missouri IncuTech, Inc.
Concept master plan: Connecticut Technology Park, a university research community. 1984. Storrs, Conn.: University of Connecticut Educational Properties, Inc.
Doyle, Jack. 1985. *Altered Harvest.* New York: Viking Press.
Fernandez-Kelly, Maria Patricia. 1983. *A cross-cultural comparison of export-processing zones in Asia and the U.S.-Mexico border.* San Diego: Center for U.S.-Mexican Studies, University of California, San Diego.
Haemmerlie, Frances M., ed. 1985. *Proceedings of the Conference on Partnerships for Rural High-Tech Incubation, University of Missouri-Rolla, August 1984.* Rolla, Mo.: Incubator Technologies, Inc.
Hartmann, Heidi I., Robert E. Kraut, and Louise A. Tilly, eds. 1986. *Computer*

chips and paper clips: Technology and women's employment. Washington, D.C.: National Academy Press.

Kenney, Martin. 1986. *Biotechnology: The university-industrial complex.* New Haven: Yale University Press.

Levitt, Rachelle L., ed. 1984. *Research parks and other ventures: The university real estate connection.* Washington, D.C.: Urban Land Institute.

Loden, Marilyn. 1985. *Feminine leadership: How to succeed in business without being one of the boys.* New York: Time Books.

Merchant, Carolyn. 1980. *The death of nature: Women, ecology and the scientific revolution.* San Francisco: Harper and Row.

Premus, Robert. 1982. *Location of high-technology firms and regional economic development.* Report prepared for the U.S. Congress Joint Economic Committee. 97th Cong. 2d sess.

Science Park Development Corporation. 1984. *Science park: Third annual review.* New Haven.

———.1985. *Science park: Fourth annual review.* New Haven.

Temali, Mihailo, and Candace Campbell. 1984. *Business incubator profiles: A national survey.* Minneapolis: Hubert H. Humphrey Institute and Department of Community Services, University of Minnesota.

Ziman, John. 1984. *An introduction to science studies: The philosophical and social aspects of science and technology.* Cambridge: Cambridge University Press.

Contributors

Eileen Appelbaum received a Ph.D. in economics from the University of Pennsylvania and is associate professor of economics at Temple University, where she is currently studying the impact of technology in service sector industries. Dr. Appelbaum serves as a consultant to the Office of Technology Assessment of the U.S. Congress and is a member of the Pay Equity Commission of the City of Philadelphia. Her book *Back to Work* (1981) is an econometric analysis of the experiences of mature women returning to the labor force.

Robert Asher is professor of history at the University of Connecticut and general editor of the American Labor History Series published by the State University of New York Press. His publications include *Connecticut Workers and Technological Change* (1983) and an edited anthology (with Charles Stephanson), *Life and Labor: Dimensions of American Working-Class History* (1986). Professor Asher is now completing *Legal Slaughter: Industrial Safety and Worker's Compensation in the United States, 1880–1980.* He is also preparing a manuscript on "Work in Historical Perspective."

Ava Baron, professor of sociology at Rider College in New Jersey, has been a visiting scholar at Cornell University's School of Industrial and Labor Relations Institute for Women and Work, a fellow of Radcliffe College's Bunting Institute, and a visiting scholar at the Center for Early American Studies at the University of Pennsylvania. Her research interests have focused on women and labor legislation as well as on the history of women and the American working class. She is a coauthor with Susan Klepp of " 'If I Didn't Have My Sewing Machine': Women and Sewing-Machine Technology," which was published in Jensen and Davidson's *A Needle, A Bobbin, A Strike* (1984).

Valerie J. Carter holds a Ph.D. in sociology from the University of Connecticut and is assistant professor of sociology at the University of Maine. She has conducted research in the areas of women and work, work organization, and workplace health and safety issues, and has presented several papers on the effects of automation. She has also studied and written about feminism, social theory, and occupational health and safety.

Kathleen Claspell received an M.A. in history from the University of Connecticut. Her research has focused on labor history and working women, and most recently she completed a project on colonial women, family life, and infanticide. Before returning to college, she worked for several years in both clerical and service occupations, where she developed a strong interest in work organization and workplace equity issues.

Katherine M. Donato, a doctoral candidate in sociology at the State University of New York at Stonybrook, is writing a dissertation on the sex composition of immigrants to the United States, and she has coauthored three articles about female immigrants. She is also interested in women and work, and is currently researching the determinants and consequences of women's entry into the systems analysis and public relations occupations.

Myra Marx Ferree is professor of sociology at the University of Connecticut. With Beth Hess, she is the author of *Controversy and Coalition: The New Feminist Movement* (1985) and editor of a new volume on feminist research in social science, *Analyzing Gender* (1987). She is also an associate editor of the journal *Gender and Society.* Her research articles focus on working-class women, the interface of paid and domestic work, and feminist attitudes.

Evelyn Nakano Glenn, professor of sociology at the State University of New York at Binghamton, has conducted research and published widely on the impact of new technology on work, especially clerical occupations. She also studies race and gender and is currently investigating black, Hispanic, and Asian-American women's work in the nineteenth and twentieth centuries.

Carol J. Haddad, associate professor at Michigan State University's School of Labor and Industrial Relations, is currently conducting research on the design of retraining programs for adults who face job dislocation or skill obsolescence due to technological change. She also develops and teaches noncredit courses for labor organizations on a statewide basis and has conducted numerous classes, workshops, and conferences on the subject of new technology and its impact on workers and their unions.

Patricia Vawter Klein is associate professor of social science at Western Michigan University and a doctoral candidate at the State University of New York at Buffalo. Professor Klein has been active in various women's organizations, including the Coalition of Labor Union Women and the National Organization for Women. Her research interests include the treatment of women in industry, biological effects on women workers in hazardous industries, protective legislation, and workers' self-management. She has also written about Josephine Goldmark and the early history of exclusionary policies.

Christine Kleinegger received a Ph.D. from the Women's History Program at the State University of New York at Binghamton, where she did research on the domestic labor of farm women and taught courses on the history of women, the family, and rural America. She was a Fellow of the Rockefeller Institute for Government in 1982 and is a founding member of the Upstate New York Women's History Conference. She currently holds a position as legislative analyst for the New York State Assembly. Her interest in rural affairs and government continues.

Linda H. Lewis holds a doctorate in adult education and is presently associate professor of educational leadership at the University of Connecticut. She has broad experience working with and teaching adults, and previously served as a manpower training specialist to the state of California. Her research in the area of high technology and education has focused on equity in classroom computer programs, and she has published numerous articles about women, computers, and adult education. She is also active in state and national organizations and has worked to improve women's status and education.

Gail O. Mellow received a Ph.D. in social psychology from George Washington University and is director of the University of Connecticut Women's Center. Her research interests include sex differences in interpersonal power; sex differences in organizational and managerial behavior; and sex equity in education, particularly regarding women's entrance into math and science courses and in relation to teenage pregnancy. With Diana Woolis she is coauthor of *Teenage Pregnancy and Education: Attrition, Achievement and Alternative Education* (1986).

Janet Polansky is professor of English and chair of the English department at the University of Wisconsin-Stout. Previously she served as director of the Women's Studies Program and directed a project to balance the professional-technical curriculum at Wisconsin-Stout, which is primarily a technical university. She is currently directing a project to empower the traditionally female disciplines. Professor Polansky received a Ph.D. from Tulane University in New Orleans and has taught numerous women's studies and interdisciplinary technology courses.

Patricia A. Roos has a Ph.D. in sociology from the University of California, Los Angeles, and is associate professor of sociology at the State University of New York at Stonybrook. In a current research project funded by the National Science Foundation and the Rockefeller Foundation, she is investigating with Barbara Reskin the determinants of changing occupational sex composition.

Frieda S. Rozen, a doctoral candidate and instructor in labor studies at Pennsylvania State University, has been interested in women and their unions since the late 1940s, when she worked as a union organizer for the Amalgamated Clothing Workers of America. Her current research focus on flight attendant unions grew out of her concern for workplace democracy and the changing role of women and minorities in unions.

Maria-Luz Daza Samper has a Ph.D. in curriculum supervision from the University of Connecticut and is associate professor at the University of Connecticut's Labor Education Center. She is an advisory board member of Women in Organizational Leadership and is active in the Coalition of Labor Union Women and the University and College Labor Education Association. Her research currently focuses on information technology and its effects on workers.

Carole Srole, assistant professor of history at California State University at Los Angeles, received her Ph.D. in history from the University of California, Los Angeles, in 1984. She is currently researching and writing a history of the feminization of clerical work.

Autumn Stanley is affiliated with the Institute for Research on Women and Gender at Stanford University. She has been a college teacher, science textbook editor, and free-lance scholar and writer in women's studies. For the past ten years, she has been researching women's contributions to human technological innovation. She is the author of *Mothers of Invention* (forthcoming).

Charles M. Tolbert II holds a Ph.D. in sociology from the University of Georgia. He is associate professor of sociology at Florida State University, where his main research interests are social stratification, and economy and society. His two most recent books are *The Organization of Work in Rural and Urban Labor Markets* (1984), which he wrote with Patrick M. Horan, and *Introduction to Computing: Applications for the Social Sciences* (1985).

Timm Triplett received a Ph.D. in philosophy from the University of Massachusetts at Amherst and is assistant professor of philosophy at the University of New Hampshire, where he coordinates the Technology, Society and Values Program. This interdisciplinary program collaborates with the University of New Hampshire Women's Studies Program, and one of Timm's research interests is integrating insights from these two interdisciplinary fields.

Sandy Weinberg is professor of computers and technology at Drexel University, specializing in the behavioral aspects of the information revolution. He is the author of numerous books, the most recent of which is *Computer Phobia* (1984). He is deeply interested in the problems of computer education for women and is currently researching gender-neutral education strategies.

Barbara Drygulski Wright received her Ph.D. from the University of California, Berkeley, and is assistant professor of German at the University of Connecticut. She has also served as the interim director of the Women's Studies Program and as co-coordinator of the Project on Women and Technology at Storrs. She has published on German Baroque drama, Expressionist politics, and foreign language pedagogy, none of which prepared her in any way for her current interests.

Index